Medical Humanities and Medical Education

The field of the medical humanities is developing rapidly. However, there has also been parallel concern from sceptics that the value of medical humanities educational interventions should be open to scrutiny and evidence. Just what is the impact of medical humanities provision upon the education of medical students? In an era of limited resources, is such provision worth the investment? This innovative text addresses these pressing questions, describes the contemporary territory comprising the medical humanities in medical education and explains how this field may be developed as a key medical education component for the future.

Bleakley, a driving force of the international movement to establish the medical humanities as a core and integrated provision in the medical curriculum, proposes a model that requires collaboration between patients, artists, humanities scholars, doctors and other health professionals in developing medical students' sensibility (clinical acumen based on close noticing) and sensitivity (ethical, professional and humane practice). In particular, this text focuses upon how medical humanities input into the curriculum can help to shape the identities of medical students as future doctors who are humane, caring, expressive and creative – whose work will be technically sound but considerably enhanced by their abilities to communicate well with patients and colleagues, to empathize, to be adaptive and innovative, and to act as 'medical citizens' in shaping a future medical culture as a model democracy where social justice is a key aspect of medicine.

Making sense of the new wave of medical humanities in medical education scholarship that calls for a 'critical medical humanities', *Medical Humanities and Medical Education* incorporates a range of case studies and illustrative and practical examples to aid integrating medical humanities into the medical curriculum. It will be important reading for medical educators and others working with the medical education community, and all those interested in the medical humanities.

Alan Bleakley is Professor of Medical Humanities, Falmouth University, UK; Emeritus Professor of Medical Education and Medical Humanities, Plymouth University Peninsula School of Medicine; Visiting Scholar, the Wilson Centre, Toronto, Canada; and President, Association for Medical Humanities. His recent publications include *Patient-Centred Medicine in Transition: The Heart of the Matter* and *Medicine, Health and the Arts: Approaches to the Medical Humanities*.

Routledge Advances in the Medical Humanities

New titles:

Medicine, Health and the Arts
Approaches to the medical humanities
Edited by Victoria Bates, Alan Bleakley and Sam Goodman

Suffering Narratives of Older Adults
A phenomenological approach to serious illness, chronic pain, recovery and maternal care
Mary Beth Morrissey

Medical Humanities and Medical Education
How the medical humanities can shape better doctors
Alan Bleakley

Forthcoming titles:

Doing Collaborative Arts-based Research for Social Justice
A guide
Victoria Foster

Learning Disability
Past, present and future
C. F. Goodey

The Experience of Institutionalisation
Social exclusion, stigma and loss of identity
Jane Hubert

Digital Stories in Health and Social Policy
Listening to marginalized voices
Nicole Matthews and Naomi Sunderland

Medical Humanities and Medical Education

How the medical humanities can shape better doctors

Alan Bleakley

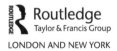

Routledge
Taylor & Francis Group

LONDON AND NEW YORK

First published 2015
by Routledge
2 Park Square, Milton Park, Abingdon, Oxfordshire OX14 4RN

and by Routledge
711 Third Avenue, New York, NY 10017

First issued in paperback 2016

Routledge is an imprint of the Taylor & Francis Group, an informa business

British Library Cataloguing-in-Publication Data
A catalogue record for this book is available from the British Library

Library of Congress Cataloging-in-Publication Data
Bleakley, Alan (Alan Douglas), author.
Medical humanities and medical education : how the medical humanities
can shape better doctors / written by Alan Bleakley.
p. ; cm. — (Routledge advances in the medical humanities)
Includes bibliographical references.
I. Title. II. Series: Routledge advances in the medical humanities.
[DNLM: 1. Education, Medical. 2. Humanities. W 18]
R737
610.71'1—dc23
2014038105

ISBN 13: 978-1-138-24367-5 (pbk)
ISBN 13: 978-1-138-77868-9 (hbk)

Typeset in Sabon
by FiSH Books Ltd, Enfield

Contents

Figures

Acknowledgements

Over the years, I have been inspired and supported by a core group of clinicians, medical humanities scholars and artists engaged with the medical humanities internationally. This group includes: Pamela Brett-MacLean, Allan Peterkin, Brian Hodges, Lorelei Lingard, Pippa Hall, Abraham Verghese, Arno Kumagai, Tess Jones, Robert Marshall, David Levine, Julie Thacker, Ian Fussell, Tim Dornan, Neville Chiavaroli, Jeffrey Bishop, John Bligh, Julie Browne, Christine Borland, David Cotterrell and Roger Kneebone. I also wish to acknowledge the commitment, enthusiasm and talent of the many medical students at Peninsula Medical School who consistently demonstrated over more than a decade that a core medical humanities curriculum 'works' and that the ideas presented in this book can be applied successfully to the undergraduate medicine and surgery curriculum.

This book is dedicated to my growing family, which offers a constant source of support, inspiration and amazement; and in particular to my wife Sue, who has patiently put up with both the enthusiasms and frustrations that accompanied the shaping of the unruly manuscript as it developed from mewling child to grumpy, growling and insistent adult.

Foreword

In his classic essay, 'The Hedgehog and the Fox', the philosopher Sir Isaiah Berlin muses on a fragment from the Greek poet, Archilocus: 'The fox knows many things, but the hedgehog knows one big thing.' Over the years, this fragment has been interpreted to mean that the fox knows many lines of attack, but the hedgehog knows only one line of defence: to roll into a protective, spiky ball. Berlin elaborates on this dichotomy between the Many and the One through a strikingly provocative proposition: that thinkers can be categorized in terms of foxes and hedgehogs. According to Berlin, some thinkers, the 'foxes', pursue many unrelated paths in order to explore the rich variety and details of life, whereas others, the 'hedgehogs', dedicate their life's work to the creation of a central, unified vision of meaning and purpose. In other words, 'hedgehogs' are individuals who spend their lives in pursuit of One Big Idea.

Taken in this context, Alan Bleakley, one of the foremost theorists of medical education on the scene today, is clearly a hedgehog, and in this insightful volume, we see him at his hedgehoggian best. And his One Big Idea? *Democratization*: to establish truly democratic interactions and practices in teaching, learning and patient care.

In *Medical Humanities and Medical Education: How the Medical Humanities can Shape Better Doctors*, Bleakley takes up several themes that he has written on authoritatively in the past, such as relationships and structures of power within the clinical and medical education environment, the use of language as a tool for dehumanization (and rehumanization) in clinical practice, the problematic nature of concepts such as global medical education, outcomes-based learning, simulation and standardization in teaching and assessment. In this book, he uses these ideas to argue that there is a 'production of insensibility' in medical education that dehumanizes students and patients and those who teach them. Bleakley frames this argument in terms that might appear foreign to those fluent in the language of competencies, milestones, and entrustable professional activities. He speaks in terms of 'the aesthetic', meaning the ways in which things, events and people are perceived, felt and defined in medicine, as well as the social processes and power dynamics that confer to privileged groups and individuals the ability to say how things are sensed, felt and named. Those who are not privileged – students, patients, non-physician health care workers – become subject to the privileged groups' objectifying gaze. Against this 'production of the insensible' is 'the political'; that is, efforts to unravel the hidden processes (the 'black boxes') that give rise to inequities and dehumanization in both medical education and medical care.

The vanguard of these efforts to 'redistribute the sensible' – to educate for democracy in medicine and medical education – is a new 'second wave' movement in the form of critical medical humanities. Instead of merely contemplating the world of doctoring and illness, critical medical humanities set out to *change it*:

> Where the humanities once studied medical phenomena from a distance, they now offer to process or remake the fabric of the medical in intimate, critical engagement.
>
> (p. 82)

Bleakley issues both an aesthetic and a political challenge to the medical education community. Using a concept borrowed from the French philosopher Jacques Rancière, Bleakley argues for the development of *dissensus*, an ability to identify inequalities of power and to act in a 'redistribution of the sensible' – to democratize and humanize interactions and activities in medicine. Part of this effort, he argues, is a shift of focus from a continual recreation of the privileged heroic, individual clinician to effective, collaborative, democratically embodied teams. Then, in a powerful demonstration of dissensus, Bleakley turns his own critical gaze to certain 'weasel words', such as 'empathy' and 'creativity', as well as popular concepts of medical education, such as art and narrative. He also critically explores (and explodes) the uses of language in the cultural production of prescriptions, drugs, and drug formularies and contrasts these uses with the all-too-human language and voices of those affected.

In an approach that is perfectly fitting for a critical medical humanist, Bleakley's conceptual reach is far and wide. One can almost sense the hedgehoggian glee with which he roots around in the intellectual underbrush in order to dig up new ideas – from philosophy, sociology, psychoanalytic theory, aesthetics, Homeric epic, avant-garde performance art and lyrical poetry – to construct entirely new (and at times disruptive) ways of looking at the humanities, medicine and medical education – all in support of his One Big Idea. Furthermore, like the hedgehog, Bleakley's spines can at times be sharp. He is unapologetic and unstinting in his assertion of the core value and central role of the humanities in the education of physicians and in his critiques of many taken-for-granted institutions in medical education, such as competencies, simulations and standardized patient exercises, all of which he contends produce insensibility in students and clinicians and objectification of patients.

Above all, Bleakley sees the role of the humanities in medical education as a critical tool in democratizing educational and clinical practices in medicine, and a celebration of all that is ambiguous, uncertain, mysterious and profound in the act of one human caring for another. In this sense, his is *the* voice to add depth and complexity to a field in education that often lacks both.

Arno K. Kumagai, MD
Ann Arbor, Michigan, USA

Introduction

Forewarned

Once a fault-line has been spotted in a culture that prevents that culture from achieving its potential, an academic has an ethical duty to critically analyse and address that fault-line. In the process, inevitably, there are unwanted casualties. The fault-line that this book is concerned with is the continuing inability for the culture of medicine to democratize in order to improve healthcare, in the face of mounting evidence that such democratization is necessary. The culture of medical education – a pedagogical culture closely aligned with clinical practice – has the role of shaping doctors of the future and, I claim, is largely responsible for failing to democratize medical culture. Indeed, I argue that medical education continues, as an unintended consequence of its methods, to produce insensibility and insensitivity in medical students. This has to change, and I argue that the vehicle for such change is the deliberate and thoughtful incorporation of the medical humanities as core and integrated provision in the undergraduate medicine and surgery curriculum.

The fall-out from this broad-brushed critique is that many excellent doctors and medical educators who are not architects of the fault-lines in medicine and medical education that I articulate, but in fact actively resist practices and views that maintain such fault-lines, will be inadvertently tarred with my general critique. Again, these are the very doctors and medical educators who are working hard to address the symptoms that I delineate in medicine and medical education as in need of treatment. Some of them, as trusted colleagues, have properly and kindly pointed out that there is a thin line between considered academic critique and polemical 'doctor-bashing' and that I sometimes flirt with that line. They also note that wider political and business interests are increasingly frustrating best medical practice and that I do not focus enough on critically addressing these other institutional influences on medicine. These trusted colleagues are right in their observations and I see them as allies in developing a better medical education through the medical humanities. I do not of course include these allies in my wider critique of the current state of medical education but see them as fellow dissenters and I celebrate their courage and conviction in championing a medical education that puts sensitive patient care and social justice at the heart of medicine.

The writer Mark Slouka (2010: 168) suggests that 'democratic institutions do not spring up, like flowers at the feet of the magi, in the tire tracks of commerce. They just don't. They're a different species. They require a different kind of tending.' But what is it that nourishes the development of an authentically democratic institution? Slouka suggests that 'the humanities, in short, are a superb delivery mechanism for what we might call democratic values'. To 'the humanities' we must explicitly add 'the arts'. Together, will the humanities and arts in medical education provide the contextual media through which democratic practices can be established in medicine, leading to improved patient care? This book sets out to address that question.

Shaping the fabric of the sensible through medical education

In Mark Haddon's (2012: 103) novel *The Red House* a rare condition that causes a mother's baby to be stillborn is diagnosed by a junior doctor. Disconcertingly, the doctor not only 'seemed pleased with himself for knowing the biology behind such a rare syndrome', but also 'gave the impression that she [the mother] was meant to feel pleased too, for having won some sort of perverse jackpot'. Haddon's observation can be seen to confirm the intuitive rationale for the inclusion of the medical humanities in medical education – to 'humanize' those doctors who place 'cases' and smart diagnoses before persons and feelings.

But this need for humanizing runs far deeper than individual doctors' practices, to the institution of medicine and the culture of medical education. Two intertwining cultures shape doctors' practices and identities – the clinical culture of medicine/healthcare and the pedagogical culture of medical education. Medical education need not act as handmaiden to normative medicine, but can formulate resistance to, and critique of, the institutional norms of medicine where these are perceived as unproductive to patient care, collaborative interprofessional teamwork and doctors' self-care. This book argues that the structure of medicine itself, its habitual practices, must be challenged and adapted if we are to produce doctors who are technically good but also deeply connected with the interpersonal aspect of their work. Further, medical education incorporating the medical humanities is the vehicle for such change. At the core of this sea-change, as I have argued in previous books (Bleakley *et al.* 2011; Bleakley 2014) is the democratizing of medicine – shifting medical practice from an authority-led hierarchy that is doctor-centred to a patient-centred and interprofessional clinical team process. This is a political challenge.

Running parallel to this is an aesthetic challenge – shifting an instrumental and technical mindset that permeates medicine, shaping it merely as technical craft, to a medicine of qualities, traditionally called the 'art' of medicine. Just what constitutes that art is what makes up the interdisciplinary field of the medical humanities in medical education: communicating sensitively with patients and colleagues; close listening in receiving the patient's history; close noticing in the physical examination; making sense of the stories that patients tell and adapting interventions accordingly; managing an identity as an expert or a connoisseur in a specialty; critically and reflexively understanding the fabric of medical culture itself; and critically and reflexively understanding historical and cultural assumptions about the body, health, disease and illness.

Medical educationalists have introduced many curriculum innovations to address the need to educate for new forms of healthcare emerging for the coming century. These include professionalism, communication skills, interprofessional teamwork, patient-centred practice, early clinical experience, structured work-based learning with briefing and debriefing and learning through simulation with actor-patients and high-tech manikins. However, some of these innovations have been counterproductive. Rather than educating and widening the sensibilities of students, such innovations can produce insensibility and narrowing of focus. As a result, we need to fundamentally reformulate medical education. Political and aesthetic dimensions are missing from medical education's current (strongly technical) profile and medical education can have unintended negative or unproductive consequences.

In the context of critical theory applied to social institutions, the French philosopher Jacques Rancière (2013: ix) describes how 'ways of perceiving and being affected' are constructed institutionally, particularly through education and popular culture. In other words, how each of us senses and how sensibilities are shaped is an issue of institutional framing. Such frames are subject to historical and local traditions ('this is the way we do things around here'). Ways of taking in the world around us and making judgements about it, such as what is noticed, appreciated and what goes unnoticed are, suggests Rancière, subject to 'modes of perception' (which I shall call 'sensibility') and 'regimes of emotion' (which I shall call 'sensitivity'). These are 'policed' by institutions and their representatives who hold power and authority to shape a fabric of the sensible. At the same time, it is possible that those who are subject to learning how to perceive and feel challenge the normative ways of being educated into these states. Rancière (2010) calls this 'dissensus'. Dissensus – the opposite of consensus – is a neologism from the 1960s. It is equivalent to the more commonly used 'dissension' that is derived from the Latin *dissensio* and *dissentire* meaning a 'difference of opinion'. Democracy relies as much on dissension or dissensus as it does on consent or agreement.

If we transfer Rancière's model to medicine and medical education, we can describe an aesthetic regime of medicine with its own expert modes of perception that are controlled and distributed by those in authority – senior clinical teachers. My argument is twofold – first that the capital of the sensible (the fabric of the sensible within medicine, or how things are perceived and felt) is not distributed fairly by senior medical teachers or clinicians in general (as representatives of normative medical culture), where it is not shared democratically with students, patients and other healthcare professionals such as nurses. Second, some current practices in medical education – both unconsciously as unintended consequences and consciously as intended consequences – produce insensibility in medical students.

The political and aesthetic structures of medical education need to be radically reformulated and I suggest that this can be achieved through incorporating the medical humanities into medical education as core and integrated provision. This is a big claim and I will justify it throughout this book. I will, of course, explain more clearly what I mean by the 'medical humanities' in this and the following two chapters, moving on to illustrate my argument in the remaining chapters. Overall, I wish to reclaim both the 'art' and 'humanity' of a medicine that is properly shaped and informed by the arts and humanities, but by a more radical version of the arts and humanities than is currently employed, where the arts in particular have generally been situated as a handmaiden to medicine rather than as a critical rejoinder (Macneill 2011).

The political aspect of this role for the medical humanities has been particularly well detailed by Arno Kumagai and colleagues (Kumagai *et al.* 2007; Kumagai and Lypson 2009; Wear *et al.* 2012) as a medical education for social justice, that treats each patient in his or her own right as a valuable human being and citizen and that aims to redress health inequalities and provide equal access to health services. Kumagai, based at the University of Michigan Medical School, is an experienced endocrinologist but also a tireless champion for the medical humanities.

A redistribution and reconfiguration of the sensible – or the capital of sensibility – would render medical students and doctors more sensible (acute) rather than more insensible (blunted) as better at close noticing, valuing, judging and offering insightful support to patients and colleagues alike. For the sake of clarity, I will again make a distinction between (1) ways of perceiving as 'sensibility', the heart of which in medical work is close noticing and diagnostic acumen; and (2) ways of being affected, or openness to the conditions of others – particularly the experiences of patients and colleagues – as 'sensitivity'.

Current ways of educating perception through medical education may be misguided or historically crystallized in the ways that they restrictively structure what is worth noticing and valuing. Through the medical humanities we can aim for a re-education of sensibility and sensitivity, where medical education again can, paradoxically, render medical students and doctors insensible or an-aesthetized. This re-education can widen to a politicizing of students, patients and healthcare practitioners to promote the democratizing of medicine.

The role of the medical humanities in addressing symptoms of a malfunctioning medical education

The aim of the medical humanities in medical education is, I suggest, a redistribution of the sensible to create a common wealth. In Rancière's (2013) phrase, the project of the medical humanities is then enormous, no less than a series of 'transformations of the sensible fabric' of medical practice. Such a reconfiguration promises to restructure performance through a reformulation of sense experience and diagnostic acumen, narrative acumen and ethical (professional) behaviour.

The single most important force shaping the structure of medical practice is work-based medical education – the clinical years of undergraduate study and the first years of junior doctoring. It is here that influential clinical teachers and teams largely shape the sensibilities of future doctors in a cognitive apprenticeship. It is experts – mainly consultants or specialists – who hold sensibility capital (diagnostic and treatment acumen: how to do a physical examination and take a history, how to diagnose and how to treat both generally and within specialties). Experts can distribute this capital as they wish to those who do not hold it – not just medical students, but also patients and other healthcare practitioners. Most clinical teachers will be generous in their intentions in sharing such capital in an equitable way. However, if they are not also expert educators as well as expert clinicians, such sharing of capital can backfire or be misplaced. As an unintended consequence of medical education, again what can result is an increase in insensibility among students – a kind of numbing or insensitivity. How does this show in symptoms?

A slide from idealism into cynicism has for too long characterized the later years of medical school as an unintended consequence of medical education. In the post-Second World War years, this slippage was pronounced, as Howard Becker described in stark detail for the 'boys in white' (Becker *et al.* 1961). Twenty years later, Robert Broadhead's (1983) description of undergraduate medical education shows the same slippage, now technically referred to as 'empathy decline' and 'moral erosion' linked to communication 'hypocompetence' or underperformance (Platt 1979). While white coats have disappeared from medicine in many countries, the permanent stains of empathy decline and moral erosion among medical students have remained – still vigorously discussed in online communities today (Remen 2012).

Paula Nunes and colleagues (Nunes *et al.* 2011: 12) show that empathy decline is a phenomenon appearing across healthcare students in general, with medical, dental and nursing students showing significant decline even in the first year of study 'with a change from idealism to realism'. Where empathy, discussed at length in Chapter 4, is usually measured by self-reports, albeit on validated scales, Colliver and colleagues (Colliver *et al.* 2010) have suggested: 'reports of the decline of empathy during medical education have been greatly exaggerated'. However, this study has been criticized on technical grounds (Marcum 2013), while erosion of empathy has been described as a wider cultural phenomenon linked with rising inequalities (McElwee 2013). Further, Colliver and colleagues' study does not account for the ongoing phenomena of moral erosion (accepting unethical behaviour as a norm), poor self-care and unacceptable rates of medical error, all of which are discussed later.

The distinguished physician and bestselling novelist Abraham Verghese (2011), now working at Stanford University Medical School in California, suggests that medical students' and junior doctors' potential empathy decline and moral erosion are best nipped in the bud through extensive and intensive bedside encounters with patients supported by highly considerate and insightful teaching faculty (Cohen 2009). It is literally in staying in touch with patients that medical students in particular can establish a powerful sensibility and sensitivity without having this drained away, blocked, or confused by established practices of bedside teaching – such as 'pimping' – that model moral erosion. The (mal)practice of 'pimping' is described by James Marcum (2013) as an attending doctor (the pimper) asking unnecessarily interrogative, demanding and gruelling questions of residents and medical students (pimpees). The outcome is often humiliation and degradation on the part of the pimpee.

Marcum (2013) draws on the Grand Round scene from Margaret Edson's (1999: 46) play *W;t* (or *Wit*) to describe how the bedside examination can be, in Edson's words, 'Full of subservience, hierarchy, gratuitous displays, (and) sublimated rivalries', in other words the very conditions that generate insensibility in medical students as medicine stutters again in its long walk to freedom or authentic democracy:

> The scene begins with the chief of medical oncology, Harvey Kelekian, and five clinical fellows, including senior fellow, Jason Posner, entering Vivian Bearing's room. Bearing is a professor of English and has stage-four metastatic ovarian tumor. She is undergoing chemotherapy and is currently receiving the second cycle. Kelekian acknowledges Bearing's presence, and Posner inquires perfunctorily how she is 'feeling' today to which she responds 'fine.' Posner then exposes Bearing's abdomen and recites the facts of her case, often palpating anatomical areas of involvement. After recitation of the clinical facts, Kelekian asks the fellows what side effects are associated with the drugs used to treat Bearing's cancer. One fellow begins to answer only to be cut short by Posner, who dismissively retorts that the side effect 'goes without saying.' The playwright notes that the other fellows resent Posner, as he belittles their attempts to list the chemotherapeutic drugs' side effects. At last, Kelekian asks if any other side effects are evident, to which the fellows are unable to answer. Kelekian asks them to use their eyes and after the fellows fail to provide the correct answer, he points out the patient's

hair loss. The fellows protest that this side effect is obvious, and Kelekian calls on Posner to expound, who then begrudgingly complies. The scene concludes with Kelekian urging Bearing to receive the 'full dose' of the chemotherapeutic drugs and to 'keep pushing the fluids.' Finally, he admonishes Posner to perform his clinical duty and thank Bearing for her cooperation, which Posner does mechanically. Bearing is left with her abdomen exposed and comments on how 'grand' the experience was...

(Marcum 2013)

This is precisely the kind of insensitive bedside medicine that Verghese wished to avoid when he designed the Stanford Initiative in Bedside Medicine, in which 25 key hands-on diagnostic techniques are taught, or, more importantly, retained (Verghese undated). But, as we shall see, for Verghese, the bedside examination is not just a technical showcase but also, if done well, a necessary and confirming ritual. Verghese's TED lecture from 2011 ('A Doctor's Touch') has been watched by over a million people, and describes what he has written about consistently, persistently and eloquently in journal articles, journalism and through the voices of characters in his fictional and non-fictional writing – again, the ritual as well as technical importance of retaining the physical examination (Verghese 2011).

Advances in technologies, such as imaging techniques, are welcomed by medicine, but have unintended consequences, threatening to make some traditional hands-on examinations redundant. Auscultation, palpation and percussion techniques are under threat. If coming generations of doctors lose these abilities, how will they teach their medical students? Verghese points out that the hands-on physical examination is not limited to these technical aspects of medicine, but affords the ritual of patient contact in which both trust is set up and a doctor's identity is confirmed. It is a context in which difference is acknowledged and celebrated. In a *New York Times* interview, Verghese says:

> The importance of the ritual of one patient baring his or her soul and body cannot be underestimated. Rituals are terribly important to human beings because they signify transformation. This is how you earn your right to say, 'I am your doctor.' If as a doctor you shortchange the ritual, you end up making patients feel you aren't interested. They lose trust.
>
> (Chen 2009)

Doctor–patient contact is also about eye contact. The philosopher Alphonso Lingis, in a biographical film – *Transfigured Night* – made by the British curator of contemporary art practices Adrian Heathfield, talks of the importance of authentic eye 'contact' as like touching, saturated with tenderness rather than practiced 'communication skill' (for a trailer, see

Heathfield undated). Yet we 'teach' medical students how to 'make' eye contact as an element of professionalism – sometimes simulated or, worse, dissimulated – rather than an expression of humanity. The 'clinical gaze', an encultured 'medical perception' – the origins of which Michel Foucault (1989) famously described in *The Birth of the Clinic* – is an echo of the traditional gaze of learning anatomy that is made on the open, dissected corpse, but is now transferred as an objectifying gaze that 'opens' the patient to 'see' the source of his or her illness, the imagined location of a lesion. The objectifying aspect of the medical gaze is not eye 'contact' in Lingis's sense, nor does it follow Verghese's recommendations to 'touch' the patient as a sign of care, humanity and respect. It is, rather, a cultivated insensibility – a product of medical (mis)education. What if we placed emphasis upon the medical gaze touching not the imagined lesion but the soul of the patient, so that the gaze is one of deep care?

The bedside examination, then, is part of a doctor's performance and learning such a performance, as a medical student, is central to the shift in identity construction from student to trainee doctor. We must then, as medical educators, be careful not to educate for misidentification (through the production of insensibility) in not exploiting the full potential of bedside teaching. Patients come to trust doctors with a good bedside or consultation manner and we know that the therapeutic relationship between doctor and patient affects the healing process (Roter and Hall 2006). So, in short, the warm bedside and consultation manner that accompanies a technically proficient physical examination diagnosis marks out a key aspect of a doctor's or trainee doctor's performance, but is in danger of being supplanted by cold and distancing technologies and testing.

Over a century ago, in the early 1900s, a similar scenario was being discussed among a community of medical educators in London. Sir Robert Hutchison noted the need to openly support the warm art of medicine in the face of an increasingly dominant cold science. Hutchison's petition concluded:

> From putting knowledge before wisdom, science before art, and
> Cleverness before common sense;
> From treating patients as cases;
> And from making the cure of the disease more grievous than the
> Endurance of the same, Good Lord, deliver us.
>
> (quoted in Shankar 2010: 2)

In Hutchison's era, the 'art' of medicine meant bedside manner and diagnostic acumen. Both were assumed to flow from character virtues, such as altruism, that in turn were an assumed product of a liberal education. Warner (2011: 92) notes that late nineteenth- and early twentieth-century 'celebrity' doctors, such as William Osler, called for 'a rehumanisation of medicine' and a cultivation of 'an ideal of the 'gentleman-physician' well versed in the classic liberal arts'. This ideal of the doctor with the 'right stuff' has lingered. As late as 1975 the UK Royal College of Physicians felt it important to say that their membership examination requirement 'remains partly a test of culture, although knowledge of Latin, Greek, French and German is no longer required' (in McManus 1995: 1144).

Science study has, however, progressively claimed and partially eroded the ground of a liberal education once thought to be an essential background for practising medicine. The benefits of scientific and technological advances in medicine are clear and we might say that the erosion of the art of medicine is a small price to pay for advances in population health. However, this erosion of the human face of medicine is a symptom of a wider structural problem – that of the continuing dominance of hierarchical clinical teamwork that favours doctors and marginalizes other healthcare professionals and patients. There is an ongoing iatrogenic (medically-caused) 'epidemic' (Starfield 2000) of medical error, where an estimated 70 per cent of such error is grounded not in technical mistakes, but in poor communication between doctors and colleagues within and between clinical teams (Xyrichis and Ream 2008). Medical error has been noted as the fourth biggest killer after cancer, cardiac disease and respiratory disease, with an estimated 200,000 deaths per year in the USA (Harmon 2009) and 40,000 per year in the UK (House of Commons Health Committee 2009; Hogan *et al.* 2012).

Medical education has, logically but mistakenly, responded to this communication 'hypocompetence' (Platt 1979) problem through intensifying instrumental training in communication skills such as empathy and breaking bad news (Bleakley 2014). However, 30 years' worth of developing communication skills in undergraduate medicine – largely through simulation, as a quasi-scientific laboratory-based training – has not addressed the continuing high level of medical error. Learning communication as an instrumental skill may be necessary, but does not offer a sufficient condition to address poor practices in clinical teamwork and patient consultations. Something else is needed. The deeper problem may be the unrealized democratization of medical culture, a shift that would challenge the root symptoms of poor communication in clinical teams – hierarchy and unproductive authoritarianism (Bleakley 2014).

Patently, educating for a virtuous character through a liberal education has never humanized medical practice – and 'humanizing' is a cloudy term in danger of slipping into piety. Now we also realize that learning communication skills instrumentally is failing to humanize medicine. It may be, however, that the medical humanities can provide the extra curriculum dimension to educate for both patient-centredness and democratic team practice. Medicine requires a medium for translation of clinical scientific knowledge into patient care and that medium may be the medical humanities. However, precisely what is meant by the 'medical humanities' is strongly debated, as we shall see.

Realizing Osler's vision

William Osler (1849–1919), perhaps the most famous doctor of his era, formally introduced planned bedside teaching of medical students into medical education. This gave an opportunity for students to learn clinical medicine first hand in collaboration with senior doctors and not from lectures. But it also gave students the opportunity to learn engaged and humane medicine from working with patients – moving beyond a professional 'bedside manner' to engage an imagination of patient-centred practice.

Osler learned medicine in Canada and later founded the Johns Hopkins University School of Medicine in Baltimore, Maryland, finally moving to Oxford as the Regius Chair of Medicine. Osler's family roots are in Falmouth, West Cornwall in the United Kingdom, close to where I live; and Falmouth hosts the University that currently employs me. Osler also initiated hospital-based specialist medical education programmes for junior doctors, known in North America as 'residencies'. It is in internship first and then residency that medical students make the transition from novices to the beginning of expertise in a specialty such as rheumatology, oncology and so forth.

Osler's vision of medicine was one of deep humanity, where 'The practice of medicine is an art, not a trade; a calling, not a business; a calling in which your heart will be exercised equally with your head' (in Silverman *et al.* 2003: 13). The book you are now reading follows the spirit of Osler's vision, arguing for the value of the medical humanities as a core and integrated element in a contemporary curriculum. By 'core' I mean including the medical humanities as major and compulsory elements in the medicine and surgery undergraduate curriculum; and by 'integrated' I mean designing a medical humanities perspective that runs through the entire curriculum provision, including science studies, without being compromised. The rationale for such a curriculum is provided by the content of this book.

Generally, medical students and junior doctors do not set out to practice medicine without using both heart and head – cognition and feeling – and imagination too; however, their practice of medicine becomes – often inadvertently – distorted. One would hope that a medical education would produce a sensibility shaping the close noticing that is required for effective diagnosis, a sensitivity shaping caring relationships with patients and colleagues and an imagination that drives innovation in practice. However, as noted above, the reality is that medical education too often works in the opposite direction, producing insensibility, insensitivity and stifling creativity.

In a famous lecture given at Pennsylvania School of Medicine in 1899, termed 'Aequanimitas', Osler (1932) suggested that doctors must maintain a degree of detachment from patients while showing deep sensitivity. Critics of Osler have jumped upon this as admittance that doctors cannot hope to show empathy for all patients in their work and indeed should not attempt to do this for fear of courting emotional burnout. Indeed, Osler said in the lecture 'a certain measure of insensibility is not only an advantage, but a positive necessity in the exercise of a calm judgement' (in Ofri 2013: 4). Osler, however, was simply following the advice that would be given to any psychotherapist – you can engage deeply with patients, but also professionally, by fine-tuning your level of involvement so that there is a professional distance. But this distance is grounded in humanity and Osler did warn later in the lecture against 'hardening the human heart'. Freud described this stance of equanimity as managing the transference and counter-transference dynamic (including management of resistance and counter-resistance). 'Aequanimitas' (equanimity) is a mental virtue that accompanies professional practice – one of internal calm. Here, Osler is surely reminding medical students and doctors that they must exercise self-care. Current medical education has not taken Osler's advice on board fully, where empathy decline, mentioned earlier, characteristically develops by year 3 in medical students and poor self-care is a common symptom among doctors. We need to return to the heart of Osler's advice to ask why contemporary medical education may not be achieving the goals that he set.

In Chapter 3, I set out in full the argument rehearsed above for why the fair distribution of the sensible through medical education is frustrated and what can be done about this. For now, however, let us continue to map the territory of the complex interdisciplinary field of study and practice collectively termed the 'medical humanities'. I will set out some of the controversies in the field and note how 'critical' versions of the medical humanities are emerging as a collective new wave of interest. My focus will ultimately be upon the medical humanities in medical education. Throughout, I use 'medical humanities' in the plural, to signify not only the multiplicity of interests in the field, but also that the field is fractured and contested rather than cohesive. This book focuses on the visual arts and literature. For those readers particularly interested in a wider remit (including music, dance, drama and performance) please see the sister publication to this volume (Bates *et al.* 2013).

1 Where do the medical humanities come from and where are they going?

The medical humanities in North America

The medical humanities first developed an identity in the USA, where the term was coined in 1948. Barr (2011) argues that American doctors in the 1870s, who had visited Germany particularly to study laboratory sciences, started a long revolution in medical education that was brought to a head by the Flexner Report in 1910 (Flexner 1910; Cooke *et al.* 2010; Bleakley *et al.* 2011). Commissioned by the Carnegie Foundation, Flexner's report exposed a lack of adequate scientific and clinical education across many American medical schools and recommended a root-and-branch overhaul, including the standardization of curricula. Unfortunately, and paradoxically, this led to closures of underfunded schools catering for minority students such that persons of colour and women would for many years find it difficult to gain entry to medical school (Hodges 2005). It is ironic that now women make up approximately 60 per cent of medical school entrants worldwide (Bleakley 2014).

Wujun Ke (2012) offers a standard critical reading of Flexner, suggesting that Flexner's emphasis on the importance of the biological sciences in early medical education led to a bias towards curative rather than caring medicine, where basic science teachers rather than clinicians have a formative influence on students. Life sciences teachers are the first to shape the identities of students, particularly anatomists who traditionally educate through the ritual of dissection, where clinicians primarily shape students' identities in the later clinical years. The voiced scepticism of many basic science teachers towards the humanities may contribute to the 'empathy decline' of students mentioned in the Introduction – a process by which medical students also develop cynicism (Neumann *et al.* 2011). New celebratory readings of Flexner, however, suggest that his interest towards ethical and humane practice has been overlooked. Flexner was an admirer of John Dewey, sharing the latter's democratic and humanitarian values. Garrett Riggs (2010: 1669) suggests that 'if history is a guide, medical education could be on the cusp of another set of great advances by renewing interest in medical humanities...The time is ripe to embrace the rest of the Flexner Report.'

In 1937, at Vanderbilt University School of Medicine in Nashville, Tennessee, E.E. Reinke (2003: 1058) called for 'leavening technical [medical] training with a liberal education'. That such a call should be made at all was a reminder of how far medical education had strayed from the ideal of the liberally educated 'gentleman-physician' described in the Introduction. Reinke's article was a call for the development of medical humanities in undergraduate medical education in order to stem the trend, described starkly by Reinke, even in an inflammatory way, of producing the doctor who is 'a healer of organs' treating patients as 'experimental animals', rather than 'a doctor in the ancient meaning of the word'.

Reinke's reminder that a more liberal medical education was sliding into tightly focused technical training is, in retrospect, even more alarming when placed against the background of North American medical schools offering graduate entry programmes. Most students entering medical schools at that time would have previously graduated with a science degree such as biology, chemistry, physics or engineering. However, most students, in the North American tradition of higher education, would also have studied a compulsory humanities introductory course in their early undergraduate career following a mini 'great books' curriculum, where critical and liberal thinking would be espoused. In other words, they would not be strangers to 'thinking with the humanities'. Currently, 15 per cent of entrants to medical schools in North America have a first degree in either social sciences or the humanities (Wershof Schwartz *et al.* 2009).

Throughout the 1970s, a series of discussion papers developed a critical debate around 'warm' humanist medicine in a time of unprecedented explosion of 'cold' scientific understanding (Clouser 1971; Banks and Vastyan 1973; Leake 1973; Pellegrino 1974, 1979; Reynolds and Carson 1976), arguing that the traditional bedside art of medicine may be eclipsed as a need for greater knowledge of science crowded out the curriculum. A further group of papers in the 1980s and 1990s brought this debate to a head, already describing a lost era not only of the art of bedside medicine, as discussed in the Introduction, but of humane practice in general, noting the 'inhumanity' (Weatherall 1994: 1671) of scientific medicine, including serial objectification of patients.

Sceptics towards the value of humanities in medicine responded vigorously towards these criticisms of medicine's perceived inhumanity. For example, Wassersug (1987: 317) cynically argued: 'real medical progress has not been made by humanitarians but by doctors equipped with microscopes, scalpels, dyes, catheters, rays, test tubes, and culture plates'. Such sceptics gained a tactical high ground by demanding that proponents of medical humanities should offer solid (scientific) evidence of impact, placing the burden of proof on the shoulders of those who would characteristically question the meaning of such instrumental 'evidence'. This challenge is discussed at length in Chapter 9.

Thus, McManus (1995: 1143) suggested that 'Any serious evaluation of the humanities in medicine...must bite the bullet of definition and measurement, even if it seems to be "defining the indefinable".' At this point, the body of orthodox medicine could readily absorb the promised critical sting of the medical humanities. From the perspective of the medical humanities, the 'bullet of definition and measurement' to be bitten was also the bullet of sterile experimental science – by definition intolerant of ambiguity – that threatened to kill the fecund and ambiguous body of art.

In this emerging debate about responsibility for providing evidence of the worth of medical humanities interventions, the lesson of Crawshaw's seminal paper 'Humanism in Medicine' was buried. Crawshaw (1975: 1320) had suggested that it was the responsibility of the medical profession to respond to the accusation that it is 'more mechanical and less human', where 'Our ears are bent, our minds filled, perhaps even our hearts weighed with the burgeoning catalogue of iatrogenic problems.' Such 'iatrogenic problems' were identified from cumulative evidence of an unacceptably high level of medical error, as indicated earlier.

Brian Hurwitz and Paul Dakin (2009: 84) note that the historian of science George Sarton 'first used the term "medical humanities" in the 1940s in the pages of *ISIS*, a journal devoted to the history of science, medicine and civilization'. In 1951, in a Canadian context, Van Wyck (1951) wrote an article on the role of the humanities in medical education. And in 1952, the first major medical humanities curriculum innovation was established in a North American medical school in the wake of Reinke's (1937) suggestion mentioned earlier. Case Western Reserve medical school in Cleveland, Ohio overhauled the medicine curriculum over a period of five years between 1952–57 and in this process introduced an optional element of study in the history of medicine (Cook 2010). Case Western Reserve had a history of innovation – in 1852 and 1854 it graduated two women, only the second and third to receive medical degrees in North America. Its curriculum overhaul between 1952 and 1957 was considered radical at the time, integrating basic and applied (clinical) sciences.

Over a decade passed before a North American medical school underwent a major curriculum development of the sort modelled by Case Western Reserve. In 1967, Pennsylvania State University's College of Medicine developed a unique undergraduate medicine programme biased towards community medicine, ethics and spiritual aspects of chronic illness and care, providing a fertile ideological ground for the establishment of the medical humanities, where the reductive biomedical model was already enlarged to a more encompassing biopsychosocial model. A Department of Humanities, the first of its kind, was established within the medical school (Hawkins *et al.* 2003), where medical students learned about religion, history and philosophy as these applied to medicine, while literature was added in 1969.

In the same year (1969) *The Society for Health and Human Values* was officially launched as a membership organization, keeping records from

1970–97 now lodged at the University of Texas medical school at Galveston (Moody Medical Library undated). This was the first professional membership organization internationally for those committed to supporting and developing human values in medicine. In 1998, the Society was merged with the American Society for Bioethics and the Society for Bioethics Consultation to form the American Society for Bioethics and Humanities (www.asbh.org), now a vigorous and flourishing organization promoting scholarship, research and teaching in the twin fields of bioethics and the medical humanities but with a clear bias towards bioethics.

Whereas bioethics and the medical humanities have traditionally been closely aligned in North American medical education, this has not been the case in the United Kingdom for example, where the establishment of ethics and law as compulsory study in the undergraduate curriculum has been seen largely as a separate stream of interest from the establishment of the medical humanities. While establishing ethics in medical schools has often been seen as an instrumental precursor to the development of the medical humanities in the UK, a careful argument has yet to be made about the pedagogical structure of an ethics curriculum being used as a prototype for development of the medical humanities in medical education.

The marriage between ethics and the medical humanities in the medical education curriculum has been more successful in a North American context. In the early 1970s, around 4 per cent of American medical schools taught formal courses in bioethics where by 1994 such courses were compulsory in the medicine curriculum (Fox *et al.* 1995). Many overlaps were noted between bioethics and the medical humanities, especially in the use of narrative. For example, Tod Chambers (1999) analyses classic ethics 'cases' regularly used in teaching as literary, rather than functional, texts. Hilde Lindemann Nelson and colleagues (1997) also outline a narrative approach to bioethics. However, just as a subject such as the history of medicine has its own specialized journals, associations and meetings, so bioethics tends to run as a parallel stream to the medical humanities. In the UK, the *British Medical Journal* publishes sister journals dedicated to ethics (*Journal of Medical Ethics*) and medical humanities (*Medical Humanities*) with little overlap. This carries through to separate associations, conferences and academic communities.

That the landmark events briefly described above occurred is one thing, but why they occurred is of course much more important. Introducing medical ethics to the undergraduate medicine curriculum can be explained as a response to a variety of new ethical problems raised by technological advances throughout the 1960s and 1970s. Advances included a proliferation of new drugs, including those for mental health such as anxiolytics (antipanic and antianxiety) and antidepressants that were appropriated as lifestyle drugs as a replacement for, or in concert with, alcohol. Other advances included in vitro fertilization, organ transplants and readily available contraception.

Beyond medical ethics, why would the humanities be of interest to medical schools during this period? The introduction of medical history seems straightforward, where students should know about the history of diseases as a background to public health and even a smattering of knowledge about the history of their own discipline of medicine – but why humanities such as literature? Drawing on the work of Kathryn Montgomery (then Kathryn Montgomery Hunter), Tess Jones, Delese Wear and Lester Friedman (2014: 2) suggest that academic literary criticism was increasingly becoming interested in the inward-looking intricacies of the text isolated from its historical and cultural contexts. This resulted, in Kathryn Montgomery Hunter's phrase, in a cadre of 'intellectually under-employed' scholars disinterested in the intricacies of intratextual analysis, so that, in the words of Jones, Wear and Friedman, 'these disenchanted faculty members, along with a growing cadre of newer scholars interested in interdisciplinary education were drawn to medical education as a fertile ground for their ideas and passions' (*ibid.*). Hunter (1991a) wrote a key article on this evolving condition ('Toward the Cultural Interpretation of Medicine') in the journal *Literature and Medicine*. But this journal was already nearly a decade old, having been launched in 1982, showing that the convergence between the two disciplines of literature and medicine was already under way. However, literary approaches had not yet gained a foothold in medical education, despite initiatives at Galveston, Texas described below.

Edmund Pellegrino (1972) saw the wave of interest in medical ethics and the first flush of interest in narrative medicine within medical education as a marriage made in heaven, where abstract issues of value (ethics) could now be given concrete focus in doctor–patient encounters and the structures of medical knowledge (diagnosis and treatment) through an ethics–humanities–medicine trialogue. An inaugural meeting of the Institute on Human Values in Medicine (*ibid.*) considered the value of humanities disciplines for medical education working in concert with medical approaches for mutual benefit. Jones, Wear and Friedman (2014) ask, in hindsight, just how this mutual benefit might work and point to two possibilities. First are the multiple nuts and bolts of narrative knowing, such as close noticing in medical diagnosis as an equivalent to close reading of texts in literature; second is the complex education of a moral practice promising the incorporation of cross-cultural perspectives and social justice into medical work – the first a perceptual sensibility, the second a moral sensibility (or, better, sensitivity). In total, the humanities can offer an education into seeing otherwise.

In 1973, the *Institute of Medical Humanities* was founded at the University of Texas, Galveston (Jones and Carson 2003) with a bias towards literature and medicine. Anne Hudson Jones joined this faculty in 1979 as one of the first literature professors to teach in a medical school. Where modern medical humanities reinvented the traditional art of medicine, it offered an extension to the study of scientific medicine, but not a critical rejoinder. The introduction of literature, however, potentially offered the medical humanities a clear critical stance, articulating a paradigm of care based on careful appreciation and use of patients' stories. Narrative-based medicine (Chapter 7) challenged the dominant values of evidence-based medicine, turning attention away from generalized population statistics to the meaning of illness for the individual in context, encouraging a felt response to persons rather than simply a clinical problem-solving mentality.

The North American *Journal of Medical Humanities* (http://link.springer.com/journal/10912) was launched earlier, in 1979, inviting articles on humanities, social sciences with 'strong humanistic traditions', cultural studies and bioethics topics related to medicine and healthcare. The journal is edited by Tess Jones from the University of Colorado at Boulder, a humanities scholar with a PhD in English and a research interest in HIV/AIDS and the arts. Tess Jones is lead editor of the *Health Humanities Reader* (Jones *et al.* 2014) published by Rutgers University Press, a landmark publication in the field. The journal she edits now calls specifically for papers from the three areas of medical humanities, cultural studies and pedagogy. This key journal formally acknowledged an academic community of scholars, researchers and teachers, who, while embracing a number of disciplines and experimenting with interdisciplinary approaches, recognized themselves as contributing to the 'medical humanities'. This formal establishment of such a community was reinforced through the publication of an influential Hastings-commissioned report in 1984 – *The Place of the Humanities in Medicine* – authored by a physician specializing in the nature and ethics of suffering, Eric Cassell.

The medical humanities community in North America by now was, in the eyes of some, achieving adulthood. In 1984, Edmund Pellegrino (1984) suggested that the medical humanities had developed into a 'movement' that had already been through a phase of evangelism, where the virtues of the movement were assumed in the absence of evidence for their effects. Pellegrino described a 'post-evangelical era' as evidence of maturity in the field. Cassell's Hastings Centre commissioned report confirmed this maturity. Cassell argued that the humanities were better placed than science and technology to develop certain functions needed to practice and develop modern medicine, such as the capacities for empathy and collaboration.

The two decades following Cassell's report were characterized by consolidation of medical humanities provision in the USA. In 1988, Arnold Gold, a physician, and Sandra Gold, a psychologist and educationalist, with colleagues at the Columbia University College of Physicians and Surgeons in New York, founded The Arnold P. Gold Foundation, a public, not-for-profit organization. The Arnold P. Gold Foundation (http://humanism-in-medicine.org), through a series of educational programmes and sponsored research, develops 'humanistic medical care'. The foundation insists:

> Humanistic medical care is not simply compassion. It is the best of medicine. When skilled physicians build caring, trusting and collaborative relationships with patients, studies reveal more appropriate medical decisions, better patient adherence with treatment plans, and less costly healthcare outcomes.
>
> (Arnold P. Gold Foundation undated)

The Sirridge Office of medical humanities, named after its physician patrons Marjorie and William Sirridge, was opened in 1992 at the University of Missouri–Kansas City School of Medicine. Coupled with an interest in bioethics, this has developed into a major medical humanities provision feeding into the later (5th and 6th) years and providing compulsory core provision, with a medicine and music provision that allows for study in Graz, Austria. The Sirridge programme promises to move medical students beyond 'superior clinical skills' to 'observe, analyze and reflect on each medical challenge they encounter' (UMKC undated). The six-year BA/MD programme requires study of the liberal arts in the first two years.

By 1994, the first medical humanities website was established at the New York School of Medicine (http://medhum.med.nyu.edu) – at the time, this was one of a relative handful of websites on a nascent Internet – followed by the establishment of the *Program in Narrative Medicine* at Columbia University directed by Rita Charon. Around a decade later, in October 2003, a special edition of the journal *Academic Medicine* (vol. 78, no. 10) was devoted to the state of the art of medical humanities in medical education – an indication that the medical humanities in medical education were now being taken seriously by the academic medicine or medical education community. Yet this edition was explicitly celebratory rather than critical. For example, programme descriptions offered scant detail on content of medical humanities provision, such as what *kinds* of literature, visual art, music, and so forth were employed; and whether or not the 'art' and 'humanities' chosen were decorative, comforting or even banal, rather than challenging and purposefully destabilizing, or constructively critical of their 'father figure' of medical culture. Finally, a North American based electronic medical humanities journal *Hektoen International* was founded in Chicago in 2009 by the Hektoen Institute of Medicine (www.hektoeninternational.org) offering a brief for eclectic publications going far beyond the world of the medical humanities in medical education.

In 1991, the bioethicist Kathryn Montgomery Hunter (mentioned earlier) wrote the first book on narrative medicine (Hunter 1991b; see also Chapter 7 of the present volume, and Montgomery 2006). She argued that medical knowledge is narratively structured – doctors learn to diagnose and treat from repeated exposure to patients' stories, thinking narratively. For example, what is the course of a patient's story, even while it is a fragment of a whole? Montgomery provocatively suggested that science education in contemporary medicine was over emphasized, where medicine is a 'science-*using*' practice

(Hunter 1991b: 25; my emphasis). Montgomery placed narrative clinical reasoning in the genre of the detective story – a pragmatic focus that appealed to doctors as they use the senses to discriminate among clues (Bleakley 2004, 2006b; Bleakley *et al.* 2003a, 2003b). It is received wisdom in medicine that doctors make their diagnoses largely on the basis of what is in a patient's story outside of the physical examination and clinical tests, and recent research confirms this (Mylopoulos *et al.* 2012).

Kathryn Montgomery's (2006) work is fundamental to understanding why the medical humanities can have a core and integrated place in the undergraduate medicine and surgery curriculum. The implications of her work are radical – medical students probably learn too much science content for the jobs they will undertake as junior doctors prior to specialization, too much of the 'wrong' science (for example complexity science is not emphasized enough), and not enough of how to 'think with science' narratively in order to understand patients' stories. The implication of this critique is far reaching for medical education – it suggests that the focus for identity construction of doctors (first as scientists and then as clinicians) is misplaced.

Rather, doctors achieve an expert identity as 'science-using' diagnosticians, where a narrative imagination and formal narrative capabilities are paramount. But they do this, in educational terms, in a haphazard and poorly designed manner, picking up expertise through immersion in expert communities of practice. Part of the design of the undergraduate curriculum is then itself misplaced as a form of what Paul Goodman (1966) called 'compulsory miseducation'. Medical education has an unintended consequence – the production of insensibility in medical students. Put another way, the sensibility capital available among expert clinicians is poorly distributed (or withheld) where medical students, patients and healthcare colleagues are not apportioned such sensibility capital as a result of a structural power-based hierarchy. To compound this issue of maldistribution of sensibility, expert clinicians may only be, at best, average clinical teachers and educationalists. This argument is set out in detail in Chapter 3.

In 2002, Rachel Kaiser (2002) suggested that identity construction through medical education was a kind of misidentification, where students were socialized into a dysfunctional community based on structural inequalities. The historically conditioned authoritarian and hierarchical nature of medicine is also patriarchal and imitates oppressive post-colonial contexts. The power structure reinforces the notion that medical students 'lack' what seniors can give them. This privileges a 'transmission' model of pedagogy in which, paradoxically, withholding information affirms seniority and power. Drawing on a psychoanalytic perspective, Kaiser (*ibid.*: 95) describes how a medical education 'limits uniqueness, squelches inquisitiveness, and damages one's self-confidence'. For Kaiser, such hierarchies must be resisted and destabilized as a political activity through students defining themselves not as different from patients and healthcare colleagues (strong identification with doctors) but outside of such differences, as for example citizens or women and men challenging a wider patriarchal and authority led power discourse.

To return to the historical conditions under which the medical humanities were made possible, Kenneth Ludmerer (1999) traces the history of twentieth-century American medical education in political terms as a cycle of erosion then regaining of public trust, in which doctors must engage with wider social concerns as well as empathy for individuals. Political consciousness-raising in the USA in the 1960s and early 1970s, spanning the Vietnam War and the Civil Rights movement, led to medical schools becoming more responsive socially and engaging with educational reform. A knock-on effect was to introduce more humanities teaching in medical education (*ibid.*: 237–59). This involved innovations such as the introduction of professional actors playing 'standardized' patients for the purposes of student learning and assessment in simulated clinical contexts (Hardee and Kasper 2005).

However, as medicine became increasingly driven by a profit motive during the 1960s and 1970s – framed as a business, with patients as consumers – so insurers became more adept at litigation for medical error in protecting consumer rights (Mohr 2000). Such litigation increasingly involved breakdown in doctor–patient communication (Huntington and Kuhn 2003). Medicine had to regain its human touch. The early hegemony of science studies and anatomy helped to desensitize medical students through objectifying the body, with such an-aesthetizing driving out any lingering interest in the aesthetic. By the 1990s the 'inhumanity' (Weatherall 1994: 1671) of scientific medicine referred to earlier was deemed to be endemic.

The need to reconnect with an alienated public expressed itself in the consulting room as a need to listen closely to patients' stories. Also, the rising wave of litigation (increasingly centred on doctors' poor communication, as noted above) demanded that medical ethics take a central place in medical education. Literature offered a rich medium for teaching ethics. Interest in the history of medicine was supplemented by an interest in restoring the art of 'taking a history' from the patient. This is why 'narrative-based medicine' (Greenhalgh and Hurwitz 1999) became the most popular form of the early medical humanities, challenging the dominant values of evidence-based medicine by turning attention away from generalized population statistics to the meaning of illness for the individual in context. Importantly, narrative-based medicine placed linguistic performance at the core of doctor–patient encounters as a key element in clinical effectiveness.

Medicine not only objectifies through language performances but also sets up a defence against uncertainty. Ludmerer (1999) reminds us that intolerance of uncertainty and refusal to admit to uncertainty are, historically, medicine's greatest wounds. Current medical education fails to prepare medical students adequately for tolerance of ambiguity in their work as doctors, blunting sensibilities. Intolerance of ambiguity not only leads to misdiagnoses and overdiagnoses, but also to bolstering the hierarchical structures endemic to medical culture (Bleakley 2014). Medicine, says Ludmerer, must learn to share its inevitable load of uncertainty with patients. I will talk much more about this in future chapters, where the indicative mood ('this *is*') is preferred to the subjunctive mood ('this could *be*') and modal auxiliaries for the verb such as 'might', 'could', 'possibly' and 'maybe' are avoided or defended against in medicine's linguistic performance (see Chapter 7).

As Jerome Bruner (in Good 1994: 153) suggests: 'To be in the subjunctive is...to be trafficking in human possibilities rather than in settled certainties.' Intolerance of ambiguity is a refusal of narrative tension and affect. The classic medical 'case presentation' formally suspends or brackets out the emotional charge characterizing clinical exchanges. John Austin (1962) refers to the ritualized functions of language, for example as used by the medical professions, as illocutionary, where the perlocutionary carries a high degree of ambiguity. French poststructuralist feminists such as Hélène Cixous (1991) point to indicative language as gendered male, typically relying on strategies of oppositional forms and authority-led statements (statements, telling, informing, ordering, confronting) rather than democratic performances of open-ended questions (asking, conversing, inviting, supporting). Indicative language is not written in what Cixous (1981) refers to as 'mother's milk' – a language (and activity) of tenderness and succour. Medical language is peppered too with masculinist, militaristic metaphors (Bleakley *et al.* 2014).

To return to the point about the link between narrative and medicine, if medicine narrates illness in indicative, martial ways, then simply importing narrative outlook into medical practice is counterproductive, another example of production of insensibility, discussed in subsequent chapters. As the anthropologist Byron Good (2000: no pagination) suggests: 'The narratization of illness draws on subjunctivizing tactics as a means of maintaining openness, sources of potency and hope.' These doors are closed where doctors objectify patients through the indicative, imagining that patients want a 'clear diagnosis'. Of course patients hope for clarity in diagnosis, treatment and prognosis, but they are more concerned to have an open and authentic discussion with a doctor who cares, in which uncertainty may loom large but is managed collaboratively.

While Delese Wear (2009) sees the first session of the Institute on Human Values in Medicine in 1972 as the primary spark for the subsequent spread of the medical humanities fire, in hindsight, the 1973 Galveston experimental curriculum innovation may have been the most important contribution to the initiative of the medical humanities in medical education in North America. Stemming from this initiative, narrative-based medicine has remained the primary topic of choice for North American medical schools, where the history of medicine has largely developed independently from medical schools in university history departments. Characteristically, since the 1973 Texas innovation, medical schools based in University settings have attracted key faculty members from departments such as English within the parent University to offer elective programmes for medical students, for the reasons perhaps that Montgomery (Hunter) and Jones, Wear and Friedman suggest above. Figures such as Kathryn Montgomery and Rita Charon in particular have made powerful arguments for the inclusion of narrative-based medicine in the core medicine curriculum to be considered on an equal footing with biomedical science. Medical students should know as much about how patients express and live their symptoms as they do about the science behind those symptoms. More importantly, medical students must learn, in the process of becoming doctors, how to perform consultations, bedside diagnoses, teamwork and the teaching of medicine.

At the time of writing, the major turn in the medical humanities in North America appears to be towards a more inclusive 'health humanities' with a recognition that health humanities can be practiced across a variety of locations, primarily medical school faculties, but also arts and humanities faculties in universities, private and charitable Trusts such as the Gold Foundation that sponsor activities within medical schools and promote medical education at events such as national and international conferences and in the public sphere through public engagement activities such as exhibitions. This differs from the current trend in the UK towards university humanities departments reclaiming ownership of the medical humanities, albeit as an interdisciplinary project, resulting in some dampening of medical humanities interest in medical schools' medical education departments, partly due to lack of funding for research.

The North American eclectic approach extends beyond embracing healthcare as a whole, to include practices beyond medicine, but also to celebrating interdisciplinary approaches and the variety of modes in which the health humanities culture's interests might be expressed – from formal academic research to informal journalistic and impressionistic writing, to literary description. The *Health Humanities Reader* edited by Therese Jones, Delese Wear and Lester Friedman (2014) offers a hefty 600+ pages of absorbing contemporary engagement with the field of the health humanities themed not by disciplines but topics, such as 'disability', 'the body', 'gender and sexuality' and 'spirituality and religion'. Poems with commentary mix easily with historical accounts, polemical essays, academic accounts laced with findings from empirical studies, comix, works of fiction and future-fantasy essays. This text marks a significant shift away from discipline-based, territorial squabbling to a genuine sense of collaboration in the development of the medical/ health humanities culture although it misses an international dimension among authors, showing a North American bias. It will, however, act as a key text in the field for many years to come and be mined thoroughly for its riches by both scholars and practitioners.

One of the editors of this text, Delese Wear (2009) conducted an interesting survey study of 15 faculty members who are experts in the field of medical humanities and their conclusions on the state of the art of the medical humanities in medical education in North America will serve as a conclusion to this section. Wear notes that medical humanities provision is rarely subject to formal assessment, has been characterized in recent times as aligned with 'professionalism' and varies considerably across local contexts. She was particularly interested in respondents' views of establishing a core medical humanities provision – discussed at length throughout this book.

Wear's expert panel focused largely on medical humanities providing a perspective for practice that not only oriented clinicians towards the human face of their work – the intimate lives of patients and their social and cultural contexts – but also contextualised practice in current political, legal and governmental strategies. Respondents were less inclined to make a direct link between medical humanities provision and the education of empathy, a common association in the medical humanities literature that is often left unexamined. There was lack of consensus on the issue of a core curriculum, but insightful comments from one participant who argued for full integration of the medical humanities with other provision to offer a critical counterweight (for example, learning anatomy cannot be disentangled from learning respect and necessary emotional desensitization).

Views on what qualifications are needed to teach humanities varied, with a general view that quality of engagement and passion for the teaching outweighed technical credentials. Interestingly, none of the sample appeared to comment on the value of team teaching, or pairing clinicians with arts practitioners and humanities scholars. Further, the article concentrates on humanities provision and does not mention the employment of arts practitioners – a prominent bias in the North American literature. This is important because Wear argues for a medical humanities that confounds disciplinary interests so that the medical humanities themselves does not come to discipline medical students but rather to liberate them from the constraints of medical disciplining. Surely the radical arts, such as performance in particular, are ready-made for such powerful pedagogical interventions? However, Wear argues too for the value of 'softer' approaches to include humility in inquiry, so that we do not merely imitate the martial stance of medicine in which we harden ourselves and armour ourselves with sharp, critical tools. Medical humanities also need not become soft relaxation (the caricature ascribed by the 'hard' anatomists for example), but can offer a necessary suppleness to a medical education.

The medical humanities in the United Kingdom

Beyond North America, the medical humanities flame was kindled most strongly in the United Kingdom, although Anthony Moore (1976: 1479), a surgeon working at the University of Melbourne, first used the descriptor 'medical humanities' in the published literature, describing a short course designed for medical students to discuss 'broader cultural, philosophical and personal issues relevant to doctorship [*sic*]' based around literature. And coincidentally, in 1976, the University of La Plata medical school in the Argentine Republic developed an optional medical humanities provision (Acuña 2000, 2003).

The poet Philip Larkin famously wrote: 'Sexual intercourse began / In nineteen sixty-three / (Which was rather late for me) – / Between the end of the *Chatterley* ban / And the Beatles' first LP'(Larkin 2003). Of course sexual intercourse did not begin in 1963, but we know what Larkin means – the conditions of possibility emerged for a sexual revolution: a generational revolution against post-war austerity, relaxation in censorship and the availability of the contraceptive pill. In the same way, 'medical humanities' as a formal celebration of the creative relationship between art and medicine did not 'begin' in the UK in 1944–45 as the nascent art therapy movement, although this offers a convenient starting point. For example, paintings had been hung in hospitals for the benefit of patients long before – such paintings were usually neither comforting nor decorative, but faced patients directly with issues such as mortality (Cork 2012). A painter, Adrian Hill, is usually acknowledged as the founder of art therapy in the UK. While being treated in a tuberculosis sanatorium, Hill introduced artistic work to his fellow patients as part of the treatment, chronicled in *Art Versus Illness* (Hill 1945). This work was then extended to long-term patients in mental hospitals. During the same period, the psychologist Margaret Naumberg and artist Edith Kramer initiated art therapy in the USA.

The arts therapy movement was not directly linked with medical education until The Wellcome Foundation organized a seminar on the arts in health, the first of its kind in the UK, almost a half century after Hill's ground-breaking work in 1993. In the same year, the General Medical Council (GMC) published the first edition of *Tomorrow's Doctors* that set out a curriculum framework for UK medical schools (General Medical Council 1993). The GMC encouraged provision of optional special study components beyond the core undergraduate curriculum. These would be mainly in sciences, but modules in history of medicine and literature were also encouraged. However, Deborah Kirklin (2002: 101) later pointed out that no extra funding was available to medical schools to support this initiative, while in 2002 'only three dedicated medical humanities academic posts exist in the UK'. Victoria Bates and Sam Goodman (2014) note that in the UK, medical humanities provision in medical schools has often relied on multidisciplinary collaboration across University departments rather than providing truly interdisciplinary, dedicated faculty job roles within medical school departments.

On the tail of the 1993 Wellcome Foundation seminar, the UK Royal Society of Medicine organized a symposium in 1995 entitled 'Art in

Hospitals: Past, Present and Future'. In 1995, I.C. McManus, based at St Mary's Hospital (Imperial College, London), wrote an article in *The Lancet* entitled 'Humanity and the Medical Humanities' (referred to earlier), pointing to what he saw as a longstanding cultural blind spot, where 'The literature is replete with pleas for the central role of the humanities in medical education, and has been so at least since the 1960s as part of a long tradition of medical humanism' (McManus 1995: 1143). McManus was presumably thinking of the literature from the USA, where little had been published in the UK at this time.

Kenneth Ludmerer (1999: xxi) suggested that 'it would be a great error to view the history of American medical education as devoid of people or personalities' and the same can be said for the development of the medical humanities in the UK. Two figures – Robin Philipp and Kenneth Calman – offered a formative influence, with particular interests, respectively, in arts in health and medical humanities in medical education. Calman was the Chief Medical Officer (CMO) for Scotland (1989–91) and then England (1991–98), a member of the Nuffield Council on Bioethics (2000–08) and had strong links with the Wellcome Trust. Philipp, a public health consultant working within the NHS, was interested in health inequalities, the area in which 'arts for health' was having its greatest impact (Coats 2004). Philipp had come from New Zealand, where he was involved in the first medical humanities conference organized outside the USA, in Wellington in 1994. In 1996, the University of Auckland, New Zealand, hosted the first Pacific Rim conference on narrative-based medicine. In the same year, the University of Otago, New Zealand, held a conference on the relationships between literature and healthcare practice and education entitled 'Health in the Writer's Hand'.

Arts for, and in, health, however, refused to be 'medicalized', supporting a range of psychological and therapeutic approaches from its association with arts therapies, and had little to do with the training of doctors (Hamilton *et al.* 2003; Health Development Agency 2000). In the wake of the GMC's 1993 initial recommendations about study of humanities for medical students – certainly influenced by Calman as CMO for England – Calman met with the Minister of Health in December 1996 to discuss the initiative of the 'humanities in medicine'. A particularly optimistic view of the arts and humanities in medicine was promoted, where Calman later suggested that the Department of Health should become a 'Department of Health and Happiness' (Ward 1999).

This idealist and utilitarian view would set the tone for the development of the medical humanities in the UK into the new millennium. It mirrored the dominant North American approach to the medical humanities as a force for wellbeing, under the sway of the philosophy embodied in the Constitution and the Declaration of Independence as 'self-evident truths' – the ideals of 'Life, liberty and the pursuit of happiness'. This offers a 'homeostasis' view of medical humanities – mirroring the conventional homeostasis model of medicine – where the purpose of the humanities is also to pursue 'health', 'happiness' and 'wellbeing'. Paradoxically, this is at odds with what many artists would see as the purpose of art (and of complexity science, to which medicine is warming), which is not to encourage homeostasis, but rather to produce a permanent state of disequilibrium as the basis for the emergence of innovation. This not only continuously challenges cultural norms and habits, but also sees value in pathology and symptom, and meaning in illness (Macneill 2011; Cork 2012). Perhaps more importantly, the medical humanities were not seen as having potentially negative unintended consequences such as the paradoxical imperative 'you will be humane!' (Petersen *et al.* 2008) as a further example of the production of insensibility.

The first major UK conference organized by Philipp and Calman, the 1998 Windsor conference (Philipp *et al.* 1999: 8), embodied a dual approach of arts in health and humanities in medical education, setting out explicitly to 'promote the arts from the margins into the very heart of healthcare planning, policy-making and practice'. It was supported by the Nuffield Trust, who later also supported the development of the first institute for the medical humanities in the UK at Durham University, where Calman was by then vice chancellor. The 1998 and subsequent 1999 Windsor conferences downplayed those aspects of the medical humanities that constituted an academic study of medicine, particularly through disciplines such as history, philosophy and literature. The lack of attention given to this form of medical humanities was ironic, as it would later become the dominant medical humanities approach attracting strong funding support from the Wellcome Trust.

While these conferences seemed ground-breaking at the time, in retrospect, in bringing the 'marginal' arts into the mainstream of medicine the radical role of the arts as marginal agitator and critic was in danger of being subsumed within a more powerful, conservative medical culture. The arts would become a tame friend and ally to medicine rather than a critical counterweight or outright pest and agitator. Given the revolutionary nature of the arts in wider culture at the time, this taming of the arts in service to medical education can be seen as the core issue in the (mal)distribution of sensibility through medical education that is discussed at length in Chapter 3. In bringing in the arts and taming them, or in bringing in tame arts (decorative rather than critical, apolitical and aesthetically unchallenging) as a 'welcome relief' from the supposedly hard grind of science studies, medical education increased the insensibility of medical students and in turn did the arts a disservice.

Political questions concerning medicine's authoritarian structure and lack of public transparency were avoided, as were ethical questions concerning the education of sensitivity (warmth, compassion, humane practice, empathy) and aesthetic questions concerning medicine as a performance and an act of connoisseurship. These were not entirely conscious acts on behalf of curriculum designers, but their effects ran deep – again to avoid the distribution of sensibility capital held by senior clinical teachers to medical students and patients as a form of consciousness-raising and democratizing politically, deepening sensibility aesthetically and educating for sensitivity ethically.

In case readers think that I am overstating the case, the report from a second Windsor conference in 1999 contained a warning from the philosopher Robin Downie that 'art can be counterproductive if it is done for the wrong reasons. The typical artist is for example, not a good health role model!' (quoted in Philipp *et al.* 2002). This stereotype is revealing, as it made the UK medical humanities initiative suddenly look reactionary (from the point of view of the cutting edge or avant-garde arts). The two Windsor conferences, under the influence of utilitarianism rather than scepticism (Bleakley 2013b), framed the medical humanities as a 'healing' force in the service of medicine, rather than problematizing the ideal of 'healing', or asking whether illness and disability can be reconfigured as strengths or personal and cultural capital.

A manifesto emerged from the first Windsor conference, with a rhetorical tone of urgency. The medical humanities would lead to medical students becoming 'more 'rounded' people' who would develop the values and skills of compassion and empathy for both patients and colleagues (Philipp *et al.* 1999: 115). The pedagogical plan, however, was confused. While medical schools 'should' include humanities such as moral philosophy, theology and literature, and perhaps history, creative writing and painting (implying core and integrated provision), it was proposed that this approach *could* be introduced through an intercalated BA degree (implying elective choice). This avoided the issue of how to design a core and integrated medical humanities curriculum, leaving the 'rounding' of medical students to the tiny handful who would opt for an intercalated degree. Further, such a degree would almost certainly isolate students from learning humanities in clinical contexts, returning them to the classroom to formally study history, literature and so forth.

Anne Hudson Jones and former graduate student Faith McLellan from the pioneering University of Texas, Galveston medical humanities programme were invited to participate in this first UK medical humanities conference and the conference proceedings referred to UK medical humanities initiatives as 'twenty years behind' the Galveston model. A second Windsor conference took place in 1999. The overall rhetoric of this conference again applauded the idealism of the arts and health movement with vacuous descriptors such as 'good health'. Yet embedded in the report is a valuable suggestion from Downie: that we can learn from the arts by '*imaginative identification with situations or characters depicted, and by having our imaginations stretched through being made to enter into unfamiliar situations or to see points of view other than our own*' (Philipp *et al.* 2002: 14; emphasis original).

This is commendable, but how does this square with the 'happiness and health' ethic? Such views are problematic for example when considered from the point of view of contemporary disability studies. It is at this point in Downie's statement that the suspicious warning mentioned earlier follows – that 'Art can be counterproductive if it is done for the wrong reasons. The typical artist is for example, not a good health role model!' (*ibid.*: 109). The reader is left wondering whether or not those students opting for an intercalated humanities degree would ever be exposed to the radical arts and their promises to challenge the conservatism of the medicine curriculum, or the introduction to the idea first proposed by Nietzsche and taken up by Gilles Deleuze, that artists are like doctors, but their work is as 'diagnosticians of culture', or the body of culture rather than the body of the individual. Artists diagnose cultural symptoms and treat them, sometimes against the grain of unexamined ideas of 'health' and 'wellbeing'.

The outcome of the two Windsor conferences was to frame the medical humanities as a 'healing' force in the service of medicine, rather than to shape its presence as a force of resistance problematizing the ideal of 'healing'. Support was sought from within the heart of the establishment, including endorsement by the president of the GMC. Such lobbying would have an effect. As mentioned above, in a 2003 publication the GMC encouraged inclusion of the medical humanities in undergraduate medical curricula – again in the service of 'wellbeing' – where literature, arts, poetry, and philosophy are thought to potentially foster the doctor's ability to 'communicate with patients, to penetrate more deeply into the patient's wider narrative, and to seek more diverse ways of promoting well being and reducing the impact of illness or disability' (General Medical Council 2003). Such a statement paradoxically positions illness and disability in opposition to (the fictions of) health and normality and as the lesser term in the opposition.

The GMC suggested that 25–33 per cent of the curriculum should include optional Student Selected Units (SSUs) or Components (SSCs) focused on the 'humanities related to medicine'. However, since that important step forward, a backsliding has occurred. The revised GMC 2009 document made no specific reference to humanities in medicine and recommended that SSCs provision be cut to 10 per cent (General Medical Council 2009: 50), while emphasis was placed upon the value of teaching communication skills to medical students rather than integrating the medical humanities into the curriculum.

At the same time as the Windsor conferences, two London-based GPs, Deborah Kirklin and Richard Meakin, established a Centre for Medical Humanities at the Royal Free and University College Medical School, London (Kirklin 2003). This began in 1998 as the Medical Humanities Unit, drawing together a group of medical educators with interest in the arts and humanities to (i) feed in to the undergraduate medical curriculum with core and optional provision, (ii) provide a one-year intercalated BSc in Medical Humanities, and (iii) offer postgraduates a continuing professional development accredited two-day course in medical humanities and an annual residential retreat open only to graduates of the course, the first of its kind in the UK. Despite its strong academic and critical approach, a decade later the Centre was controversially closed in a strategic 'rationalization' by the host university, indicating that the medical humanities were still regarded as marginal. A strong, expanding network had failed to form. Fault-lines were evident in the culture.

In 1999, the Nuffield Trust also helped to establish a Centre for the Arts and Humanities in Health and Medicine (CAHHM) at the University of Durham (where Kenneth Calman was to become vice chancellor) and a new Institute of Medical Humanities. The latter was developed as the Association for Medical Humanities (AMH) whose primary functions have been to run annual conferences to develop the field and to lobby grant awarding bodies such as the Wellcome Trust and Arts Council England (ACE) in strategic development of the medical humanities nationally.

In June 2000, the BMJ publishing group launched a new journal – *Medical Humanities* – as a sister publication to the established *Journal of Medical Ethics*. In the same year, a research colloquium on the medical humanities was set up through the University of Swansea. This meeting led to the first UK publication to describe the emerging field of the medical humanities (Evans and Finlay 2001), also discussing how the medical humanities could be integrated into the core curriculum in undergraduate medical education through meeting learning outcomes set by the UK GMC. A second colloquium was run in 2001 at Powys, Wales, sponsored by the Nuffield Trust and the University of Wales, where 'The purpose of the meeting was to provide the opportunity for an intensive exploration of how the medical humanities could, as a recently emerging field of inquiry, best be developed into a worthwhile area of university-based teaching and research' (Evans and Greaves 2001b: 93).

The University of Wales Swansea had been at the forefront of development of the medical humanities for some time, having offered a MA in Medical Humanities since 1997 (*ibid.*). Martyn Evans, a philosopher, and David Greaves, a doctor with a PhD in ethics, were instrumental in setting up the programme that had a bias towards ethics and philosophy. Evans would become the President of the Association for Medical Humanities and co-editor of the journal *Medical Humanities* and later would move to Durham University where he was instrumental in successfully bidding for Wellcome Trust funding to support a Centre for Medical Humanities and was then appointed as co-director of the research programme along with Jane Macnaughton. Anne Borsay, a medical historian, took up the baton at Swansea and became the director of the Health Humanities programme (see www.swansea.ac.uk/humanandhealthsciences/research/centres-and-groups/health-humanities).

In 2002, the inaugural meeting of the UK Association for Medical Humanities (AMH) was held at the University of Birmingham (the AMH conference has subsequently been run annually at differing venues). In an account of that meeting, Martyn Evans and David Greaves asked 'how "medical humanities" would be – and *should* be – understood' (Evans and Greaves 2002: 1; emphasis added). This is a prescription rather than a request, as if the authors had already made up their minds that there was a definitive answer. 'Medical humanities' were not framed as problematic. The authors suggested that the descriptor 'medical' is not exclusive to doctors, but covers all aspects of health and illness, and in any case 'has already gained international recognition'. Evans and Greaves recognized 'an alternative title such as "Humanities in Health Care"' but felt it to be superfluous (*ibid.*). Dr Robert Marshall, a consultant pathologist and medical educator from Truro, raised an objection at the Birmingham meeting to the title 'medical humanities' on the grounds that it could be seen as exclusive, but this objection was ignored. Further, the inaugural AMH conference group decided that both the medical humanities in medical education and the arts in healthcare 'were not its central concern'. The medical humanities were defined rather as 'the literary, anthropological, historical, or philosophical engagements (among others) with medicine' (*ibid.*). This view was later strongly contested within the Association and its executive committee, and debated at subsequent AMH annual conferences.

In the same year, 2002, the most innovative programme in medical humanities in any medical school internationally was launched with the first intake of students at the new Peninsula Medical School – the fruit of collaboration between the Universities of Exeter and Plymouth (Bleakley *et al.* 2006). This initiative certainly thought, against the grain of Evans and Greaves above, that 'the medical humanities in medical education' was indeed a central concern. The curriculum innovation was designed during 2001–02 as a core and integrated programme.

The medical humanities programme was 'core' in the sense that all students had to study compulsory medical humanities input such as workshops and Special Study Units, one of which was longitudinal in Year 4 and required all students to plan and run a conference to showcase the arts- and humanities-based work that they had produced across that year. Over time, a portfolio of over 100 special study unit offerings has been developed. The programme is 'integrated' in the sense that all curriculum provision was encouraged to include a 'thinking with arts and humanities' perspective. This was basically a major staff development challenge and was undertaken with vigour and enthusiasm, resulting in science and clinical skills in particular being taught with the help of artists, social sciences and humanities scholars.

Workshops were developed not just for students but also for staff and medical humanities were formally included as a curriculum development group along with science studies and clinical and communication skills. Key patient-centred practices were educated, including: doctoring as performance (with the help of actor patients); close looking in clinical skills (with the help of life drawing and visual artists); education for tolerance of ambiguity as key in clinical work; and explicit attention to language, such as 'receiving' a patient's history rather than 'taking' a history, and development of facilitative language of discussion, debate and support rather than authoritative language of prescription and confrontation.

Medical humanities components are now common across UK medical schools although no UK schools have been able to develop a core and integrated model in the way that Peninsula has. Peninsula split into two separate medical schools – Plymouth University Peninsula Schools of Medicine and Dentistry, and Exeter University Medical School – in 2012, with a first intake of students in 2013. Both schools continue with the tradition of the medical humanities provision established at Peninsula but the future of that provision at the time of writing is uncertain. There are also neighbouring dedicated medical humanities initiatives – such as Exeter University's (see www.exeter.ac.uk/research/inspiring/keythemes/hass/medicalhumanities) – that operate outside the medical school structure.

In the UK, universities and medical schools in the following locations have medical humanities programmes or research interests:

* Aberdeen (www.abdn.ac.uk/smd/medical-humanities)
* Belfast (www.qub.ac.uk/schools/SchoolofModernLanguages/Research/LatinAmericanStudiesForum/MedicalhumanitiesPGskillsworkshop)
* Birmingham (www.birmingham.ac.uk/research/activity/mds/domains/health-pop/healthcare-evaluation-and-methodology/ethics-and-medical-humanities/index.aspx)
* Bristol (www.bristol.ac.uk/philosophy/courses/undergraduate/ibamh)
* Canterbury (www.kent.ac.uk/history/centres/medicine)
* Durham (www.dur.ac.uk/cmh)
* Falmouth (www.falmouth.ac.uk/academy-of-music-theatre-arts)
* Glasgow (www.gla.ac.uk/schools/medicine/medicine/medical humanitiesunit; see also the Medical Humanities Research network run by Dr David Shuttleton, www.gla.ac.uk/schools/critical/research/fundedresearchprojects/mhrns)
* Keele (www.keele.ac.uk/hums/medicalhumanities)
* Leeds (www.leeds.ac.uk/arts/info/125123/centre_for_medical_humanities)
* Leicester (www2.le.ac.uk/research/current-research/medical-humanities-research-centre)
* London, King's College (www.kcl.ac.uk/prospectus/graduate/medical-humanities)
* London, Birkbeck (www.bbk.ac.uk/study/2014/postgraduate/programmes/TMAHUMED_C)
* Manchester (www.chstm.manchester.ac.uk/postgraduate/taught/courses/routeintercalatedmscformedicine)
* Nottingham (www.healthhumanities.org/pages/view/home)

- Sheffield (http://mhs.group.shef.ac.uk)
- Southampton (www.southampton.ac.uk/medu/curriculum_design_ and_delivery/humanities.page)
- Swansea (www.swansea.ac.uk/undergraduate/courses/human-and- health-sciences/bschonsmedicalsciencesandhumanities)

Postgraduate and intercalated degrees are offered at Birkbeck, Manchester, Leicester, King's College, Swansea and Bristol (see links at www.amh.ac.uk).

This landscape is developing and there is a need for a critical and systematic review of provision across the UK. I will not pursue detail here as specific provision comes in and out of focus so rapidly, but the list above is enough to show a developing and healthy set of activities across UK universities. How these activities will be effectively networked is another matter.

After intensive lobbying over a period of five years, in 2008 the UK Wellcome Trust awarded two large grants to set up centres for research in the medical humanities, widening their medical history remit to include the medical humanities. Both of the successful centres focused upon themes of health and wellbeing, again aligning with utilitarianism rather than scepticism. The University of Durham Centre for Medical Humanities addresses the themes of 'health', 'wellbeing' and 'human flourishing', while the University of London King's College centre – headed by Brian Hurwitz – is the 'Centre for the Humanities and Health'. The Durham Centre has been particularly influenced by Martyn Evans's background in philosophy, evident in developing research programmes in topics such as 'human wonder'. For example, the medical humanities in medical education can develop 'a sense of wonder at embodied human nature and embodied consciousness, leading to medical education that is, in its essence, reverential' (Gordon and Evans 2014: 214). The sentiment is to be applauded, but this is perhaps precisely the kind of language to be avoided in winning over hard-headed medical students to the medical humanities!

Controversies, contradictions and fault-lines have thus gradually emerged within the medical humanities movement in the UK, which originally tried to contain and rationalize the interests of three disparate groups: arts in health practitioners who aligned with psychological views of health and illness and refused to be 'medicalized'; humanities scholars who took medicine as their topic and were not necessarily interested in medical education; and medical educators, often clinicians, who were interested in how medical practice could be humanized, but were not interested in either psychological therapies or academic scholarship. In the following chapter, I will track how these controversies have led to the emergence of two distinct streams of a 'critical' medical humanities, suggesting that an expanding network of the 'medical humanities' as a stable interdisciplinary field may not be possible. Rather, it is likely that the medical humanities will be composed of several interacting networks, sometimes in potentially disruptive tension and sometimes allowing for exchange and translations that promote common expansion.

This book provides an introduction to the development of the 'critical' medical humanities in medical education. A forthcoming edited collection (Woods and Whitehead forthcoming) will provide a comprehensive introduction to the development of a 'critical' medical humanities that is not primarily engaged with medical education but with the culture of medicine and the medical – ranging from population health to cultural conceptions of the body. A third edited volume from North America attempts to circumvent the tensions between the two emerging cultures of 'critical' medical humanities that I outline in the following chapter through inclusivity, to describe the scope of an eclectic 'health humanities' (Jones *et al.* 2014).

A key factor in expansion of the medical humanities in the UK is the recent widening scope of Wellcome Trust research funding, which has changed from 'history of medicine' to 'medical history and humanities', and may serve to broaden the field in coming years. Following a review in 2008–09, the Wellcome Trust has presented a new vision that explicitly embraces critical conversations between artists, academics and practitioners, promoting a more critical form of medical humanities (see www.wellcome.ac.uk/Funding/Medical-humanities).

The medical humanities internationally

My aim in this book is not to consider the medical humanities in detail in terms of an 'international' or 'global' curriculum text. That is another book in its own right, facing the kinds of problems that global medical education faces – how will we avoid an imperialism or colonialism of medical humanities, where Western/North American values embodied in medical humanities curricula are exported to dominate globally? Alan Bleakley, John Bligh and Julie Browne (2011) have considered some of the issues of exporting a Western brand of medical education globally, for example the attempted introduction of practices such as small group problem-based learning into Japanese medical education where authority-led and lecture-based education is the norm and long periods of eye contact are considered rude and uncomfortable, even distressing. Claire Hooker and Estelle Noonan (2011) have argued that the medical humanities too can act in this neo-imperialist and exclusive way, as 'expressive of Western culture'.

Medical schools providing courses on 'cultural competence' for medical students often address such neo-colonialist/ imperialist dangers and these courses are seen as legitimate members of the medical humanities portfolio. However, as Linda Raphael (2013) from George Washington University School of Medicine suggests, a more sophisticated offering of the medical humanities is to stimulate reflection on 'cultural difference' as represented in the arts and humanities. The important issue here of course is 'whose' arts and humanities? Raphael suggests for example that medical students should critically study accounts of indigenous peoples' and immigrants' encounters with the American health system. The focus is not on how North American medical students might accommodate the views of the Other, but on what these views can teach in terms of disrupting worldviews and habits.

As mentioned earlier, the University of La Plata medical school in the Argentine Republic developed an optional medical humanities provision in 1976, one of the first of its kind internationally and well documented (Acuña 2000, 2003). This innovation has developed into a thriving medical humanities community, especially in Buenos Aires, including the development of a journal entitled *eä* (see www.ea-journal.com/en/about-us/about-ea-journal) that covers the intersections between the medical humanities and social studies of science and technology. Interestingly, this intersection is invisible in the UK, for example, where 'science studies' rarely engage with the medical humanities and medical education, despite strong potential such as the development of actor-network-theory from Bruno Latour's original work in the sociology of science (Bleakley 2014). It is interesting to note how broad the remit of the journal's understanding of 'the medical humanities' is:

> The Medical Humanities are an academic interdisciplinary field in the intersection of health and medicine with the humanities (philosophy, ethics, history, and religion), the arts (literature, theatre, visual arts, and music) and the social sciences (sociology, anthropology, psychology, political science, economy, law, communication, cultural studies). Disciplines that are often included under this category are history of medicine, bioethics, medical epistemology and scientific research methodology, medical esthetics, medical pedagogy, medical sociology, medical anthropology, economy of health, medical law, health politics, and medical communication, among others.
>
> (*eä* undated)

Canada in particular is developing a strong medical humanities culture with pressure on curriculum designers in medical schools to include medical humanities components (Banaszek 2011). Some schools have a long history of introducing medical students to medical humanities opportunities – for example, Jock Murray (2003) has reviewed the development of a vigorous medical humanities programme inaugurated in 2003 at Dalhousie University Faculty of Medicine, Nova Scotia.

Kidd and Connor (2008) conducted a systematic, key-informant review of medical humanities provision at 14 of Canada's 17 medical schools, describing what they saw as an 'anarchic' approach to medical humanities teaching in comparison with teaching of clinical science. The authors noted that the medical humanities are commonly marginalized, and urged providers to consider how they might close this gap. On the back of the success of an established journal (*Ars Medica*) run from Toronto since 2004 with a tag line of 'what makes medicine an art?', a well-networked annual conference has run in different Canadian venues since 2011 (the Canadian Health Humanities Network), and this nascent movement has taken up Kidd and Connor's challenge. Allan Peterkin and Allison Crawford were among the founder editors of *Ars Medica* and Crawford remains editor-in-chief (see www.ars-medica.ca/index.php/journal). Both are psychiatrists, although Peterkin also trained as a family medicine practitioner and has a first degree in the humanities. Peterkin has fought tirelessly to make the health humanities inclusive and liberal, reflecting his own eclectic range of work – besides his clinical work he has published 14 books for adults and children (see www.adpeterkin.com), including a 'how to survive' manual for junior doctors and a clinical guide to caring for lesbian and gay people, co-authored with Cathy Risdon (Peterkin and Risdon 2003). Pamela Brett-Maclean (2012) has worked tirelessly to establish a distinctive medical humanities programme at the University of Alberta Faculty of Medicine and Dentistry in Edmonton, with a focus on the arts.

In Australia, as noted above, Anthony Moore, a surgeon working at the University of Melbourne, first described the medical humanities (Moore 1976: 1479). Moore had developed a short course designed for medical students to discuss 'broader cultural, philosophical and personal issues' relevant to medical practice based largely around literature. Jill Gordon at the Faculty of Arts, University of Sydney (http://sydney.edu.au/medicine/humanities), initiated the first serious wave of medical humanities interest in 2003 as a postgraduate programme. In 2005, Gordon claimed that the medical humanities 'are now integrated into many medical curricula in Australia' (Gordon 2005: 5), although she does not specify detail and the descriptor 'integrated' is probably too strong. 'Attached to' curricula may be more accurate. The Australasian Association for the Medical Humanities was inaugurated in November 2004, where:

> The medical humanities are concerned with 'the science of the human', and bring the perspectives of disciplines such as history, philosophy, literature, art and music to understanding health, illness and medicine. The medical humanities are designed to overcome the separation of clinical care from the 'human sciences' and to foster interdisciplinary teaching and research to optimise patient care.
>
> (Gordon (2005: 5)

This encompassing brief has subsequently been sharpened and clarified by medical humanities scholars in Australia, such as Claire Hooker and Estelle Noonan in Sydney, and Neville Chiavaroli in Melbourne (Chiavaroli and Ellwood 2012). In the context of Jill Gordon's legacy, the medical humanities have now morphed into the 'health humanities' and changed location:

Medical Humanities is now known as Health Humanities and is a specialisation in the Sydney School of Public Health's Bioethics program. The health humanities specialisation allows you to explore the humanistic side of health care. The health humanities are broad and diverse, encompassing everything from arts and health to history and literature.

(Gordon (2005: 5)

Sydney University's Centre for Values, Ethics and Law in Medicine (VELIM) hosts the health humanities and is a sister institution to the Wellcome Centre for Medical Humanities at the University of Durham, UK. Neville Chiavaroli has been instrumental in setting up interest in the medical humanities at the University of Melbourne Medical School. A physiotherapist with a further education in medieval literature, Chiavaroli is active in developing an international medical humanities culture, spending a sabbatical in 2014 looking at provision of medical humanities in UK medical schools.

As noted earlier, initiation of the medical humanities in the UK was partly due to Robin Philipp's earlier experience of developing conferences in New Zealand in the mid-1990s. Valerie Grant (2003) describes later developments in the field at the University of Auckland. However, as with developments in Australia, Pacific Rim medical humanities have not as yet flowered with the kind of momentum modelled by US, UK and now Canadian initiatives. Ireland is also at this level of initial interest with a developing programme at Trinity College, Dublin, where longer-term goals include a research centre (see www.tcd.ie/trinitylongroomhub/projects/medical-humanities).

There are also isolated examples globally of established medical humanities networks, such as Italy (Fieschi *et al.* 2013) and single school developments such as a medical humanities unit at Istanbul University Faculty of Medicine, Department of History of Medicine and Ethics, Turkey, under the direction of Rainer Brömer who originally supervised the medical humanities at Peninsula Medical School. In Italy, the Centre for Advanced Studies in Ethics in Padua, the Chair of History of Medicine at the University of Padua and the Chair of Medical Humanities at the Marmara University in Istanbul have collaborated to run a week long Summer school in Padua and Venice in the medical humanities. Sifa University, Izmir, Turkey hosts the online *Journal of the History of Medicine and Medical Humanities* (www.johmmh.org).

The issue concerning medical humanities development globally being 'expressive of Western culture' (Hooker and Noonan 2011), or a potentially neo-imperialist 'one model suits all as long as it is our model' is, perhaps, secondary in Europe to how 'medical humanities' translates across cultures. 'Medical humanities' is to some extent a meaningless descriptor within French medical education where medicine is traditionally preoccupied with the humanities as well as the sciences, while Fieschi and colleagues (Fieschi *et al.* 2013: 59) point out that 'medical humanities' does not translate readily into Italian for similar reasons. In Italian medical schools, a combination of logic and moral knowing is better understood as a 'humanistic' approach to medicine. Further, notions such as 'empathy' are culturally contingent. Empathy in an Italian context is not, suggests Fieschi and colleagues, understood as a technique, but rather a 'cultural outlook of consideration and attention' that is modulated according to cultural, and even local, flavours and habits (*ibid.*).

Batistatou and colleagues (2010: 243) suggest that medical education in Greece would benefit from the introduction of the medical humanities, although the suggested pedagogy is a series of lectures on topics such as ethics, history of medicine, literature and clinical observation. They assume that the medical humanities can be packaged up as a 'course' for early years medical students that can serve as a 'zone of creative relaxation' that may 'counteract burnout'. The connection between the two is based on the assumption that the humanities may provide a space for reflection and that learning about empathy for others may also translate into self-care. But this is a false assumption. Relaxation is not the same as reflection – the former implies switching off, the latter switching on. Again, the arts are in danger of being reduced to soft entertainment rather than disturbance and trouble. The arts and humanities set out to stress as much as relax, to question rather than provide answers and to problematize the taken-for-granted. This approach merely returns us to Sir Ken Calman's 'Department of Health and Happiness' discussed earlier. The authors do, however, propose that the humanities might turn ordinary medicine into an 'exceptional medicine', and I would certainly support this.

Richa Gupta and colleagues (2011) point out that while the medical humanities are new to Asian medical schools generally, they were introduced in Nepal in 2009. A journal – *Research and Humanities in Medical Education* (www.rhime.in) – was established in 2014 in India, while the *Formosan Journal of Medical Humanities* (www.researchgate.net/journal/16065727_Formosan_journal_of_medical_humanities), with a bias towards medical ethics, has been set up in Taiwan. The claim by Gupta and colleagues that the medical humanities might 'perk up' the communication skills of Indian medical students does not exactly provide a rigorous vision for a culturally sensitive form of medical humanities in medical education. Given the wealth of writing on post-colonialism and globalization that focuses on the Indian subcontinent, medical schools would seem ripe for development of theoretical and practical concerns with a culturally sensitive medical humanities. Again, the pedagogy for the initiative that Gupta and colleagues introduced in Delhi is underwhelming – largely a lecture format, although supplemented by film and visual exhibition, with the more innovative approach of students presenting a 'Street Play', a piece of critical theatre about increasing workloads in medical schools.

Radha Ramaswamy (2013) extends this use of theatre to describe an innovative and successful 'Theatre of the Oppressed' intervention to improve patient–doctor interactions. The author ran seven workshops for medical students and faculty across four Indian and Nepalese cities between 2010 and 2012 with over 200 participants. The drama-based workshops facilitated greater understanding not only of doctor–patient communication but also of faculty–medical student communication. P. Ravi Shankar (2008) describes setting up a medical humanities module in a medical school in Nepal. The project was hit-and-miss, with very little thought given to cultural sensitivities. Indeed, Shankar, against the local traditions of hierarchical education, simply ploughed on with 'imposing' small group work, open discussion and debate, apparently with some success. We are back to un-reflexive introduction of both pedagogies and medical education strategies that 'work' at some level, but in no way are carefully and sensitively designed with stakeholders as local curriculum interventions.

Michael Clark (2013), discussing the use of film in the medical humanities, wonders 'whether it is possible...to imagine a distinctively Chinese version of the medical humanities'. This comes from an experience of teaching a course at King's College, University of London, on 'Chinese Film and Body' in a MA in Chinese Health and Humanity (see www.ucl.ac.uk/chinahealth/teaching/chinese_film_and_the_body). The issue for Clark is that the Western biomedical model infects the medical humanities in medical education and is not compatible with other cultural models of health, illness and disease.

In short, to talk of 'global' medical humanities is to describe – to borrow a phrase from Jacques Derrida who spoke of a 'democracy to come' – a 'medical humanities to come'. Despite the fact that the 2013 Association for Medical Humanities annual conference (University of Aberdeen) took as its theme 'Global Medical Humanities', it would be fair to say that such a notion has not at the time of writing gained full traction. Of the 78 papers presented at that conference, fewer than half were about medical education. The majority addressed medical history and public health topics.

Canadian, Australian and New Zealand medical schools are in what can be seen as a privileged position to be able to learn from the cultures of indigenous peoples. Shaun Ewen (2013: 33) from the University of Melbourne for example asks if 'there is an opportunity for indigenous health medical educators to team with medical humanities educators to develop a mutually beneficial curriculum'? Many medical schools have developed programmes in so-called 'cultural competence' and the medical humanities have readily aligned with such programmes. But, as Arno Kumagai and Monica Lypson (2009) point out, we must go beyond cultural competence to engage a critical consciousness, social justice and multicultural education. The authors note that critical consciousness is not the same as, although can be allied with, critical thinking. Critical consciousness is essentially political, involving awareness of power structures that privilege communities, ethnic groups and individuals, where such power structures can be resisted to foster social justice. I have called this process the democratization of medicine (Bleakley 2014) and see it as the main goal of medical education.

Arno Kumagai and colleagues (2007) do not stop at diagnosing medical education's ills in the field of cultural awareness and social justice, but have developed medical humanities interventions that address these symptoms, particularly the use of interactive theatre to promote critical consciousness as a basis to social justice. Here, Kumagai focuses on faculty development to educate facilitative capabilities to run small group activities with medical students in assimilating and reflecting on the issues of social justice raised by their clinical placements. These involve issues of privilege, exclusion, marginalization, gender, race, sexual orientation and so forth. 'Forum Theater' techniques were successfully used in workshop settings to raise the consciousness of faculty and equip them with more democratic, liberatory pedagogies (Freire 1996).

Such theatre techniques – primarily David Diamond's (2007) 'Theatre for Living', which employs community-based dialogue to empower minority groups – have been used, for example, at the University of Alberta medical school, Edmonton by Pamela Brett-Maclean (2012) in exploring 'professionalism' with medical and dental students. Brazilian theatre director Augusto Boal created Forum Theatre to promote dialogue between performers and audience, where a scene is first played then replayed with audience interventions and participations. This format is ideal for use with reflective small groups in medical education, post-clinical placement, for example in critically interrogating behaviours such as 'pimping' in bedside teaching, discussed earlier.

It is perhaps not surprising that the cutting edge work on addressing issues of social justice in medicine is being carried out in democratic 'Western' medical education. But we should remind ourselves that within both urban and rural contexts of medical education in North America, Canada, UK, New Zealand and Australia there are vibrant multicultural communities as well as issues of marginalization of indigenous communities. The medical humanities need not be exclusively expressive of Western values in such contexts although it remains the case that recruitment to medical schools remains heavily biased towards white, middle-class persons.

2   What are the 'medical humanities'?

Definitions and controversies

Defining the medical humanities: 'what's in a name?'

The medical humanities are undergoing a transition from what might be termed a naïve and celebratory 'first wave' – often attracting raw enthusiasm rather than reflexive scholarship – to a 'second wave' of more critical approaches. Let us call this first wave 'medical humanities lite' and the second wave a 'critical medical humanities'. This second wave has brought both maturity and complexity to the medical humanities culture, but not necessarily coherence. Interesting fault-lines and contradictions have appeared in the culture and are the subject of this chapter. In summary, the descriptor 'medical humanities' accommodates three distinct approaches: first, the study of medicine and the medical by humanities scholars usually based in university humanities departments; second, arts and humanities interventions in medical education; and third, arts practitioners engaging the public with issues of the body and illness through literature, performance, theatre and the visual arts in particular. Such practitioners may be based in art schools or performance and humanities departments of arts universities.

In their 2008 review of the state of play of medical humanities in Canadian medical schools, Kidd and Connor described the field as 'anarchic'. Many took this as a backhanded compliment, but the authors warned that a lack of cohesion in the field merely played into the hands of sceptics towards the medical humanities who pointed to what they saw as a scattergun approach to curriculum interventions. While a frontier spirit pervades the medical humanities this has been accompanied by a lack of rigour and discrimination. For example, surprisingly little work has been done on mapping the territory of the medical humanities in the face of unquestioned assumptions about the field's interests and limits.

Johanna Shapiro and colleagues (Shapiro *et al.* 2009: 193) wrote a perceptive article in 2009 summarising 'medical humanities and their discontents'. This focused on the medical humanities as 'an intriguing sideline in the main project of medical education' (*ibid.*). The authors point to studies showing that medical students typically critiqued medical humanities content as irrelevant; teaching as untrustworthy and personally intrusive; and curriculum design as misplaced where content was core rather than elective. The issue for these authors is a pedagogical one – simply, medicine is not taught as a process of critical thinking and reflection but one of direct, pragmatic application. The humanities bring pedagogical process as well as content, such as critical dialogue and theory as 'sense making'. Ways of learning that are more critical could be introduced, aligned with use of media such as reflective portfolios that allow for meaningful integration of clinical experiences rather than a cataloguing of activities such as clinical skills. Humanities should not be 'add-on' but integrated.

Finally, 'applied humanities scholars' without clinical experience could work collaboratively with clinicians adding a critical dimension introduced from the arts and humanities. Prior to Shapiro and colleagues' article, since introducing a core and integrated medical humanities curriculum in 2002, Peninsula Medical School (Universities of Exeter and Plymouth, UK) had successfully introduced much of what these authors suggested to the undergraduate medicine curriculum, including an 'applied humanities scholars' faculty under the directorship of myself and Dr Robert Marshall, a consultant histopathologist with a first degree from Oxford in Classics. Marshall is a passionate advocate of the arts and humanities in medical education and provided the initial impetus for considering such a high profile for the medical humanities during the first wave of curriculum planning for Peninsula Medical School. Those humanities and social science scholars at Peninsula who had no previous clinical experience underwent staff development to gain an appreciation of clinical environments through observational placements prior to working collaboratively with clinical teaching staff. Importantly, the Peninsula curriculum plan was grounded in the assumption that the biomedical sciences are intrinsically aesthetic.

Hal Cook (2010: 3), a historian, sees the medical humanities as a way of exploring the 'complexities and ambiguities of the human condition' as these relate to medical practice. He also uses the metaphor of 'borderlands' to describe the medical humanities' position in relation to established academic disciplines. Cook's view is from the humanities looking in on medicine. In contrast, Deborah Kirklin (2002, 2003, 2005), a doctor and medical ethicist, works from within the overall field of the medical and healthcare, seeing the application of the arts and humanities as a kind of fine-tuning of sensibility allowing us to develop a far more subtle and nuanced appreciation of the context within which illness is experienced and healthcare delivered. Kirklin then looks out from the practice of medicine and healthcare towards the arts and humanities. The two positions generated by Cook and Kirklin are not incompatible, but suggest differing lines of flight.

Following Cook's definition, we might see 'the medical' as one historically and culturally determined dimension of human experience. This may lead us to ask questions such as that raised by Ivan Illich (1977) of how does a culture become so thoroughly 'medicalized'? Illich's focus is not on the rise of technical biomedicine but rather on the deskilling of the layperson, whose capability to offer everyday healthcare is put into question as health practices are professionalized. Michel Foucault (1989) asks a different set of questions, but they are still historically and culturally grounded. Using examples from French historical archives, Foucault asks how the focus of medical practice shifted from the home visit (with its bias towards the patient and family and its restrictions on the doctor as guest in another's house) to the patient attending a clinic (with its bias towards the clinician and its restrictions on the patient as a visitor to the hospital)? What conditions emerged that legitimated intimate examinations ordinarily taboo in everyday social exchanges (legitimated in the clinic but not necessarily sanctioned in the patient's house)? What is different about the way that a doctor and a layperson gaze on, or at, a body? These are questions from outside medicine looking in.

Following Deborah Kirklin's view of the medical humanities, we would pose different questions and pursue differing methods of inquiry. Looking out from medicine and healthcare to the worlds of the arts and humanities, the most pressing, and problematic, question is then how might we improve healthcare with the help of the medical humanities? Kirklin's position is ultimately embedded in pedagogy – how can medical education be designed with medical humanities in mind?

Here, we might draw on the engagement of the radical arts with contemporary medicine as a response to Kirklin's prompt, noting that such an arts intervention is not located within the medical school and teaching hospital, nor within the University humanities department, but within a gallery engaging the public. In this case, it happens that the gallery space within a museum of art simulates a hospital ward. Bob Flanagan was an American performance artist who died in 1996 from cystic fibrosis. He was also a masochist who derived sexual pleasure from being dominated by his partner Sheree Rose. A film, released in 1997, about Flanagan's complex relationship with terminal illness – *Sick: The Life and Death of Bob Flanagan, Supermasochist* – won the Special Jury Prize at the Sundance Film Festival in 1997. With Sheree Rose, Flanagan made a performance piece called 'Visiting Hours' (shown at Santa Monica Museum of Art in 1992–3, the New Museum New York City in 1994 and the Museum of Fine Arts Boston in 1995) in which museum spaces were transformed into a hospital ward with waiting room and X-rays. Flanagan lay in a hospital bed at the centre of the installation.

Flanagan's performance dramatically challenges what the hospital expects of the supine and conforming patient, and what culture may expect of playing the 'sick' role, in what he termed 'fighting sickness with sickness'. The performance climaxes with Flanagan being tied by the ankles and winched out of the bed by Sheree Rose to hang upside down, literally inverting the supposedly proper and normal relationship of patient with clinic, of sick patient with medicine (see www.youtube.com/watch?v=vgWyxjjecOw).

Such radical art questions notions of what is 'healthy' and positions medical education as, potentially, a pedagogy of difference. Here, if authentic 'patient-centredness' is practised many of the conventions of medicine reinforced through a traditional medical education must be questioned.

Flanagan's work brings together the medical humanities as (i) a perspective looking in on medicine and healthcare from the outside to critically examine historically and culturally determined assumptions about the body and illness, and as (ii) a perspective looking out from within medicine and healthcare to critically examine how apprentice practitioners are socialized, gain and consolidate identities – or learn. From docile and supine 'patient' (literally 'one who suffers') to hanging, inverted above the bed – having metaphorically transcended suffering through inflicting even more pain – Flanagan points to critical positions that both look in on and look out from medicine and healthcare simultaneously. Importantly, Flanagan, an against-the-odds survivor of cystic fibrosis (he outlived medical mortality predictions by around 35 years) problematizes descriptors such as 'health', 'wellbeing' and 'quality of life'.

Paul Crawford and colleagues (Crawford *et al.* 2010) see the 'health' humanities as the 'future of medical humanities', objecting to the implied exclusion of wider healthcare when using the descriptor 'medical'. Yet Deborah Kirklin's approach to the medical humanities from 2006 is certainly inclusive, specifically referring to 'healthcare'. In the UK, this debate goes back to at least 2002, when an editorial in *Medical Humanities* by Martyn Evans and David Greaves suggested that the 'medical' in 'medical humanities' was not being used just to refer to medicine, but the term 'medical humanities' had already gained currency and traction internationally and that it was effectively too late to attempt to introduce the potentially more inclusive descriptor 'humanities in healthcare'. Evans and Greaves (2002) asked, rhetorically: '"Medical humanities" – what's in a name?' This related to the development of an Association for Medical Humanities (for which Evans twice served as president, and for which I am currently president at the time of writing).

The authors apologized for potential exclusivity in sticking with the term 'medical', both for healthcare practitioners such as nurses, and for non-medical participants in the medical humanities culture such as social sciences, arts and humanities academics and practitioners (Evans himself is a philosopher and not a clinician). But this issue really only matters to those who align the medical humanities with medical education. Here, non-clinical academics and artists will meet healthcare in general even as they work with doctors, where they see doctors working with patients and in multiprofessional clinical teams. On the other hand, for humanities scholars or artists working outside of medical schools in humanities or arts departments, 'medical' humanities is an appropriate descriptor, as these scholars engage mainly with the subject of medicine or with the roles and identities of doctors.

Certainly in Canada, with the development of the health humanities network and an associated annual conference, the health humanities is now the preferred term, displacing the medical humanities. The decision to publish a comprehensive compendium of articles on the state of the art of the medical humanities under the title *The Health Humanities Reader* (edited by Tess Jones, Delese Wear and Lester Friedman), as noted in the previous chapter, makes a significant statement: that 'health humanities' may become the preferred term in North America (Jones *et al.* 2014).

My concern with the health humanities, as indicated in the previous chapter, is the privileging of 'health', generally linked with optimism and wellbeing, now extended also to 'safety'. Artists such as Bob Flanagan – while his work was extreme even for contemporary performance art – seek to critically challenge assumptions about 'health', 'illness' and 'disease' and the role of the patient. Flanagan did not seek to challenge western biomedicine per se, but rather assumptions about the status of the human body as it encounters the cultural process of medicalization as normalizing. Ironically, medical education itself has historically offered a distinctly sado-masochistic model of apprenticeship. Combinations of punishing work schedules, learning on the job through ritual humiliation and plunging junior doctors in at the deep end at the limits of their competence have led to doctors having higher rates of suicide and burnout than the average population (Wible 2014) and medical students also showing high rates of suicide ideation and burnout (Dyrbye *et al.* 2008) and produced 'survival' guides for residents (Peterkin 2012). This is coupled with a lack of formal support structures for the psychological wellbeing of doctors who traditionally resist self-help, make poor patients and dislike treating other doctors (Garelick 2014). Further, our cultural models of 'health' and 'wellbeing' are ambiguous. On the one hand we are asked to adopt lifestyles that promote health, but on the other, we do so in ways that court danger and risk, such as extreme sports. 'Quality of life' does not necessarily equate with medical models of 'health' or health-care models of 'wellbeing'.

The 'medical' and 'health' descriptors in medical/ health humanities are then problematic, but I am equally concerned with the potential exclusivity of the 'humanities' descriptor in 'medical humanities', where 'humanities' are assumed to include the arts. Also, do we include the humanities-facing social sciences? In my own work in medical education, I have often used the term 'medical aesthetics' as a composite descriptor, but recognize that this must also encompass politics and ethics (Bleakley 2014). The concern of Martyn Evans and David Greaves (2002) to address 'what's in a name?' in a 'first wave' of medical humanities is far from resolved, but we cannot simply leave things to rest. The beehive must be stirred and we must be stung into action to consider that a 'name' does matter.

A multidisciplinary or interdisciplinary field?

The descriptor 'medical humanities' has been applied to the following five fields of activity:

- The humanities studying medicine (such as history of medicine or the critical evaluation of medicine in literature).
- Arts and humanities intersecting with medicine in medical education – often called 'medicine as art'.
- The arts engaging with medical themes in public engagement.
- Arts for health (for example, art in hospitals and arts activities with patients – often called 'arts as medicine').
- Arts therapies (sometimes linked with arts for health, but usually associated with mental health interventions using arts media within a psychotherapeutic framework).

While the medical humanities in the UK may have its roots in arts therapies, the arts as therapy culture now has its own academic meetings, journals and societies and has limited overlap with the other four areas above. Arts for health, like the arts therapies (with which it has resonance) also has its own networks, conferences and publications that are separate from medical humanities. Medical humanities, rather, has flourished in three places – university humanities departments, through the formal study of medicine; university medical schools, teaching hospital and community clinics, through medical education; and public galleries, museum spaces and theatres through arts engagement with medical themes.

Claire Hooker (2008: 369–70) echoes the fields described above, where the medical humanities offer:

1 'a field of academic inquiry';
2 'the intersection of medicine and the creative arts'; and
3 creating 'more compassionate, more capably communicative doctors' that may 'lead to better health outcomes for patients'.

Hooker's rhetoric, however, sets out to persuade that medical education (3 above) is less sexy than the field of academic inquiry into medical culture and history (1 above) where she gives an example from the University of Auckland, New Zealand: 'researchers who investigate such things as illness narratives, death and dying, mental health and incarceration, and the semiotics of disease, are primarily charged with the task of training doctors to be more likeable and trustworthy for their patients' (*ibid.*).

This is an unfair reading of the complexity of medical education as it draws on the arts and humanities, as I hope Chapter 3 will demonstrate. Democratizing and politicizing medical culture – both of which are necessary aims for the medical humanities in medical education – is a far more onerous task than that of 'training doctors to be more likeable and trust-worthy for their patients'. For example, educating doctors in teamwork in order to reduce medical error – one key strand in democratizing medicine – seems to me to be a key outcome and reason for including, say, illness narra-tives and the semiotics of disease in a medicine curriculum. Further, a reflexive medical education does not set out to 'train' doctors but to educate them, for example in how to deal with disgust (see the extract from Gabriel Weston's semi-autobiographical 2014 novel *Dirty Work* that opens Chapter 4), or with erotic and sexual attraction to patients and colleagues.

An evolving area in the medical humanities is how contemporary arts practitioners can engage critically with medical education to shape new practices, moving clear of the territory of arts therapies and arts in health (where the art is a medium for working with patients, and not primarily a cultural object or artefact that has independent impetus to challenge the 'health' of a culture). For example, the Scottish artist Christine Borland was appointed as Visiting Professor of Visual Art at Peninsula Medical School precisely to challenge the habitual use of artists as handmaidens to medicine (such as life drawing classes for anatomy learning or medical illustration). Borland, a Turner Prize nominee in 1997, has worked consistently in the areas of medicine and forensic science to provide critical visual commen-tary. She is interested in how exposure to the medical can depersonalize, where art interventions can reconstruct and personalize.

Borland reformulates issues of social justice, ethics and representation of the 'human' through complex visual art projects, often involving collabora-tions with scientists, doctors, anatomists and forensics experts. In making the 1994 piece 'From Life' (Borland 2006), Borland sought out a human skeleton sold through an anatomy catalogue. She imagined that skeletons would be plastic and was shocked and intrigued to find that, at the time, she could buy a real human skeleton. In the setting of the medical school's anatomy laboratory, the skeleton is simply a passive teaching object, acting not only to depersonalize the human who once inhabited this skeleton, but acting as a signifier for medicine as a whole as a depersonalizing institution. Borland aimed to reconstruct and repersonalize the human who once fleshed the skeleton. Through tracing ownership of the skeleton and through forensic reconstruction of the face Borland discovered that this was an Asian female. This forensic art process offers a model for a humane medicine that does not strip us back to anonymous skeleton but refleshes us and builds meaningful relationship layer by layer. Such a process too is transdisciplinary where it is powered by moral dilemmas. While the medical humanities in medical education may draw from several disciplines, the worry is not how we knit those disciplines together, but whether or not we can find compelling topics that act as encompassing vehicles for collabora-tion between differing approaches of thinking and making.

Of the five fields of activity referred to above, arts for health and arts therapies have activities, organizations and publications that are distinct from the medical humanities, although there is overlap, particularly with the arts for health field. Of the other three approaches, two – the medical humanities in medical education and the medical humanities as the discipline-based study of medicine and the medical – are, however, in tension and not readily interdisciplinary or transdisciplinary. Both of these traditions have passed through an historical 'first wave' and are entering a 'second wave' of interest. Both claim the descriptor the 'critical medical humanities' for this second wave of activity. The passage from first to second wave in both cases can also be described as from 'celebratory' to 'critical', or from the naïve to the reflexive.

In the development of the medical humanities in medical education, a first wave of interest saw the medical humanities introduced to medical students as modules in ethics and the history of medicine, while this gradually expanded to include narrative-based medicine and topics such as how looking at art may help medical students to look more closely at patients. Given that medical students gain an identity as a doctor through performing like their seniors, medicine developed an interest in drama, and this was reinforced through the widespread use of actor patients in learning clinical skills through simulation. However, in this first wave the introduction of the medical humanities was characteristically 'lite' educationally – as a supplement within the curriculum, as optional learning, as light relief from biomedical science and even conceived as 'edutainment'.

A second wave has reformulated the medical humanities as a critical educational intervention. Here, the 'critical' medical humanities can act as a counterpoint to reductive biomedical science from within the curriculum, as core and integrated provision. This extends technical interest in diagnosing and treating the chief complaint (disease) to a wider appreciation of the illness in the context of the patient's life, as the chief concern (Schleifer and Vannatta 2013). This critical role for the medical humanities is pedagogical where it educates for a more reflective and reflexive imagination than the literalism encouraged by other aspects of the curriculum.

The medical humanities are no longer supplementary or complementary but actively reformulate what clinical thinking and clinical practice – or the clinical imagination – might be. The arts and humanities are given a central role (i) politically – in democratizing medicine, where they also educate for tolerance of ambiguity, and (ii) aesthetically – in providing the necessary media for learning how to communicate professionally and sensitively through a moral imagination and learning how to engage close noticing in physical examination and diagnoses. In short, within medical education, the medical humanities have come to configure a radical and primary educational intervention, shaping practice aesthetically and politically (Bleakley 2014).

In a parallel development, a first wave of interest in humanities disciplines studying medicine, such as the history of medicine, often left medicine untouched. Medicine was a passive object studied by an active discipline.

The aim was not to *transform* medicine or indeed to trace the vicissitudes of 'the medical' but merely to *describe* and *understand* medicine. In a second wave of interest, as noted, a 'critical medical humanities' has emerged (Woods and Whitehead forthcoming). The project is now to not just engage with, but also contribute to, the medical understanding of individuals and populations in terms of potential transformation. Where the humanities once studied medical phenomena from a distance they now offer to process or remake the fabric of the medical in intimate, critical engagement.

Proponents of this kind of 'critical' medical humanities have emerged from the Wellcome-funded Centre for Medical Humanities at Durham University, UK, including Angela Woods and Corinne Saunders and Anne Whitehead at the University of Newcastle. The 2009 online manifesto describes the medical humanities as:

> the name given to a so-far rather diverse field of enquiry. Its object is medicine as a human practice and, by implication, human health and illness, and the enquirers are, basically, people working from the perspectives of humanities disciplines. Thus 'medical humanities' denotes humanities looking at medicine, looking at patients, and – crucially – looking at medicine looking at patients. At present, history, literature studies, theology, anthropology and philosophy are promi- nent among the disciplines that engage in medical humanities. If they act separately and in isolation from one another, then 'medical human- ities' is just a list. But it becomes far more interesting when these disciplines' perspectives are combined in a genuinely interdisciplinary way.
>
> (Durham University 2009)

There is nothing here about pedagogy, or medical education as an arts- or humanities-led intervention; nor about the arts operating as 'diagnosticians of culture' (Smith 2005). The 'critical' medical humanities are described as diverging away from centres developed in medical schools to:

> a new generation of research groups emerging from humanities depart- ments. [Where] critical social and cultural theories ... direct and infuse our work to unpick the hidden assumptions underpinning the use of key concepts, lines of policy argument and characterisations of partic- ular bodies or groups of bodies.... We have a particular interest in collaborating with the creative arts and the arts and health community in exploring the radical potential of the arts within a critical medical humanities.
>
> (Durham University undated)

As mentioned earlier, just as Foucault (1989) suggested that the movement away from doctors visiting patients at home to patients visiting doctors in clinics changed the nature of the relationship between doctors and patients, for example in legitimating the intimate examination, so the Durham manifesto suggests that a shift in location from medical schools to humanities departments can herald a revolution in medical humanities by ushering in the critical approaches common to academic study, particularly in an era of critical theory. This moves in the opposite direction to Johanna Shapiro and colleagues' idea of an 'applied medical humanities scholar', who would work alongside clinical faculty and gain knowledge of clinical environments rather than working out of humanities departments (Shapiro *et al.* 2009). The key aspect of such a role is to critically engage with clinicians, medical students and patients in clinical spaces to expand, for example, awareness of the limits to practice, or of values informing practice.

As noted above, at Peninsula Medical School, from its inception in 2002, this model of non-clinical arts, humanities and social science scholars working closely with clinical teaching faculty in clinical spaces was developed. Non-clinical faculty underwent socialization into clinical environments such as hospital wards, operating theatres, laboratories, morgues and community general practices, and teaching spaces such as simulation suites, working alongside clinicians, often in interprofessional team settings. For example, Christine Borland, mentioned above, appointed as Visiting Professor of Visual Art at Peninsula, set up a project in which she worked alongside clinicians, actor-patients, technicians and students in critically examining learning clinical skills through simulation. Critical questions were asked, for example, about the male gendering of manikins, the ready slippage of simulation into dissimulation as medical students learned roles and scripts within a structure of performance and the lack of aesthetic in simulation suites. Borland made film, installations and artefacts exploring aesthetic, ethical and pedagogic contradictions and controversies in clinical skills learning, and presented this to a public audience in a gallery context over an extended period (e.g. *With Practice*; *Sim Bodies, NoBodies and Me*; see, for example, www.gsa.ac.uk/life/gsa-events/events/c/christine-borland). The work was continued and extended with students and faculty at Glasgow medical school's 'communication suite' where professional clinical communication is first learned with actor patients in simulation.

The final line from the Durham Centre website quoted above shows confused thinking and is rhetorical. It persuades us into thinking that a second wave critical medical humanities engages with the avant-garde in the arts, but in the same sentence adds the 'arts and health' community into the mix. The latter certainly does not have a track record of 'exploring the radical potential of the arts' in the way as, say, the Peninsula Medical School experience with Christine Borland as faculty (along with Visiting Professor of Music and Medicine Paul Robertson and Visiting Professor of Medical History Helen King).

Importantly, the approach of the humanities as applied to medicine in this second wave does position the medical humanities not as additive, as

handmaiden, or supportive friend to medicine but as a constructively critical intervention that sets a climate for medicine's reformulation of its aims
including how it configures embodiment. This role of interlocutor is vital to
the development of medical practice and knowledge, but also to how poli-
cymakers frame their social interventions (for example in public health
education).

Proponents of this 'second wave' of medical humanities have suggested
that the first wave was the application of the medical humanities to medical
education, but this is misconceived and historically inaccurate. As I suggest
above, there are two streams at work. These two streams of the critical
medical humanities – one situated in medical education and the other in the
humanities engaging with medical understanding – do, however, have
common concerns. For example, from within the humanities-based critical
medical humanities 'second wave' have emerged sophisticated interroga-
tions of taken for granted notions such as 'empathy' (Macnaughton 2009)
and 'narrative' (Woods 2011). In the second wave of medical humanities
within medical education, critiques of the unquestioned notions of 'empathy' (Marshall and Bleakley 2009) and 'narrative' (Bleakley 2005) have also
emerged, but these have had explicitly educational aims, those of improving patient care and safety through medical education.

I suggest that while a first wave of the medical humanities promised to
counter medicine's scientific conservatism (appearing in practice as the
dehumanizing of patients), and authoritarianism (appearing in practice as
the depowering of healthcare colleagues), this wave is already being
absorbed into the mainstream of medicine, where its revolutionary potential is being sublimated. Such sublimation is readily achieved where the
kinds of arts and humanities that this first wave draws on are conservative,
pointedly avoiding the liberal avant-garde. Further, this wave of medical
humanities aligns with the dominant discourse of medicine as homeostasis
(health and wellbeing, or human flourishing) grounded in utilitarianism.

Paul Macneill (2011) is one of the few commentators in the field of the
medical humanities who has engaged with this problem of avoidance of the
avant-garde. Macneill calls for a more 'muscular' approach to the medical
humanities – perhaps an unfortunate metaphor in light of the other major
issue in the medical humanities being one of ignorance of gender issues.
Macneill sees the arts and humanities as pressed into service by medical
humanities and remaining as 'benign' and 'servile' in relation to medicine
and the health professions. While humanities interventions may critically
address the limits of the biomedical model of medicine, it may also 'challenge quiescent notions of the arts'. Macneill considers the work of
performance artists such as Stelarc (see http://stelarc.org/?catID=20247)
and Orlan (see www.orlan.eu), who have subjected their bodies to modifications and extensions. Such work questions assumptions about the
normative medical model of the body and extensions to this in what is
considered a normal appearance. For Macneill, it is difficult to simply graft

on the more radical arts to medical education without medicine questioning its foundational assumptions about what constitutes a 'normal' body.

Carrying the burden of the medical humanities

The development of the critical medical humanities within academic humanities departments does carry a danger – of distancing itself from the clinical coalface and of passing the responsibility for evidence of impact of medical humanities interventions to those still working within medical school medical education, humanities and ethics departments. Some of the ghosts from the more 'anarchic' days of medical humanities experimentation still linger. Geoffrey Rees (2010: 267) speaks for many in the medical humanities community when he talks of the 'slights endured by persons who labor under the rubric of the medical humanities'. This aligns with the assumption by sceptics towards the medical humanities that burden of proof of impact rests with those who support the medical humanities. And, of course, such proof must be provided under the terms set out by sceptics as evidence gained from empirical studies following a scientific or quasi-scientific experimental paradigm. In Chapter 9, I address this demand in detail and suggest that 'proof' cannot be reduced to an 'either it exists or it does not' scenario. Further, as Neville Chiavaroli and Constance Ellwood (2012) note, Ousager and Johannessen's (2010) review of the impact of research in the medical humanities suggests that 30 per cent of studies are justifications or 'pleading the case' for the inclusion of the medical humanities in the undergraduate medicine curriculum – again with backs to the wall.

Rees notes that the quality of a humanities intervention in medicine is more likely to be judged by those who make the intervention on the basis that it is ethically important – the intervention makes for a more caring medicine. This, however, may apply to medical humanities more oriented to the wider critical engagement with the goals of biomedicine and the medicalizing of the body. It does not so readily apply to medical humanities engaged primarily with pedagogy in medical education. Here, some pragmatic value is expected from medical humanities interventions, even if this is paradoxical, such as adding value to sensibility (for example, educating for close noticing, such as Chapter 6 details).

Jeffrey Bishop (2008, 2011) bemoans the fact that the medical humanities are commonly reduced to a medical 'humanism' that is an anaemic, technical version of the complex historical project of the arts and humanities. For example, proponents of the medical humanities may find themselves justifying curriculum models that set out to include medical humanities on the weakest of platforms that turns out to be the best understood by medical school pedagogical cultures. Here, instead of being able to celebrate the patent richness, complexity and critical challenge of the arts and humanities in the life of humanity as a starting point for a (usually minor) curriculum reform, champions of the medical humanities find them-selves arguing, for example, from the platform of a functional 'professionalism', the arts and humanities running away like sand through their fingers as they speak. Bishop warns of getting into divisive debate about separating 'fact' (science in medical education) and 'value' (ethics and humanities in medical education) and then trying to stitch them together through medical education, when they are inseparable at root and should be considered as such – the medical humanities in principle cannot then be separated from learning biomedical science. This returns us to the argument we made when developing the curriculum at Peninsula Medical School – that the 'medical humanities' issue does not start with a battle between science and the arts but rather with a recognition that good science is intrin-sically aesthetic, ethical, complex and necessarily ambiguous, where science's 'truth' claims are historically and culturally determined.

Delese Wear and Julie Aultman (2005: 1056) describe a course for fourth-year medical students called 'Family Values' in which they used a range of required reading and written response to critically engage 'with violence, illness and end-of-life matters, and issues related to race, social class, gender and sexual identity'. The class, they report, 'fell flat'. In trying to understand why, Wear and Aultman suggest that the reading matter was not contextualized and too challenging. Where fictional characters fell out of the compass of tradition and normative values, students found difficulty in engaging with the issues that these characterizations brought up. Students then resisted the text. The authors suggest that the focus should be shifted away from individuals (representing types of patients that medical students may meet as future doctors) towards structural issues of the social, political, economic and cultural conditions that may affect health.

In defence of their original method, Wear and Aultman wished to apply Megan Boler's 'pedagogy of discomfort' in challenging preconceptions of medical students about wider cultural practices that deprive persons of 'their full humanity' to help doctors to 'reduce the social causes of suffer-ing' (*ibid.*) – hence the choice of challenging texts such as Alice Walker's *The Color Purple*. Resistance took three main forms: blaming individuals for not achieving or failing to work hard enough (recognized as an American cultural trait); discounting content as irrelevant (for example, equality of treatment is ingrained in medical oaths, so why learn about inequalities?); and distancing – social issues are beyond our control, we treat disease on a patient-by-patient basis. Boler makes a distinction between 'passive empathy' and a 'semiotics of identity'. Medical students may read a text and empathise with an 'other' through a passive identifica-tion. However, how will students recognize that they may be part of the oppressive forces that alienate, marginalize or impoverish others, who remain 'different' and beyond interpersonal empathy? Students must recog-nize complicity in a status quo that maintains inequalities of opportunity and inequities.

It may be that these American medical students are also resistant to university medical school classes that appear to be similar to University humanities classes they attended (but also resisted) as compulsory in their undergraduate careers, such as a liberal arts 'great books' course. An alternative pedagogical approach is to always aim for relevance in teaching while incorporating meaning. In Chapter 8, I provide a case study illustration of a way that I introduced, collaborating with medical colleagues, study of contemporary fiction to analyse 'prescription culture' or the way that prescription drugs have now become part of the fabric of everyday life in North American cultural contexts. The students had no difficulty in engaging with the idea of an 'alternative' drug formulary that considered a small group of anti-depressants and anti-anxiety drugs as having 'character' when linked with case studies of real patients observed through their publicly accessible YouTube confessional videos.

Casey White, Arno Kumagai and colleagues (White *et al.* 2009) looked at the concept of patient-centred care with medical students through experiences of these students on clinical clerkships. Students reported that supervisors modelled behaviours antithetical to patient-centred care and this confused them. A programme was launched in 2003 at the University of Michigan medical school called 'the Family Centred Experience' that facilitated longitudinal placements and followed these up with small group class discussions (10–12 students) to integrate experiences. In 2002 at Peninsula Medical School, UK, 'jigsaw groups' were first developed for students to integrate clinical placement experiences and reflect on these in small group discussions with clinical tutors. The point about these pedagogical innovations is that structural issues such as social justice and equality are taught through reflection upon clinical experiential or work-based learning. Arts, humanities and social science scholars can readily be integrated into these reflections, for example through co-facilitation of reflective small groups. But, for these collaborative medical humanities opportunities to be successful, all participants must have first-hand experience of an issue such as 'patient-centredness' and 'patient-centred practice'. This again invites development of faculty along the lines of Johanna Shapiro's 'applied medical humanities scholars'.

At the heart of Arno Kumagai's (2009) 'Family Centered Experience Program', inaugurated for first-year medical students, is social justice. This shifts the frame of reference for medical humanities away from what can be read as more abstract notions, such as empathy and humanism, to the concrete acts of treating patients as complex and rich human beings whatever their social circumstances. Students work in pairs on a longitudinal placement with a patient volunteer suffering from a chronic or serious medical condition. The focus is then primarily political – setting medicine as a resource or capital to be fairly distributed across a community within a democratic framework. This framework is reinforced through fostering non-authoritarian faculty-student relationships. The primary method of inquiry is narrative – there is a focus upon stories told and heard and subsequent assimilation and reflection. Key to the process is recognition and appreciation of difference.

Kumagai's brave medical education innovation runs against the grain of the typical processes of rendering medical students insensible through power structures. Inviting students into a democratic space of participation with their patients and their teaching faculty resists the traditional medical educational processes of marginalization and impoverishment that makes them – temporarily – the poor and dispossessed in the medical hierarchy. Such temporary conditions of marginalization are part of apprenticeships with quasi-militaristic training including the law and learning to be an airline pilot. But, while apprentices are held in this state of relative contempt, can they not engage more readily in acts of resistance? Will they not, when their false consciousness is revealed, be more willing to reflexively consider their part in later oppression of others such as patients and healthcare colleagues? As Wear and Aultman (2005) suggest, this is an invitation for medical students to engage not just with patients as allies, but with the historical, cultural and social structures that position individuals as marginal.

The first wave of the medical humanities can be seen to have subscribed to the same value system as orthodox medicine, presenting a 'tame' (Macneill 2011: 86) approach offering students 'soft' relaxation, celebratory supplement, or diversion from the 'hard' stuff of biomedical science and evidence-based clinical practice. For example, Geoffrey Rees (2010) notes that the medical humanities can be employed non-critically, serving medical dominance rather than used in an interventionist manner. Where the functional limit of the arts and humanities has been to nuance medical practice, rather than fundamentally critiquing such practice, the form of the arts and humanities drawn upon has, as noted, avoided the critical, and political, (liberal) avant-garde that Felix Guattari (1995: 106) describes as 'the incessant clash of the movement of art against established boundaries'.

To be cynical, examples of this uncritical first wave can be seen time after time as medical schools advertise their medical humanities wares with great gusto and pride, for this to be an elective programme attracting few students who write some (often bad) poetry or make some music as a diversion from core studies. This is then self-evaluated through a satisfaction score while self-selected students are still on a high. This is some way from the kind of hard-won, self-taught pedagogy of resistance that the 15-year-old adolescents model in Peter Weiss's (2005) novel *The Aesthetics of Resistance* as they grow up in the face of the Nazi regime committed to aesthetics as the framework for democracy.

What does the future hold for the medical humanities?

Where medicine aims for homeostasis or relief from symptom, it also aims to reduce uncertainty or is intolerant of ambiguity. However, medical practice is laced with uncertainty. Art, however, is tolerant of ambiguity. Indeed, the liberal avant-garde in particular aims to generate ambiguity and uncertainty in order to questions certainties, habits and conventions, or to promote social critique. Good medical practice implies not simply tolerance, but also connoisseurship, of conditions of uncertainty (Luther and Crandall 2011) and the arts are where expertise in such connoisseurship rests. Medicine must collaborate with the arts and humanities if only to reap the rewards of learning about tolerance of uncertainty and ambiguity, such as awareness of the cultural habit to repress or deny uncertainty that is also a symptom of the high rate of medical error.

The 1998 Windsor Conference (Phillip *et al.* 1999: 26), discussed in the previous chapter as a landmark occasion for the development of the medical humanities in the UK, linked a classic definition of the humanities, as 'the study of human nature and the practice of compassionate concern for the advancement of mankind's welfare', with 'the WHO definition of health' that described 'a balanced relationship of the body and mind and complete adjustment to the external environment'. 'Balanced' and 'complete adjustment' echo the utilitarian rhetoric of normative, idealistic wellbeing, failing to see that by denying and repressing the potential of illness things may get worse, where, as Freud suggested, the repressed returns in a distorted form.

Utilitarianism sees life's purpose as the pursuit of happiness and the greatest good for the greatest number of people. 'Life, liberty and the pursuit of happiness' are ideals embedded in the American Constitution and Declaration of Independence. That happiness is preferable to misery is held to be 'self evident'. The empiricist John Locke in 1693 wrote that 'the highest perfection of intellectual nature lies in a careful and constant pursuit of true and solid happiness' (Locke 1975: 2.21.51). Modern medicine, with its central notion of homeostasis, follows this philosophical position, but the arts and humanities in general tend to diverge, often wildly, from such a philosophy.

That the pursuit of happiness is always preferred to misery must be qualified as relative. Utilitarians describe the best possible state of happiness for the greatest number of people, but again, whose 'happiness' are we describing? One person's happiness – say, misogynist hip-hop, 'death metal' music or radical performance art, is another's pain or disgust. Masochists and sadists gain pleasure from receiving and inflicting pain. Himalayan mountaineering affords huge risks, but still attracts its devotees, including doctors. Giving birth and parenting are mixtures of pain and pleasure. Love may be the most beautiful pleasure but is always close to the pain of loss. Importantly, illness is a way into rich experiences that health denies. Further, notions of pain and pleasure change historically and culturally (Elias 2000).

Voltaire, Nietzsche and other philosophers of 'pessimism' disagree with utilitarianism and the optimism of philosophers such as Leibniz who see life as the 'best of all possible worlds'. This is not simply because they are realists and accept the inevitability of human suffering, but because they recognize value in such suffering. Nietzsche (1984) articulated a philosophy of life from within his own illness, suggesting that suffering artists make sensitive diagnosticians of a suffering culture, a notion expanded by the philosopher Gilles Deleuze (1993; see also Smith 2005). Could Beethoven have composed the sublime late quartets without his deafness, or Chekhov have written such insightful literature without contracting tuberculosis that afforded empathy for the suffering of his patients? Importantly, Nietzsche, Beethoven and Chekhov did not invite or cultivate suffering, but turned misfortune into opportunity.

This philosophy of 'pathologizing' (Hillman 1992) does not square with Ken Calman's desire to set up a 'Department for Health and Happiness', where the function of art is to please and to heal rather than to challenge homeostasis for transgression, instability and education into tolerance of ambiguity and paradox as a permanent revolution, thus refreshing culture. The potential implications of this run deep – art can be anti-fascist in its desire to educate for tolerance of ambiguity, where intolerance of ambiguity is the mark of the authoritarian personality (Adorno *et al.* 1950), again combining the aesthetic with the political.

Where 'hospital' and 'hospitality' have the same root, Jacques Derrida (2000) notes the aporia, or puzzle, of hospitality – that those who provide hospitality must at the same time exert control over their household, thus providing a challenge as well as a welcome to visitors who cross the threshold. A hospital is an aporia, where healing and hospital-induced illness, such as 'avoidable' medical error and hospital-acquired infections, go hand in hand. Richard Cork's (2012) history of art in hospitals reveals a similar conundrum. While contemporary art in hospitals tends to be decorative and bland, certainly not challenging or upsetting, Cork shows that since the Renaissance art in hospitals had traditionally been shocking and challenging. It is only relatively recently that such art has become mundane. Art hung in hospitals, up to the time of Hogarth in eighteenth-century England, often included challenging motifs such as displaying symptoms suffered by patients, who would have to cathartically confront the reality of their conditions rather than be distracted or comforted by palliative images.

Belling (2010) refers to the more radical stream of thinking within the medical humanities exemplified by Wear and Aultman (2005), who show that exposing medical students to narrative approaches can produce discomfort, defensiveness and resistance to confronting political issues such as inequality and oppression. Students readily tolerate benign plots and characters in literature, where transgressive and challenging plots and characters at first produce resistance rather than empathy. This again offers a reminder of what is, arguably, the central purpose of art, certainly of the avant-garde – consciousness-raising through creating discomfort, challenge or ambiguity.

Such consciousness-raising is a three-step process: first, producing disruption through challenging habit; second, allowing typical patterns of resistance to emerge; and third, analysing such resistance to develop new awareness, as one suffers the uncertainty produced – as a resource rather than a hindrance. Belling concludes:

> Wear and Aultman articulate the limitations of treating [medical] humanities merely as a palatable reprieve from 'hard' work. They argue instead that we must attend to resistance, *even provoke it*, if [medical] humanities teaching is to promote critical inquiry as well as neutral reflection, where rigorous humanities teaching can develop an orientation toward uncertainty, knowledge, and action that characterizes the best physicians.
>
> (Belling 2010: 939; emphasis added)

Further, Alan Petersen and colleagues (2008) do not see the medical humanities as necessarily benign or liberating, but as affording an unintended form of governance, where the invitation to be 'humane' becomes a paradoxical imperative – 'you will be humane!', as in 'have a nice day!'

Some of the purported benefits of teaching medical humanities include: the promotion of patient-centred approaches to medical care; counteracting professional burnout; and equipping doctors to meet moral challenges not covered by biomedicine. In other words, the medical humanities are conventionally seen to redress a *deficit* in medicine: to act as a counterbalance to the relentless reductionism of the biomedical sciences – this, rather than reminding scientists of the aesthetic riches in their worlds. By contributing to the creation of a reflective practitioner who will exhibit empathic understanding of the patient, it is claimed (or simply assumed) that the medical humanities are necessarily good for doctors. While this sounds like good news, there is a dark side, an unintended consequence to the development of the medical humanities, where they may come to serve as a tool of governance. 'Governance' has multiple meanings with positive and negative connotations, but broadly refers to the process of steering or guiding others' or one's own conduct – in Foucault's succinct description 'the conduct of conduct'. Several questions arise from a more sceptical approach to the value of the medical humanities. For example:

1 Who is asking whom to be 'humane'?
2 What kinds of subjectivity are assumed and formed through the teaching of the medical humanities and are these welcome identity constructions?
3 What kinds of thinking and knowledge are produced by the medical humanities and how may these serve to guide action? For example, if the medical humanities are driven by the desire to 'humanize' individual practitioners, will this take our eye away from systemic failures

caused for example by poor management? Will we end up compensating structurally induced overwork and poor management with the arts and humanities?

4   How will unintended negative consequences of medical humanities interventions be noted, or indeed measured and evaluated?

The new subculture of resistance within the medical humanities culture briefly outlined above has several other foci, questioning assumptions of conventional and benign medical humanities approaches. For example, Johanna Shapiro (2011) warns against narrative medicine becoming inflated through smart textual approaches that question the authenticity or reliability of patients' stories. Shapiro then calls for 'narrative humility' from researchers. As noted in the close to the previous chapter, Claire Hooker and Estelle Noonan (2011) point to the medical humanities' largely unexamined western imperialistic tendencies, an observation that has been made about medical education in general (Bleakley *et al.* 2011). Again, Paul Macneill (2011) suggests that the arts and humanities employed in medical education are in danger of being brought into the service of a more powerful biomedical science and then tamed, as pleasant diversions for students rather than industrial strength tools for learning involving critique of reductive biomedical models.

However, what needs to be further developed is a focus upon a radical political project – that of democratizing medical culture. Democracy itself of course is a complex project. For example, Derrida *et al.* (2004) again points to the inherent paradoxes, aporias, contradictions, and ambiguities in the practices of democracy, preferring to imagine a 'democracy to come'. 'Shaping' such a horizon democracy is both an aesthetic and an ethical project (Weiss 2005). For Martha Nussbaum (2010) and Mark Slouka (2010), democracy generally is impossible without the arts and humanities, for these are the media that imaginatively allow us to educate for, and develop, the necessary and sufficient conditions for empathy, or tolerance of 'otherness', as a foundation to debate. As Slouka (*ibid.*) argues, 'the humanities are a superb delivery mechanism for what we might call democratic values'. The humanities diagnose social ills, such as unproductive authoritarian behaviour grounded in intolerance of ambiguity; and suggest cures, such as tolerance of difference through open debate and collaborative activities.

Following the detention of the internationally celebrated Chinese artist Ai Weiwei by Beijing police in April 2011, ostensibly for tax evasion but more likely as a consequence of persistent political dissidence through his art, *The Times* newspaper in London published responses from high-profile public figures as a collective open letter of protest to the Chinese government (O'Connell 2011). Sir Nicholas Serota, the Director of the Tate Gallery, observed in his response (*ibid.*) that:

The health of a society is indicated, in part, by the freedom of its artists and writers to express their views without fear of suppression. Diversity of view generates creativity and occurs through meeting of opposing ideas, a respect for differing viewpoints and the expression of distinctive visions. A society that tolerates difference will remain creative as its values are challenged. A society that cannot accommodate points of view will stagnate and become an empty husk.

The first part of what Serota suggests – that the mark of 'health of a society' is its level of democracy – is familiar to proponents of 'open' societies (Popper 2002). The second part, however, is more radical – that it is particularly the work of artists that protects a liberal democracy. The philosopher Gilles Deleuze (1997), in his last work before his death – *Essays Critical and Clinical* – developed Nietzsche's cultural analysis to suggest that artists are physicians in another realm, as 'diagnosticians' and 'symptomatologists' of the body of culture (Smith 2005). Thus, perhaps artists are closer to doctors than we think.

3 The distribution of the sensible

Introduction

In the Introduction and Chapters 1 and 2, I discussed *what* the medical humanities are and some of the controversies surrounding definitions. In this chapter, I discuss *why* the medical humanities are needed in medical education. In subsequent chapters, I show *how* the medical humanities can work effectively as key medical education interventions.

I draw on one main theoretical framework to inform the discussion of why the medical humanities are needed for medical education. I adapt a post-Marxist model developed by Jacques Rancière (2006, 2010, 2013) exploring the distribution of the fabric of the sensible (or sensibility) in culture to argue that current habitual practices in medical education may paradoxically restrict, rather than enhance, quality of learning. This perspective was introduced earlier in the book and will be explained more fully here. The argument links a political call to democratize medical practice with an aesthetic call to promote education of the sensible, or sensibility. If medical education produces insensibility, either consciously to maintain existing power structures, or unconsciously as, say, a form of defence against ambiguity, how might this be countered? The overall argument of this book is that the medical humanities offer a primary form of resistance to production of insensibility; or, there are various ways of employing the medical humanities to redistribute sensibility capital held by expert clinical teachers fairly among students, patients and marginalized healthcare practitioners. The medical humanities even out or redistribute lumps in the fabric of the sensible produced by unfair concentration of capital; or – the medical humanities repair and restore rents in the fabric of the sensible produced by interested parties, sometimes violently and unfairly, appropriating sensibility capital.

I also draw briefly on a psychoanalytic model developed by Donald Winnicott and expanded by Martha Nussbaum to argue for the value of the arts and humanities in educating for sensibility and sensitivity in clinical practice. Finally, I introduce the poststructuralist feminism of Hélène Cixous to suggest that education for compassionate medicine amounts to a cultivation of a necessary tenderness, even where tough-minded medical culture refuses such language and sentiment as 'soft and fluffy'. This remains the case despite the fact that more women than men are now entering medicine worldwide.

In each of these arguments, a block to effective practice is analysed. It is not of course that medical education in general intentionally goes out of its way to create conditions that stifle creativity, imagination, sensitivity and sensibility in the work of medical students. Rather, the production of insensibility is a largely unintended consequence, or paradoxical effect, of dominant and unexamined practices in medical education that amount to a medical 'miseducation'. I borrow this awkward, but compelling, term from Paul Goodman's (1964) classic *Compulsory Mis-education*, first published in 1964 as a scathing attack on the American schools system.

In medical education, dominant discourses and habits of practice lead to symptoms that include:

1   The production and distribution of insensibility, or institutional 'dulling' through medical education. A contemporary characteristic of this is the trend towards abandoning teaching of hands-on physical examination for medical students with the rationale that machine-based, remote testing has now largely replaced hands-on diagnoses as the most reliable method. As a consequence, the arts of auscultation, palpation and percussion are fast disappearing (Verghese 2011). This is discussed at length in Chapter 6. This, partially conscious and partially unintended, consequence of medical education is exacerbated by typically having to learn and work in dulling clinical environments that are tolerated rather than critically refused as part of the symptom pattern of medical education's machismo.

2   Mistaking complex and nonlinear medical work for the complicated and linear. This centres on attempting to translate the generalizations of population-based and evidence-based medicine into treatment of the individual patient. Where a jigsaw mentality pervades evidence-based generalizations (work out the parts and they will add up to the whole), the individual's complex needs may be misjudged (the whole is greater than the sum of the individual parts).

3   Medicine's literalism – a combination of reduction of the nonlinear complex to the linear complicated, the abstract to the instrumental, and problem stating to habitual problem solving. These factors add up to an intolerance of ambiguity and uncertainty, the central feature of both an authoritarian institutional structure and personality type. Literalism – the need to translate the conceptual into the concrete and the abstract into the instrumental – shows in the typical reductive 'case presentation', where the 'chief complaint' diagnosed by the doctor replaces the more complex 'chief concern' of the patient; and where the certainties of indicative thinking and language ('this is'/'certainly') replace the

admittance of ambiguity characteristic of subjunctivizing ('this may be'/ 'possibly/ maybe').

4   Arrested development of medicine, in psychoanalytic terms, as an 'anal' culture and institution with associated character types, typified by authoritarian structures such as hierarchies and the need to control and be controlled. This has a subset of symptoms that can be characterized as paternalism, or what Alfred Adler (2009) called the 'masculine protest'. An outcome of these symptoms is the inability for medical culture to progress towards authentic democratic forms of work (Bleakley 2014).

5   Iatrogenesis, where medical interventions cause unintended harm. This is relatively rare for technical interventions such as surgery or side effects of prescribed drugs, but far more common in terms of mistakes arising from the non-technical side of medical work, such as poor communication with colleagues in clinical team settings or between doctor and patient.

6   Empathy decline and moral erosion in medical students.

7   Poor self-care among medical students and doctors.

In order to resist this slippage into production of the insensible, where medical education adds to a general anaesthetizing and depoliticizing of students rather than an aestheticizing and politicizing, I will argue that the medical humanities in medical education can promote:

1   Redistribution of the sensible to allow for new ways of noticing and appreciating. This is fundamentally a re-education of the senses.

2   Development of practice from an 'anal' arrested stage to a 'genital', collaborative and progressive stage in which tenderness and collaboration are seen as strengths rather than weaknesses, in a challenge to the dominant and controlling patriarchy gripped by an outmoded ideology of heroic individualism.

The distribution of the sensible is a historical phenomenon

What we do, say, think, imagine and even feel is regulated historically, culturally and socially (Elias 2000). For example, spitting in public was once acceptable but is now frowned upon; how and when we cough, sniff, blow our noses, or eat our food are subject to layers of cultural habit. We blush even when we are not in company; we dissimulate in order to not lose face or offend another. 'Manners' in a culture develop historically and become normalized and habitual – Norbert Elias (*ibid.*) refers to this as 'the civilizing process'. Ivan Illich (1985) describes the history of the water closet, to show how the private toilet was developed not out of concern for hygiene but for the growing practice of privacy (hence the 'privy'). Privacy in turn is part of a major discourse centred on the forming of the 'individual', giving rise not only to the cults of autonomy and celebrity, but also psychiatry and psychology as the institutional regulation of personality (Foucault 2006).

Practices and behaviours arising from the historical dominance of discourses (such as respecting somebody's 'personal space') become 'black boxed' – taken for granted and not examined. Michel Foucault (2002) famously suggests that these cultural practices are effects of 'biopower', authority that reaches right into the very finest ways in which our bodies are controlled, resulting for example in blushing in private at an embarrassing memory, thought or reflection. Importantly, for Foucault, we have not 'liberated' ourselves from power and authority, or lead a more enlightened life (such as not spitting in public taken as a more 'developed' cultural position). Rather, patterns of control, domination and resistance change forms historically. Biopower – social production and control of bodily functions (including illness) – is always there, but expressions differ historically. At any one point historically, as 'sovereign' power is exerted as authority and *reproduced* through institutional structures, so 'capillary' power is also *produced* and runs through any system or any body, showing fine regulation. Further, as sovereign power is exerted through dominant discourses, so it may be resisted by a countermovement.

While the capacity to sense, imagine, feel, talk, work, consume, form relationships and so on is available to us as birthright, how these capacities are realized then depends upon a prior (historical) condition of possibility. For example, beyond the biological fact that one senses, how, what and even where one senses are culturally determined through pre-existing structures (Corbin 2005). At an institutional level, such as medicine, patterns of sensing become historically determined habits remaining largely unexamined. They have a logic of course: this is how a physical examination is carried out, this is how bedside teaching is done. But that logic can grow to be counterproductive, such as the habit of interrupting patients too early in the consultation, or of talking 'over', rather than with, patients.

Patterns of sensing can go through Kuhnian revolutions – historically rapid paradigmatic shifts in ways of practice and learning. For example, the introduction of simulation into teaching both clinical and communication skills has revolutionized the ways that medical students learn how to insert a urinary catheter or communicate bad news. But, as these modes of learning become habitual, so they begin to produce insensibilities. For example, students can simulate, or worse, dissimulate effective communication (Bleakley *et al.* 2011). Currently, as discussed earlier, students spend less time in bedside physical examination and more making sense of the results of tests and scans, potentially leading to overdiagnoses (Welch *et al.* 2011) and depriving the student–patient relationship of the ritual of professional contact. Students' senses are dulled in the process because the opportunity to sharpen them is withdrawn through new forms of medical education. Typical habitual production of insensibilities includes objectifying the patient as cynicism is modelled among seasoned clinical educators. Let us look a little more closely at the dynamics of production of professional insensibilities.

Inattentional blindness

In a seminal experiment, James Potchen (2006) asked radiologists to review standard cases as if for an examination and introduced chest X-rays but with the clavicle or collarbone removed. Sixty per cent of those in the study failed to notice the missing clavicle, simply because that is not what they were focusing upon. That 40 per cent of the radiologists did note the missing clavicle means that the radiologists would characteristically scan the entire X-ray prior to focusing on the specific part relevant to the diagnosis. However, the power of attention to the specific generally cuts out the meaning of the overall image, so that the majority did not see the obvious.

Does this matter? Well, selective attention may lead to the doctor missing information that is vital to a correct diagnosis, and this may then result in a misdiagnosis. Many misdiagnoses do not lead to harm, but some do. Of medical errors that lead to unnecessary death or serious harm, it is estimated that between 10–15 per cent are due to misdiagnoses (Sanders 2010).

Potchen's study used a standard 'single slice' medical image. Contemporary radiology, however, deals with far more complex imagery such as hundreds of slices in a chest CT scan. You would expect that an expert scrolling through a stack of images might more easily avoid error. Further, not seeing something that should be there is not the same as being 'blind' to something that is there but is missed (psychologists call this phenomenon 'inattentional blindness'). Evidence shows that it is harder to note the absence of what should be there than to detect the presence of something. A more striking and sophisticated recent experiment by Trafton Drew, Melissa Võ and Jeremy Wolfe (2013), at the Visual Attention Laboratory of Harvard Medical School, again shows that experts making visual diagnostic judgements are highly selective in their attention and perception. These researchers changed the conditions of Potchen's study by providing multiple images and introducing something which was plainly in the image but could be missed through focused attention.

That experts in visual acuity in medicine (primarily radiologists, pathologists and dermatologists) use selective attention in making standard expert judgements is something we already knew (Bleakley 2004, 2006b; Bleakley *et al.* 2003a, 2003b), but the results of Drew and colleagues' experiments raise to awareness the implications of such selective attention for foreclosing on clinical reasoning, or making a hasty diagnostic judgement. The authors asked 24 expert radiologists to perform a standard and familiar lung-nodule detection on a standard X-ray. They scrolled through stacks of five chest CTs looking for evidence of nodules, that appear as light circles. Typically, a stack contains 100 to 500 slices. In the final of the five stacks, a large image of a gorilla was introduced. This stack contained 239 slices. The gorilla faded in and out of perception across five slices (each 2 mm thick) within this stack. At the size of a matchbook, the image of the gorilla was 48 times the size of the nodule and was inserted in the last case presented.

Of the 24 radiologists, 20 (83 per cent) did not see the gorilla, although eye tracking showed that they had looked directly at the location of the gorilla – again showing 'inattentional blindness'. All the radiologists saw the gorilla clearly when it was pointed out to them. A non-medical control group was set up. These 25 individuals were trained to see the lung nodules. None of them saw the gorilla and this group, as expected, showed poor recognition of the lung nodules. However, this confirms that novices, who are looking 'harder' than experts or in a sense straining their attention, also showed selective attention. A naïve group of 12 observers was shown a movie with the frames of the movie corresponding to slices of the stack, so that the gorilla was plainly evident on some of the frames. Eighty-eight per cent of this group were able to see the gorilla, showing that it was plainly visible also to the other two groups, but not 'seen'. This experiment also shows the phenomenon of 'satisfaction of search'. When what is expected is seen, the search is discontinued. This is an example of premature closure, and is one of the main causes of misdiagnoses.

The authors conclude that

> even this high level of expertise does not immunize individuals against inherent limitations of human attention and perception. Researchers should seek better understanding of these limits, so that medical and other man-made search tasks could be designed in ways that reduce the consequences of these limitations.
>
> (Drew *et al.* 2013: 5)

But there is another way and that is the substance of this book. Why not educate the perceptual or sensory acuity of doctors and healthcare professionals generally as core activity? Who better to do this than artists and humanities scholars – visual artists working with medical students and doctors to improve visual acumen; writers working to improve narrative intelligence; and actors and performance artists working to improve communication performance and management of identity? Indeed, this collaborative model can be extended to perfumier and oenophile (wine taster) educating the smell and taste of medical students (a successful and longstanding fourth-year special study unit at Peninsula Medical School, UK).

Of course, in some areas, such as the use of actor-patients (introduced by Howard Barrows in 1963 at the University of Southern California), we might say that such actors have long taught performance to medical students and even assessed such performance. However, medical educators have managed to turn this opportunity into production of insensibility through an insistence upon standardizing actor patient-student interactions for the sake of fairness in assessment. No patient is 'standard' – this is a form of objectification. Before moving on to recommend how, for example, visual artists and doctors might work together to create a new kind of pedagogy within medical education, we need, first, to thoroughly understand the reasons why such a pedagogical intervention is needed at all. And second, we need to adequately theorize the pedagogical intervention of the medical humanities.

The social organization of perception

The German literary critic, social theorist and philosopher Walter Benjamin (1968) first described preforming of the sensible in the early 1930s, where 'the manner in which human sense perception is organised, the medium in which it is accomplished, is determined not only by nature but by historical circumstances as well'. The fact and consequences of perception includes the field of aesthetics. At root, aesthetics simply means 'sense impression'. How perceptions are preorganized through historical discourses is, however, a matter of power or politics. Benjamin thus initiated an important dialogue between aesthetics and politics.

The French philosopher Jacques Rancière is the primary contemporary exponent of Benjamin's idea of the socio-historical preforming of perception (see Deranty 2010; Bowman and Stamp 2011). Rancière adapts Karl Marx's original insight concerning inequalities not only in the distribution of material wealth, but also in the distribution of the immaterial such as sensible and emotional capital. This is often referred to as the production and distribution of 'knowledge capital' in a 'knowledge economy'. Medicine produces, for consumption by patients and doctors, a range of material goods such as hospital buildings, ambulances, surgical instruments and pharmaceuticals. However, medical education deals largely with immaterial capital such as knowledge, practices and values, where the economy in which medicine works is largely that of talk and performance. How then is the collective capital of knowledge, practices and values distributed in medicine? Are there blatant inequalities in distribution and is 'counter-capital' produced that is counter-productive to effective medical practice?

The meeting of aesthetics and politics in the distribution of the sensible

Benjamin and Rancière, like many of Rancière's contemporaries in French postwar intellectual life in particular, have adapted Marx's legacy to explore contemporary social existence. Marx's main concern, in a rapidly industrializing world, was with how capital produced by factories (raw goods and their cash equivalent) would be distributed; and with who owned the means of production (factories, machinery, raw materials). Just as labour had been exploited through slavery to harvest raw materials such as sugar, or to dig metals from mines, so labour was exploited in factories or steelworks in refining the sugar or turning the metal into ingots. The owners of the means of production (capitalists) would cream off the major part of profit for themselves and exploit the workers by paying low wages, treating them as mechanical parts in a production process and threatening that they could readily be replaced if they rebelled. Workers were treated as dispensable objects or as units in production, stripping them of sensibility.

Marx's socialism promised to fundamentally reorganize the industrial process to give workers shares in the means of production such as factories, and to not exploit their labour but provide them with fair remuneration. Profits would be ploughed back to improve work conditions and living standards in a redistribution of wealth. What, however, of a post-industrial world in which consumption of the immaterial (Gorz 2010) – ideas, symbols, education, advertising, entertainment and so on – is more important than the production and consumption of material goods such as televisions and cars? Post-Marxist analyses have taken Marx's ideas into the realms of the immaterial world by treating experiences such as human emotions or affect and human sensibility, or aesthetic responses and cultural taste, as capital open to manipulation by vested interests. For example, what we consider to be aesthetic 'choices' in life, such as our manners, the clothes we wear, the colours of our cars, the art, or the music, cinema and television we enjoy, are manipulated by vested interests. Control over production and consumption of goods is paralleled by control over production and consumption of symbols, signs and knowledge such as entertainment, education and psychological therapies.

Where Marx focused on the fair distribution of material wealth and the ethical use of labour, Rancière considers the fair distribution of aesthetic and emotional capital and ethical use of aesthetic and emotional labour. Rancière notes that the 'sensible' in life – what is worth noticing and appreciating and the processes by which sensing, noting and appreciating are socially legitimated – does not simply occur as a transparent or natural process. Rather, what is considered worth noticing and, more importantly, who is given the privilege to notice and appreciate, is determined socially. There is a process through which the sensible and sensibility are apportioned and applied that is fundamentally unfair or shows inequalities. Some (many) are considered insensible, or are denied participation in legitimate judgements about what is worthwhile noticing and appreciating. Aesthetics, or sense impressions, the basis for perception and appreciation, form a value system, but a dominant minority decides what these values shall be. This minority also further decides that some members of society shall be insensible, kept ignorant in terms of sensitivity and sensibility, implying that these members of society have blunt affect. The majority – who are left insensible – are the underprivileged, the poor and the disaffected (Vollman

2007), but in professions such as medicine this group includes those low on the hierarchy, primarily medical students. Aesthetics is then closely tied to politics – what shall be judged worthwhile to notice is inseparable from power. What is worth noticing (and requires close noticing) in medicine is symptom expression and this is often at the expense of noticing the person who expresses the symptom(s) and the contexts in which symptom expression occurs.

Rancière (2010: 36; 2013: ix) describes a historical transformation of the forms of sensible experience or 'ways of perceiving and being affected'. Aesthetics is described as a 'mode of intelligibility' through 'reconfiguration of experience'. Again, we do not experience 'raw' or directly, rather our perceptions are first formed, shaped and refined socially (and such social engineering is necessarily a political forming); and second, perceptions are adjusted through forms of education, themselves subject to the relationships between power (politics), knowledge and sensing. This leads to 'ways ... of being affected', in which persons, groups, societies and even cultures might be sidelined or conceived as 'insensible' as they are denied participation in sensibility (see Panagia 2010). Again, this can range from a privileged group deciding on what constitutes legitimate 'art', 'humanities' or 'education' on behalf of excluded groups, to medical students as uninitiated 'novices' being denied access to medicine proper until certain initiations have occurred and a level of expertise has been demonstrated. The sensible (again, the aesthetic realm) is first partitioned or parcelled off, and then apportioned or distributed (the realm of power). However, such partitioning and distribution, once raised to awareness, can be resisted. A major role for a radical and critical medical education is to show how redistribution of the sensible may be achieved through resistance and primary media for such distribution are the arts and humanities within medicine and medical education – as primary forms of the medical humanities.

The 'police', 'politics' and 'dissensus'

Rancière (2006, 2010) suggests that power affecting the partition and distribution of the sensible operates through two channels: 'the police' and 'politics'. The functions of 'the police' (a general descriptor and metaphor for legitimized authority and control in a society) are (i) to fill a potential void ('move along, there's nothing for you to see here'), and (ii) to deny 'supplement' (there may be another way of thinking about this, or of acting on that thought). Again, by 'the police' Rancière does not mean just the police force. Rather, it is a general term for a legitimate authority's structuring of the sensible that distributes this capital selectively.

Rancière insists that the essence of the police does not rest in oppression, repression or control. Rather, 'the police', as dominant and legitimate institutional practices, represent the privileged way of distributing the sensible. Just as wealth is distributed according to privilege – and then, in Marx's critique, reinforces inequalities – so the sensible (what is sensed and how it is sensed) is distributed through prior power structures. Again, perceptions, as modes of participation in the world, are contingent upon prior historical conditions. What shall be sensed and how it shall be sensed are pre-patterned.

'Politics', on the other hand, is a form of resistance to the police. Politics describes any intervention that attempts to redistribute the sensible, or to uncover the 'black boxes' that insensibility produces – habitual practices that normally remain unexamined. Most importantly, politics gives a voice (subjectivity) to those who are normally excluded from participating in deciding how the sensible shall be distributed (again, the poor, the under-privileged, or those lowest on the hierarchy such as medical students in a medical culture). The process through which politics is mobilized as a redis-tribution of the sensible is 'dissensus' (Rancière 2010). As Rockhill (2006: 85) suggests:

> A dissensus is not a quarrel over personal interests or opinions. It is a political process that resists juridical litigation and creates a fissure in the sensible order by confronting the established framework of percep-tion, thought, and action with the 'inadmissable', i.e. a political subject.

By a 'political subject', Rockhill means a politicized person – someone who has seen through the processes by which sensibility capital is unfairly distributed or withheld, or, conversely, insensibility is produced. The politi-cized subject acts in resistance to such dominance. This suggests that medical students can (or should) be politicized as well as aestheticized through medical education, gaining a legitimate identity as an active rather than passive learner and an authentic voice in their medical education. Patients and 'other' healthcare practitioners should become part of this process of dissensus.

Predetermination of what and how one shall engage with the world percep-tually is of two kinds: first, separation and exclusion; and second, allowance of participation. Thus, says Rancière 'what is visible and what not' and 'what can be heard and what cannot' is not an issue of persons naively entering the world and perceiving in a 'raw' state, but rather the consequences of a set of preconditions that already shape perception. When 'the police' say 'move along, there's nothing for you to see here', a 'partition of the sensible' occurs that 'is characterized by the absence of void and of supplement'. Occupations and places are already predetermined such that there is no place for a void or doubt, uncertainty and ambiguity. Thus, *this is how a doctor shall perceive* (as in clinical judgement) is a matter of the distribution of the sensible through the efforts of 'the police' – as those at the top of the medical education hier-archy in any local context (the chief clinical teachers).

The practice of 'policing' is one of legitimating 'what is' by repressing 'what is not', or what is *possible*. In contrast, the essence of 'politics' is to reveal what is possible, through engagement with the ambiguous and uncertain. Politics 'is an intervention in the visible and the sayable' (Rancière 2010: 37) to redistribute sensibility. In essence, this is to change the conditions of possibility for sensing. Again, Rancière (2010) terms this 'dissensus' – a form of resistance against the police. Dissensus (Panagia 2010) is a dissent from inequality and insensibility – the latter not only referring to how or what may be encompassed by the senses, noticed or discriminated, but, crucially, *an inability to be sensed, noticed or accounted for.* Of course, this 'inability' is not an issue of agency, of wishing or choosing to be able to be noticed, but one of structure – of marginalization, exclusion and ineligibility.

If we take the example of the 'birth' of democracy in fifth-century BC Athens – women and slaves were not part of this democratic experiment. They were 'policed' as unsuitable for political involvement and then stripped of the opportunity to experience through the senses what men could. The distribution of the sensible was unequal. If this example is transposed to modern medicine, the conditions of possibility for sense experiences are highly regulated or policed by an elite authority of consultants or experts. What presents itself to sense experience in medical education is then preconfigured by this historical tradition (also, a male gendered body of expertise). Indeed, the sensible is ill-distributed where what is traditionally valued is the expertise of the autonomous individual – the heroic figure or the rogue diagnostician, caricatured in the most successful of all television medical dramas: *House*, starring Hugh Laurie.

The distribution of the sensible can be equated with delimitation (drawing of boundary) of spaces and times and of the visible and invisible, as Michel Foucault (1989) traces in *The Birth of the Clinic*, where certain historical conventions apply such as the tight, focused case presentation (time) in the setting of the clinic (space) determining what can and cannot be said and performed. In medical education, patients are objectified as 'cases' presented crisply and concisely within a limited time, where the 'chief complaint' overshadows the 'chief concern' (Schleifer and Vannatta 2013). This distribution of the sensible can again be read as production of the insensible, adding to the historical tradition of the bluntness, literal stance and materiality of the medical culture, with its suspicion towards the intellectual, the baroque and the tender-minded.

Further, the clinic legitimizes what is not permissible in ordinary discourse, such as intimate examinations necessary for diagnosis and treatment. Here, the patient is again potentially rendered insensible. But such intimate interactions are complex. While the senses are focused and channelled for diagnostic acumen, a parallel insensibility is produced linked to ethical and professional behaviour, in which 'normal' responses of sexual arousal, curiosity and disgust are suspended or dulled, while ethical boundaries are sharpened. In communication, professional 'empathy' can be seen to be a result of the regulated balance between the sensible and the insensible in terms of ordinary human compassion being balanced by professional distance. The problem, again, is that historically the dominant discourse has been biased towards the – in relational terms – insensible, where empathy decline and moral erosion occur.

Rancière's model then accounts not only for how medical students' learning is preformed through an historically established tight distribution of the sensible, but also accounts for why medical students do not have an authentic 'voice' in the practices of clinical learning. While pedagogies appear to become outwardly more 'student-centred' and medical practices more 'patient-centred', this does not necessarily disrupt the underlying structure of the distribution of the sensible, where forms of perception (aesthetics) and modes of relations (politics) resist redistribution shaped by equity (fairness and justice) and equality of opportunity.

Of course, medical students are novices learning clinical expertise from senior doctors and the gradual accrual by novices of expert clinical practice and knowledge offers a legitimate and standard form of appropriate distribution of sensibility capital. This is not what I am questioning or critiquing. Rather, my focus is on the supposed pedagogical expertise of clinical experts in promoting accelerated learning, student- and patient-centredness and professionalism and interprofessionalism. And, more importantly, in how democratic practices stemming potential empathy decline and moral erosion can lessen production of insensibility and insensitivity. To return to earlier points in this chapter, forms of 'inattentional blindness' are endemic to medical education, as are resistances to democratic structures. Medical students gain identities as doctors through socialization into these skewed forms of the distribution of the sensible. Enlightened medical educationists should be applauded for their work in developing student-centred learning for patient-centred practice, but they are constantly working against the grain of the institutional and structural conditions of the production and reproduction of insensibility in medicine.

Tampering with this system will not change it. In order to democratize the processes of production and distribution of the capital of sensibility and sensitivity, the system of medical education needs root and branch changes. Dissensus, or dissent, requires a fundamental redistribution of the sensible. While I argue throughout this book that the medical humanities may provide the vehicle for such a fundamental redistribution of the sensible, this does not readily address the issue of how the medical humanities may be introduced into an undergraduate medicine curriculum. Wholesale introduction of generative medical humanities in medical education requires a revolution in medical education similar to that of Abraham Flexner's reforms of 1910 in North American medical education (Cooke *et al.* 2010; Bleakley *et al.* 2011). However, as Rancière himself points out, dissensus is a slow and permeating process and not an overnight radicalization of practices.

The redistribution of the sensible through a new medical education that draws on the medical humanities

So what does Rancière's model tell us about the value of the medical humanities in medical education? Rancière insists that art's (and the humanities') function is to change or repair, through redistribution, the sensible fabric of the world. Art makes us rethink our lives, to look and think again, to think against the grain. The medical humanities do this for medicine – redistributing the sensible fabric of medical practice to make medical students and doctors think again. Medical humanities interventions in medical education set out to – often disruptively – change the perception of students but also to politicize them, forming an identity of resistance (Weiss 2005). To dwell on the process of dissensus, let us equate Rancière's 'the police' with a scientific medicine that is sceptical of the value of the medical humanities. Redistribution of the sensible is denied through design and implementation of a curriculum that excludes the arts and humanities and produces insensibility. Further, the burden of proof of the value of the medical humanities is placed on the shoulders of its protagonists (see Chapter 9), rather than sceptics having to demonstrate the value of their scepticism. Again, the medical humanities can offer a medium for resistance or dissensus, inviting a (re)distribution of the sensible as a dual political and aesthetic gesture. This gesture counters the production and reproduction of the insensible through medical education.

To draw on Rancière's example, 'the police' do not interpellate (demand an explanation and give an identity to) demonstrators, but, cleverly, refuse to offer an identity to demonstrators simply by breaking up the demonstration ('there's nothing for you here, please move on'). By not recognizing the medical humanities through moving the demonstration (resistance) on, sceptics treat proponents in the same way as the men in the Athenian democratic experiment treated women and slaves – as non-citizens or barbarians. To the sceptics, the medical humanities are, literally, a 'non-sense' as distribution of sensibility is refused and insensibility is produced. Dissensus challenges such a partition and distribution of the sensible. This political intervention makes what was unseen visible and renders what was merely noise as speech. Dissensus challenges the notion that students do not have a voice in medicine until they have gained requisite technical expertise (actually, they may be highly capable morally, ethically and in communication and this may show in challenging perceived unethical practices of seniors). Juniors may well practice the art of medicine as well, or better than, more cynical and hardened seniors, even if their applied clinical science is as yet undeveloped. Historically, the Flexnerian legacy has deprived medical students of the early clinical experience that may accelerate learning clinical judgement because it insists on first forming the identity of 'scientist'. This deprivation is a form of production of insensibility as opportunities for early forming of pattern recognition are frustrated.

Rancière (2010: 38) says that dissensus is 'not a confrontation between interests or opinions' but rather 'the demonstration (*manifestation*) of a gap in the sensible itself' (emphasis original). What Rancière refers to as a 'gap in the sensible' I refer to as production of insensibility (either conscious or unintended). Importantly, here is the creation of an identity – as a humane practitioner who has acquired a slice of the sensible by speaking out against its repression. Again, this revolution is not an overnight coup, but a slow process of realization of the power of the medical humanities as a medium through which redistribution of the sensible is possible. When Rancière (*ibid*.: 92) says politics and 'the police', respectively, refer to 'two ways of framing a sensory space, of seeing or not seeing common objects in it, of hearing or not hearing in it subjects that designate them or reason in their relation' we can apply this directly to the doctor's relation to her patients and colleagues. This is not seen as a revelation, but rather reclamation, of what is suppressed by 'the police' in terms of a denial of democratic distribution of the sensible.

While Jacques Rancière has been our main guide in this chapter, I will refine his argument with reference, briefly, to the work of the psychoanalyst Donald Winnicott as developed by the philosopher Martha Nussbaum in arguing for the value of the arts and humanities in culture. I transpose this argument to medicine to argue for the value of the arts and humanities in medical education. Second, I will briefly draw on the work of the feminist writer, philosopher and literary critic Hélène Cixous to argue that one of the main purposes of developing the medical humanities in medical education is to counter the dominant patriarchal discourse with one informed by contemporary feminisms.

The production of insensibility can be aligned with authoritarianism and intolerance of ambiguity: Donald Winnicott and Martha Nussbaum

There is a thread that runs through the work of psychoanalysis and literary criticism that provides an explanatory model for the value of the medical humanities in medical education. Medicine has traditionally been patriarchal and hierarchical; has overvalued autonomy of the profession and of individuals at the expense of transparency, public scrutiny and collaboration; and has been doctor-centred rather than patient-centred. Medicine and medical education are both undergoing a major transformation that will counter this historical situation.

Psychoanalytically, medical culture has been in a state of arrested development – stuck in an anal stage of development (irrational need for control) without transition to a genital or adult stage (letting go of neurotic control for authentic interprofessional collaboration or interprofessionalism). The genital stage is one of adult collaboration and sharing of resources, or a democratizing of medicine and healthcare. Under anality, hierarchies, coercion and autonomy as self-interest flourish, while co-operation, collaboration and understanding of the positions of others (empathy) are never fully realised. Democracy, as informed participation in a collaborative discussion, is then impossible to achieve, as various forms of autocracy flourish. These may be strict, as authoritarian behaviour, or softer, as autocracy disguised as meritocracy. They may call on legitimate authority (merit through knowledge or skills) that is not exercised in order to educate others, but is again exercised for control. Of course, this is a generalization that excludes the innovative clinical and pedagogical work of many individual doctors who show dissensus and resistance to medical culture's and medical education's normative patterns and I applaud and celebrate their vision, generosity and sacrifices.

Development to a 'genital' stage is Freud's way of describing the potential for an adult relationship that is consensual and warm, indeed erotic in the sense that such a relationship is fuelled by eros or life force, rather than thanatos, or a 'death' force – metaphorically one person strangling another's voice through unfair dominance. Anality can be readily linked with intolerance of ambiguity – an inability to cope with uncertainty and a fear of chaos. A more mature outlook demands taking on board disturbing, unsettling and even opposing views, values and behaviours of others in a climate of debate. Such debate involves critique and argument, but not oppression. This is again the basis for democracy as a developmental project. Doctors are faced with uncertainty or ambiguity daily in their work. Their work might also be characterized as reducing uncertainty – attempting to get a right diagnosis and treatment and making sure that the patient is compliant with the best possible attempted cure, while respecting the patient's view and accommodating this in the process of treatment. Doctors then need to tolerate ambiguity first in their own practices, second in the patient's responses and third in how uncertainties are best discussed with patients. Medicine – and surgery in particular – has historically been marked by intolerance of ambiguity (Ludmerer 1999).

Artists and humanities scholars, however, on the whole cultivate ambiguity and uncertainty and open this to public scrutiny. Their worlds are ones in which certainties are constantly questioned and problem setting is more important than problem solving. It would seem appropriate then to introduce arts and humanities practices, values and thinking to medicine as an educational project, to educate for tolerance of ambiguity.

Finally, intolerance of ambiguity is the principal distinguishing feature of the authoritarian personality – of people who wish to be in control and to control others (or to be controlled by those who they see as superior). The web of connecting factors described above suggests that there is another way to do medicine than the one that has been historically established, but is, as suggested, already in deep transition. Medicine could shift from its historical focus on autonomy to collaboration, from authority-led models to democratic models, from objectivity to empathy and from patriarchal values to feminist approaches. This is not to cleanse medicine of tough-mindedness, but to shift the balance of power, so that tender-minded medicine can be properly tested for its efficacy as we move into a community-centred, patient-centred and team-based healthcare for the twenty-first-century.

In culture generally, Martha Nussbaum (2010) argues for the humanities (including the arts) as the chief force for promoting democracy (see also Mark Slouka 2009, 2010), where the humanities diagnose social ills, such as groundless and unproductive authoritarian behaviour. The humanities also suggest cures for social ills, such as tolerance of difference through open debate and collaborative activities. If we transpose Nussbaum's argument for the humanities as a democratizing force in wider culture to medical culture in particular, the medical humanities may play a bigger role in medical education than we imagine. What is a possible theoretical model for this process of democratization? Drawing on the psychoanalytic psychiatry of Donald Winnicott (1971), Nussbaum argues that social play is essential to developing empathy – tolerance for others and appreciation of their vulnerabilities. Where imaginative play is curtailed, children fail to learn how to collaborate, and retain controlling behaviour as a means of dealing with uncertainty (the very symptom that medical culture grapples with). Transition to democratic participation as adults requires what Winnicott calls 'potential space' – the humanities as an adult equivalent of play – where tolerance of ambiguity, as the basis to learning respect for others by resisting premature closure on judgement, is reinforced. In contrast, authoritarianism is characterized by intolerance of ambiguity.

Luther and Crandall (2011: 799–800) point out that while practising medicine demands high tolerance of ambiguity, 'the culture of medicine has little tolerance for ambiguity and uncertainty'. Kenneth Ludmerer's (1999) seminal history of American medical education notes 'a century-long defect in medical education: the failure of medical education to prepare learners to deal with uncertainty', where medical culture shows 'inordinate zeal for certainty', echoing Luther and Crandall above. For example, doctors who are less tolerant of ambiguity tend to order more (often unnecessary) tests and additional treatments for patients, placing a burden upon both patients and health care systems (Luther and Crandall 2011).

The purpose of the humanities is to create and debate uncertainty and ambiguity, which is also central to the democratic project (Nussbaum 2010). From a survey of 313 graduating medical students over a period of 10 years, those who scored high on an intolerance of ambiguity scale were also found to show significantly greater negative attitudes towards underserved and poor patients (Wayne *et al.* 2011). Again, intolerance of ambiguity is the central characteristic of the 'authoritarian personality' (Adorno *et al.* 1950), discussed above, and authoritarian behaviour is characterized by poor communication, with a tendency to employ monologue rather than dialogue, where dialogue again is the core of democratic behaviour. Boyle, Dwinnell and Platt (2005) see 'high-physician-control' as the main factor in communication 'hypocompetence', or poor communication with colleagues and patients. Again, decline in both empathy and tolerance of ambiguity present two faces of the same symptom – communication hypocompetence or underachievement.

A constellation of factors then accrues around authoritarian behaviour to do with lack of 'play' space opportunities for developing empathy through fantasy. Winnicott and Nussbaum suggest that 'adult play' is necessary to compensate for loss of play space as a child. Translating this to the developmental phases of a culture, an extreme way of putting this would be that medicine has never properly grown up, but remains stuck in anality where play space was never allowed, but hard-headed dominance was encouraged. The role of the humanities, suggests Nussbaum, is to educate for empathy and I am suggesting that this insight can be transferred to medical education as a form of resistance to production of insensibility in medical students and the unfair distribution of sensibility capital.

Finally, the developmental personality features scrutinized here through a psychoanalytic lens also form a distinct kind of paternalism central to the production of insensibility where it refuses more feminine approaches of kindness, tenderness and touch in doctor-patient encounters. The continued regular use of martial metaphors in medicine (such as 'waging war on disease') is a symptom of such paternalism (Bleakley *et al.* 2014), ironic in an age where more women worldwide are entering medicine than men.

The redistribution of the sensible can be aligned with promotion of a tender-minded medicine

I will draw briefly on the work of Hélène Cixous (1991, 2004; Cixous and Clément 1986) to advertise the value of dissensus towards a patriarchal and paternalistic medicine, where nourishment and tender-minded practice might challenge tough-minded habits. Cixous is one of a number of women thinkers, writers and social activists (including Julia Kristeva, Luce Irigaray and Catherine Clément) who are typically grouped together under the title of 'French post-structuralist feminists'. The kind of feminism they advertise is grounded in social inequalities as a product of language, where masculinity is dominant but can be countered – hence the use of their descriptor 'phallogocentric' as a summary of the dominant discourse in the construction of meaning (phallus + logos, or the logic of writing and speech), to be challenged by an eros of language.

As post-structuralists, these feminists challenge the primary view of structuralism that language and meaning work through binary oppositions. This has led to forms of oppression, where male dominates over female, white over black, adult over child, human over nature, and so forth. Language, however, cannot be contained in this way and is highly ambiguous so that it is destructuralist, or deconstructs. Language surprises, upsets and reconfigures. Briefly, as this will be part of the content of Chapter 7, doctors tend to use language in diagnoses and consultations in an objectifying, reductive and indicative way – to tell, point to, or circumscribe in an attempt to reduce uncertainty ('this is'). Objectification and dehumanizing are used as a way to, paradoxically, keep patients at arms' length so that they do not contaminate the process of clinical judgement. Poets tend to rely more on the subjunctive – where language is uncertain and ambiguous ('possibly, maybe'). What if doctors were taught by writers to think subjunctively? Would this educate for tolerance of ambiguity?

Cixous's own work explicitly challenges 'phallogocentric' writing and speech – language that is masculine in intent and performance, that objectifies, circumscribes and tells (forms of insemination) through logic rather than feeling. Such writing has inscribed not only Western culture, particularly its scientific enterprise, but also inscribes bodies. The process of medicalization of the body then particularizes by breaking the body down into organs and systems – a way of thinking about the body that does not match experience particularly well, where symptoms are often fuzzy, diffuse and mixed up with psychological effects and feelings.

Medicine wants precise locations, characteristic episodes and scales of pain, where patients may experience uncertain feelings, mixtures of diffuse symptoms and idiosyncratic episodes of discomfort. The distinction that Gilles Deleuze and Félix Guattari (2004a, 2004b) make between 'territorializing' and 'de-territorializing' is helpful here. The 'body without organs' is a metaphor for a 'smooth' space, one that is unconquered, has not suffered from a conquering imperialism or a dominant force (such as patriarchy). A body that is mapped, articulated, territorialized, is a 'striated' space and is domesticated (Bleakley 2014). In treating, doctors want to inscribe the patient's body with specific help – a prescription to match the 'chief complaint'. This is informed by maps and territorializing – a need for clear diagnosis or pinning down the issue. This is understandable but the patient has a wider 'chief concern' within which the complaint is embedded. To treat only the presenting complaint is to miss its context. Cixous describes 'writing with mother's milk' as a feminine form of writing (*écriture feminine*) – this conjures up images of succour and tenderness, an inscription of care rather than simply treatment.

Of oppositional categories within the structuralist library of binaries, the most important is self/Other. Identity within this model is that of knowing the self, or selfsame. Within post-structuralism, identity is realized in the mirror of the Other, as difference. In values, there is no essential truth, but a play of differences. It is through difference that meanings are generated and not from the supposed essence of a thing. To produce insensibility in others is to not respect difference. Medical education is preformed through historical habits such as valorizing the autonomous hero, but in the age of collaborative clinical teamwork such an outlook is dated and not helpful for the majority of episodes of patient treatment and care.

4   Empathy and its discontents

By choice they made themselves immune
To pity and whatever moans in man
Before the last sea and the hapless stars
                              (from 'Insensibility' by Wilfred Owen)

Introduction

In Gabriel Weston's semi-autobiographical novel *Dirty Work*, she describes calling for the help of a consultant surgeon while on ward duty as a senior medical student:

> When I knocked on the door a man answered, 'Come in,' and I recognised Mr Hanforth's voice. I put my head round the door and he beckoned me in, saying, 'Have a seat. I'm just finishing my dictation.' His manner was level, and I admired this, the democracy of his approach. I had already become so used, as a medical student, to being treated like the scum of the earth.
>
> (Weston 2013: 59)

In the previous chapter, I made an argument that an unintended consequence of medical education may be to produce insensibility in students, those in power (such as consultant surgeon educators) failing to distribute capital of sensibility appropriately and fairly among the (even if temporarily) 'poor' and 'disenfranchised' ('scum of the earth') – students, patients and healthcare colleagues such as nurses. The fragment by Wilfred Owen that heads this chapter is from a poem that discusses whether or not insensibility is something that soldiers have to cultivate to tolerate the horrors of battle, drawn from the poet's own experience as a soldier in the First World War (Owen 1994). The poet too recognizes that long-term insensibility, or 'shell shock', is a product of war. Owen equates insensibility with insensitivity – soldiers also making themselves immune to 'pity'. But, while doctors, too, in a sense see combat and also suffer a kind of shell shock in 'burn-out', how will they relate authentically to the suffering of patients if they harden to an insensibility and a lack of pity?

Weston, like Owen, puts her finger on the problem – Mr Hanforth shows 'democracy' in his 'approach'. But this decency, a moment of politeness and civility, does not add up to what we might understand by 'empathy', moving well beyond mere politeness and sympathy ('feeling for', rather than empathy's feeling 'with'). Weston's heroine, a senior medical student, unable to remove stitches from a patient without causing pain and distress, asks for Mr Hanforth's help. He simply approaches the task as a functional one and with no apparent feeling for the patient brusquely pulls the clips and stitches out in the face of the patient's evident pain and distress: 'When he was finished, Mr Hanforth grabbed some swabs and blotted them over the bleeding, sob-trembling woman and nodded to me as if to say, you can take it from here, at least? Surely? And he was off' (Weston 2013: 61). This 'cruel to be kind' act, easily read as sadistic, seems to be drained of empathy, even of sympathy, or it shows a perverse kind of sympathy.

Weston's heroine, now a junior doctor at the front line, is faced with the task of manually evacuating the bowels of a patient with learning difficulties and it is here that she has an epiphany concerning empathy or deep humanity for patients, something that had, perversely, been missing during her undergraduate medical education. It is worth telling the story at length:

> I tried to ascertain what was wrong with the man lying in the bed . . . His sheets had been pulled back. . . . His pyjamas had been pulled down, his knees hitched up. . . . I didn't understand why no one was talking to him, explaining what we were doing . . . I squirted jelly on to my own index and middle finger and smoothed it over the rest of my hand. . . . Feeling my hand curl around solid excrement . . . I brought out a mass of faeces into the bowl . . . and I retched, tasting stomach acid in my mouth, only just managing not to vomit. . . . I knew my job was far from done, and was galvanising myself to try again, to detach myself, when my eyes happened upon my patient's bedside table. On it was the hospital phone, the regulation hospital tissues, a maroon flannel in a blue dish. But just behind this I saw something that interested me more. It was an old-fashioned hairbrush, like my granny used to have. . . . Perhaps, had I not been thinking about my granny, I might not have made the connection that my patient was about the same age as my dad. But I did, and I felt sad to see a man of that age with his hands at his face like a child. And the weight in my mind of the hairbrush and the hands and my dead granny and dad was such that I rested my left hand on my patient's back for relief. As I did this, I felt him relax. . . . With five or six passes I managed to clear my patient's rectum. . . . And I looked at that damn wonderful hairbrush and thanked it in my head for making me realise something important that had been beyond me until that time. That it would never work for me to

disengage from my patients ... that no patient of mine would ever again feel that they had been treated like a piece of meat.

(Weston 2013: 70–73)

Here, it is fiction that does the work for the reader of educating for empathy. One cannot help but identify with both the junior doctor heroine and the passive patient, for whom we must feel pity. For Weston, empathy is finally kicked into gear through a subtle and serendipitous combination of factors – identification with close members of one's own family linked to nostalgia for a life fully lived (which this patient in front of me is not realizing). Further, it is the simple act of touch that creates the bridge between doctor and patient ('I felt him relax').

As noted previously, Abraham Verghese (2011) has tirelessly campaigned for retaining the full catalogue of the bedside physical examination for medical students, in the face of apparent obsolescence of auscultation, palpation and percussion techniques as technological imaging and tests have come to displace these manual skills. The primary reason, however, for Verghese's plea is that doctors in training will lose the capacity for confidently touching patients and then being 'touched' by patients in return or feeling for them, where in such mutual touch, empathy is shown and rapport established. This touch is quite different to Mr Hanforth's no-nonsense 'handling' of the patient in which rapport is considered to be an active block to getting the clinical job done. Weston's heroine, through touch, recovers the confidence of her patient as she discovers the depth of feeling she has for him as a person in the epiphany of empathy. Verghese argues that the touch proffered by the medical student or doctor is not simply an instrumental act of connection or the beginning of a diagnostic process of the physical examination, but is a significant ritual in which doctor and patient engage in a pact through which mutual trust is established.

Johanna Shapiro (2008: 9) notes that 'One of the major tasks of medical educators is to help maintain and increase trainee empathy for patients', however 'research suggests that during the course of medical training, empathy in medical students and residents decreases'. This is commonly referred to as 'empathy decline' (Neumann *et al.* 2011) and sits beside 'moral (or ethical) erosion' – the tendency for medical students and junior doctors to become increasingly cynical and to sweep less pressing ethical dilemmas under the carpet, researched by Chris Feudtner, Dimitri Christakis and Nicholas Christakis (1994) over two decades ago. Typically, empathy is measured through self-reports on psychometric scales such as the Jefferson Scale of Physician Empathy (JPE) (Hojat *et al.* 2002a, 2002b, 2002c) and the student version (JPE-S), and the Interpersonal Reactivity Index (IRI). There are reliability issues with such self-reporting and, as discussed in depth below, 'empathy' itself is a contested term with differing definitions, so that such scales also potentially have validity problems as empathy becomes instrumentally defined as that which an empathy scale measures.

Yet we cannot overlook the fact of consistency in reports of medical students' loss of self-reported empathy between the preclinical and clinical years (Hojat *et al.* 2004; Pedersen 2010; Neumann *et al.* 2011, 2012). Further, again on the basis of empathy scales measures, empathy is declining in the general population, where its opposite psychological trait, narcissism, is increasing. Sara Konrath and colleagues (Konrath *et al.* 2010) found that North American college students' self-reported empathy scores showed a significant decline over 30 years, with a steep dip in the decade between 2000 and 2010. Jean Twenge and Keith Campbell (2009), meanwhile, showed that self-reported narcissism showed a significant increase in the same period.

Raymond Mar and colleagues' research on reading habits of Americans over the past decade shows that less than 50 per cent of adults now say that they read for pleasure – a significant drop from previous years and with the most significant drop occurring among the university-level age group (Mar *et al.* 2010). Importantly, Mar found a correlation between reading habits and empathy – adults who read less fiction report themselves to be less empathic than those who read more fiction. This new wave of psychological research on empathy suggests two important things: empathy is not necessarily a personality trait but is sensitive to social context, and reading fiction may educate for empathy. This has obvious ramifications for medical education.

The highly acclaimed American surgeon and writer Richard Selzer describes his own training as a medical student and then a surgeon as brutal and quasi-militaristic, where:

> the brutality was handed down from the chiefs of surgery all the way to the chief resident, the intern, the medical students, and the nurses. We learned to pass on the brutality because it had been done to us and if you quailed or if you showed any kind of fear or sense of having been embarrassed, then you lost points and you were subject to further ridicule. It was a bad way to become a doctor because it was inhumane. You were brutalized emotionally, and sometimes physically, and it still goes on.
>
> (Selzer 2001: 6)

Ben Rich (2006) suggests that the process of medical education itself is not all to blame for empathy decline and moral (or ethical) erosion. Rich suggests that medical students are initially recruited to medical school precisely because they show what in other people's eyes may be pathologies, a condition known as 'premedical syndrome'. Medical education does not redress such symptoms, but exacerbates them. Coombs and Paulson (1990) asked not if medical education was dehumanizing, but if pre-medical education was 'overachieving, excessively competitive, cynical, dehumanized, over-specialized, and narrow'. In other words, the majority of those students who plan to enter medicine are already educated for insensibility and this process is reinforced by pre-clinical undergraduate medical education, where Rich (2006) asks: 'How could any rational person, not to mention an entire profession, ever expect to fashion humane, compassionate, caring physicians in an educational environment characterized by harshness, rigidity, and cynicism?'

However, Rich's observations are already nearly a decade old at the time of writing and a decade is a long time in medical education. The past two decades have seen the rise of 'professionalism', a blanket term referring to students' abilities to learn act in a humane and ethical towards patients and colleagues, and to senior clinical educators' abilities to act sensitively with students, overthrowing the brutalizing regime referred to by both Selzer and Weston above. Professionalism, like empathy, is now subject to varieties of measurement (Stern 2006) despite the fact that professionalism too is a contested term.

Strip back the many guises of empathy and, suggests Johanna Shapiro (2008: 10), you will find a 'true empathy', but this cannot be readily accessed because of the prevailing dominant discourse in medicine. The dominant epistemological paradigm in medicine refuses imperfections in oneself as a doctor and in treatments as these are increasingly refined through biomedical research. The Other is not just the patient, but the other of sickness and identification with this infirmed other runs against the grain of idealistic Western values of health, wellbeing and mastery (heroic individualism). This idealistic position is patently unrealistic yet it persists in the face of medicine's uncertainties and failures such as its patient safety record.

The structures of medicine do not facilitate a relationship with empathic care but rather, suggests Shapiro, medical students 'stumble' towards such a relationship against the grain. Paradoxically, the very values that shape medical practice as a scientific pursuit aiming to eradicate illness are also the values that undermine a moral medicine, producing doctors who objectify patients, where 'controllability and safety' overshadow empathy. In other words, there is a misplaced focus upon disease and its eradication as medicine refuses the abject. Paradoxically, empathy may be easier to show for those who are in recovery from medicine's magic bullets than for those who are suffering without a diagnosis or cure in sight.

As the quote from Gabriel Weston above shows, empathy and disgust sit side by side. It was only at the point of retching in disgust that Weston had her epiphany about what it is to care for patients and not objectify them or treat them like 'meat'. Shapiro suggests that medical students, in the face of the suffering of patients, fear losing control, of being swamped by their patients' conditions. Attempts at empathy merely serve to feed the students' fears of losing their own equilibrium. In short, students may insulate themselves against contamination by patients through emotional distancing.

However, where the biomedical paradigm frustrates the development of empathy, Shapiro suggests that a narrative paradigm may educate for 'true' empathy but the narrative of restitution and recovery must not dominate. Can students then develop empathy without feeling at risk themselves? Drawing on the work of David Morris, Johanna Shapiro (2008) suggests that students need to be educated about an 'ethics of imperfection', which

> requires role models who express vulnerability, share mistakes, incorporate not-knowing; who are aware of and transparent about their emotional reactions to patients and about working the edge between intimacy and detachment; and most importantly who acknowledge common bonds of humanity with their patients.

Jane Macnaughton (2009: 1940) is sceptical about the whole business of empathy, warning generally of 'the way in which medicine can hijack complex ideas, confining and defining them in its own terms, and changing their meaning and impact'. Specifically, she warns of the appropriation of the term 'empathy'. In previous chapters, I have already suggested that medicine has confined and defined the arts and humanities in such a way that their meaning and impact has been changed, indeed their *pharmakon* or 'healing poison' has been drawn out and rendered benign.

Macnaughton is sceptical not only of measurement of empathy but also of the value and possibility of emotional identification (the most common definition of empathy) in doctor–patient encounters. She allows that empathy may be possibly physically (I can relate to a pain or a feeling of numbness), but asks whether it is really possible psychologically. As we have seen from Gabriel Weston's work above, literature provides a means of empathizing with another's condition – but this is short-lived, claims Macnaughton. Once the novel is left, it does not necessarily leave a lingering emotional connection as a flesh and blood person might. Actually, the image of that man having his faeces manually removed and the touching moment of the connection with the bedside hairbrush described so graphically by Gabriel Weston have remained with me as powerfully as any live relationship.

But Macnaughton makes an important point about empathy being short-lived. Even when we empathize with patients, ten minutes later we can be joking with colleagues about a different matter entirely and the patient contact has already dissolved. Macnaughton, like Shapiro, talks of 'true empathy' and suggests that this is not possible in a doctor-patient relationship because the bonds are professional, generally short-term (with the exception of general practice and psychiatry) and not deeply intimate. The best that can be achieved is sympathy: 'feeling for not with the patient' and 'a need to respond'. Further, 'It is potentially dangerous and certainly unrealistic to suggest that we can really feel what someone else is feeling', because 'we cannot gain direct access to what is going on in our patient's head' (Macnaughton 2009: 1940), unlike the kind of access that is provided through characterization in literature.

Macnaughton's critique concludes with: 'A doctor who responds to a patient's distress with 'I understand how you feel' is likely, therefore, to be both resented by the patient and self-deceiving' (*ibid.*: 1941). These are strong words and it is easy to critique Macnaughton's view if we focus on her choice of descriptors for empathy – that we cannot know what is going on in a patient's 'head' or '*understand* how you feel'. This suggests that empathy is cognitive rather than affective, where we might want to know instead what is in the patient's heart. Macnaughton does, however, refer to feelings, or an affective dimension to empathy, but does not distinguish between the two or suggest how they might interact.

This interaction is taken for granted by most psychologically oriented workers in the field of empathy, yet the major self-report scales for measurement of empathy in medicine (the JPE and JPE-S, mentioned earlier) state emphatically that empathy is 'a cognitive (as opposed to affective) attribute that involves an understanding of the inner experiences and perspectives of the patient, combined with a capability to communicate this understanding to the patient', where the 'affective domain is seen as a key component of sympathy, rather than empathy' (Hojat *et al.* 2002a: 58). For the authors of this scale, the key element in empathy is cognitive 'understanding' and not affective identification. This conceptualization of empathy is worrying, primarily because the majority of claims for 'empathy decline' among medical students are based on longitudinal scores on self-reporting scales such as the Jefferson Student version. Yet if these scale items are focused upon empathy as cognitive understanding, are we getting any closer to appreciating empathy as affective identification in the way that Weston describes her heroine's epiphany above?

We should then approach outcome studies utilizing empathy scales with caution. For example, Neumann and colleagues (2012) report 23 outcome studies showing that empathic practice produces clinical benefits, including one study that showed how the exercise of empathy by general practitioners is a reliable predictor of the duration and severity of symptoms of the common cold, related to immune system changes in immune cytokine IL-8 (Rakel *et al.* 2009). Other associations are less specific yet meaningful, such as increased patient compliance, diagnostic accuracy and reduction in symptoms of depression. Across these studies a variety of empathy measures are used. For example, Rakel and colleagues' study used an empathy scale especially constructed for the general practice consultation, the Consultation and Relational Empathy (CARE) measure developed across Glasgow and Edinburgh Universities (www.caremeasure.org). This is a less robust measure than the Jefferson scales, but easier to administer and containing a mixture of items based on a conceptualization of empathy as having both cognitive and affective dimensions. Psychologists have been in general agreement for some time that empathy is multidimensional and should include both affective and cognitive as well as behavioural components (Feighny *et al.* 1998).

Empathy, then, is complex. We expect 'compassion' and 'empathy' to be at the heart of why we introduce the medical humanities into medicine – to humanize practice – but we are unclear as to what these terms describe. In the remainder of this chapter – written in collaboration with a senior consultant histopathologist and medical educator, Dr Robert Marshall, who first studied classics at Oxford before embarking on a career in medicine – we will unpack 'empathy'. Robert Marshall was a key figure in introducing the medical humanities into postgraduate medical education at the Postgraduate Medical Education Department at the Royal Cornwall Hospitals Trust, Truro, UK, in 1998; and as core and integrated provision in the medicine curriculum at the newly inaugurated Peninsula Medical School in 2002, and remains a champion of the medical humanities in both undergraduate and postgraduate medical education. As we have already indicated a strong link between empathy and reading literature, what better way to interrogate the problematic term 'empathy' than to return to the root ground of Western literature in Homer?

The death of Hector: pity in Homer, empathy in medical education

For many, if one word captures what the medical humanities are all about it would probably be 'empathy'. Yet this word, as we have seen, also signifies for many precisely why the medical humanities are problematic. It is a modern, ill-defined word yet surely we must admit that it points to something important in practitioner–patient and practitioner–practitioner relationships. 'Empathy' is then a weasel word in the medical humanities. It is used as if it had a commonly understood meaning or transparency. In fact, empathy is a contested term in disciplines such as psychology, where it has its modern origins. Empathy seems to carry authority, but this is false or hollow. It creates an impression of certainty but actually carries a good deal of ambiguity.

'Weasel word' is used to refer to something that is tricky or shifty. The origin of the term is sometimes attributed to Shakespeare, who describes weasels sucking eggs dry in both *As You Like It* and *Henry V* – biologically incorrect, but a good metaphor for a hollow word or phrase. Empathy can be seen as a 'black box' – we know the input and we know the output, but we are guessing what happens in between. In the remainder of this chapter, 'empathy' is critically interrogated from within the humanities themselves, by drawing on Homer's account of 'pity' in the *Iliad*. While 'pity' has taken on new connotations in the English language, Homer's original use, in context, seems to us to better capture the combination of mind and heart that characterizes the ability to temporarily stand in another's shoes. Empathy must surely be both affective and cognitive, but is there a better, deeper term? Both Shapiro and Macnaughton above claim a 'pure' empathy. What might this be?

Communication: skill, or style for life?

Where medical students' learning of communication has been reduced to performance of atomized, instrumental skills (competencies), the complexity of real clinical encounters is lost (Marshall and Bleakley 2008). Such encounters are contextually sensitive and ethical acts. Educationally, they could be grounded more in reflection on life experiences than feedback from actor patients in simulated settings. Communication skills are usually considered a-historically and as transparent and unproblematic activities. A 'return to Homer' – as a rich background against which to interrogate contemporary versions of interpersonal communication as part of a doctor's 'professionalism' – offers an alternative.

Consider the adaptability in communication that, for example, a community-based practitioner must develop: in multicultural settings, with children, with the elderly and confused, and with persons across a spectrum of disabilities, including mental health issues. This same doctor will also engage with the 'autonomous patient' (Coulter 2002) who properly rejects paternalism, with patients' advocates including family members, and with the savvy, internet-informed patient. How shall we best prepare medical students for such intense and contrasting work of relationship? It is important that we do this well, as there is a growing body of evidence demonstrating that quality of relationship between doctor and patient does have an effect on health outcomes beyond, simply, patient satisfaction (Roter and Hall 2006).

While communication skills are included in learning outcomes (General Medical Council 2007) across the spectrum of medicine curricula globally and are at the heart of recommendations concerning good medical practice (General Medical Council 2006), just how to best teach such skills is debated. There is an emerging trend towards use of 'safe' simulated settings with both actor patients and expert patients, involving videotaped encounters and direct feedback in custom-built clinical skills laboratories or communication suites. Proponents argue that this offers both 'standardization' of experience and possibility of standardized assessment (Klamen and Williams 2006).

Assessment is usually through a station of an objective structured clinical examination (OSCE). In such undergraduate assessment contexts, typically a set of skills, such as 'shows empathy', 'maintains eye contact', and 'communicates information clearly and precisely', are atomized as 'competencies', serve as learning outcomes, and offer assessment criteria. This instrumental approach is now seamless with postgraduate education. For example, the UK General Medical Council's *The New Doctor* (2007: 86) specifically lists competencies to be achieved for a Foundation (Junior) doctor to progress to registration, including demonstrating 'empathy and the ability to form constructive therapeutic relationships with patients'. Empathy trips off the tongue as readily as 'patient' or 'illness', remaining unexamined as a patient itself showing symptoms of confusion.

'Empathy', then, is a problematic term. As Veloski and Hojat (2006: 119–20) warn, 'the theoretical investigation of physician empathy has been hampered by ambiguity in its conceptualization and definition', where 'there is no agreed-upon definition of the term'. Worse, empathy may be an operational term for a psychological state that 'may not even exist'. In other words, empathy could be treated as a metaphor. Indeed, the key contemporary text on empathy in medicine, *Empathy and the Practice of Medicine: Beyond Pills and the Scalpel* (Spiro *et al.* 1993) is, paradoxically, replete with authors' uses of metaphors to describe empathy in a collection that is otherwise characterized by the desire to represent empathy as an empirical phenomenon. Metaphors of transportation, site and resonance are common and commonly occur together, describing placing oneself in the lived experience of the patient's illness and entering the perceptual world of the other, as cognitive events of understanding and insight, rather than compassion. In a book-length empathic treatment of 'sympathy', Lauren Wispé (1991) discloses the core metaphor for empathy as that of travel, or crossing over. This raises questions concerning the motives for that travel, from anthropological study, to the morbid curiosity of the tourist, to the desire for conquest and control of the imperialist or colonist.

Such (in our view, necessary) conceptual ambiguity places us in the same position as the circular operational definitions of ambiguous psychological notions such as 'intelligence' – that 'intelligence is what intelligence tests measure'. Empathy may be what empathy scales measure, or is a *construct*, a useful heuristic, rather than a tangible state of being. Yet we undeniably feel and reflect in the presence of suffering and here, we argue that a better descriptor for this duality of feeling and reflection is 'pity' as described by Homer. Substituting pity for empathy is not merely a semantic sleight of hand.

The dictionary definitions of 'empathy' and 'pity' reinforce our argument that empathy is a modern, operational term, grounded in technical–rational thinking, where pity is an ancient term grounded in aesthetics. *The Shorter Oxford English Dictionary* defines empathy as 'The power of projecting one's personality into, and so fully understanding, the object of contemplation.' In contrast, pity is defined as 'A feeling of tenderness aroused by the suffering or misfortune of another, and prompting a desire for its relief.' The first definition implies mastery, the second, a contemplation and appropriate action, importantly qualified by the descriptor 'tenderness'. This is a more feminine response of *discrimination* – hence our claim that this is grounded in the aesthetic, rather than the instrumental. Does this second definition, of pity, not chime well with the description that Gabriel Weston gives of her heroine's epiphany?

You would think that the dictionary definition of pity is hard to beat, but the word has been corrupted in modern usage, as a kind of sneering. The novelist Graham Greene (1993: 218) starkly captures this view: 'Pity is cruel. Pity destroys. Love isn't safe when pity's prowling round.' And Michael LaCombe (1993: 60), writing to a junior colleague, recommends using pity to pervert empathy: 'permit them to see their patients as simpering fools, helpless wrecks of humanity with whom they could never identify. Let this pity grow, spread like a cancer within them, and you need not worry.' Such an understanding of pity is idiosyncratic. It requires a distancing from the object and a feeling of superiority that, we suspect, most would not think was implicit in the term. We have indeed tipped over into instrumental empathy. Definitions matter. Or perhaps this is a matter of understanding and experience rather than definition.

The roots of empathy and compassion appear superficially similar: -pathy and -passion derive from words to do with suffering (one Greek, the other Latin). Their difference lies in their prefixes – suffering 'in' ('em-') or 'with' ('com-'). In fact, the Latin word *patior*, from which 'passion' derives, had a meaning largely confined to suffering or tolerating unpleasant experiences, whereas *pathos* was a much more neutral word meaning experiences both good and bad. *Chambers Dictionary* subconsciously reflects this ambiguity by translating the '-pathy' of empathy as 'feeling' and of sympathy as 'suffering'. The word sympathy existed in classical Greek times with a meaning very similar to today's, while empathy had different meanings, either a physical affliction (in Galen for example), or to mean a state of emotional engagement (the opposite of apathy). 'Pity' derives from the same word as 'piety', the Latin *pietas*. In Old and Middle English, the two senses were intermingled, only separating in the sixteenth century, when both words took on negative meanings – as a kind of knowing superiority.

Paradoxically, when empathy entered modernist thinking, it was wholly grounded in aesthetics, but has since lost this foothold. Although Jodi Halpern (2001) finds echoes of the term in Hippocrates, it is a twentieth-century invention, formally coined by the German psychologist Titchener in 1909 as a translation of the German *einfühlung* – literally meaning 'aesthetic sympathy'. Indeed, Titchener's description only provides further ambiguity, where he says of empathizing with another's expressions or qualities, such as pride, that he 'feels them in the mind's muscle' (in Wispé 1991: 78). The metaphor is again one of movement, of crossing over, of a paradoxical 'at-a-distance' proprioception, but now we are in the body of the mind, an unfamiliar territory for contemporary cognitive models of empathy.

The German philosopher Theodore Lipps (1851–1914), who had a formative influence on Freud's model of the unconscious, used *einfühlung* as early as 1903, originally in the field of aesthetics, to describe a process of the observer 'entering into' a work of art and it is only later that such language was used by him to describe entering into the mind of a person. Importantly, in these early formulations, the passions are clearly engaged and this differs greatly from contemporary definitions of empathy as the cognitive or knowing partner to affective 'compassion'. Our conclusion is that there is not only conceptual confusion concerning 'empathy', but that the modern word carries an inherent paucity.

Communication, virtue, virtuosity

'Communication' is now widely regarded within medical education as a component of medical 'professionalism', a learned set of skills and attitudes exhibited in performance, and open to objective measurement or assessment (Stern 2006). Communication includes not only doctor-patient interactions, but also working with colleagues (usually in team settings), educating students and communicating generally with the public. Policy documents typically prescribe how doctors should behave and communicate as professionals and list the virtues that inform these behaviours. For example, the UK General Medical Council's regularly updated *Good Medical Practice* (2006: 27) includes 'probity' (being honest and trustworthy) among its recommendations, suggesting that 'probity' and 'acting with integrity' are 'at the heart of medical professionalism'.

We should begin, then, as did the ancient Greeks, with such virtues. We follow the well-trodden path that there is a direct link between ancient Greek and current Western thinking (Fredrick 2002). Discussions of virtue thread through Plato, particularly *Meno*, *Protagoras*, *Republic* and *Laws*. *Meno*, a dialogue between Socrates and a young aristocrat (Meno), opens with Meno's question to Socrates: 'is virtue something that can be taught? Or does it come by practice? Or is it neither teaching nor practice that gives it to a man but natural aptitude or something else?' (Plato 1956: 115). Socrates' rhetorical strategy is to not answer the question, but to direct attention to the key prior question: what is virtue? In answer to this, Socrates says: 'The fact is that far from knowing whether it can be taught, I have no idea what virtue itself is.'

Over 2,400 years later, Louise Arnold and David Stern (Arnold and Stern 2006: 19–21) graphically model medical 'professionalism' as a classical Greek temple, where the supporting base (as three steps) is composed of 'clinical competence' (knowledge of medicine), 'communication skills' and 'ethical and legal understanding'. The roof is 'professionalism' and the pillars supporting the roof are four virtues: 'excellence', 'humanism', 'accountability' and 'altruism'. The authors explicitly equate professionalism with 'virtue'. 'Excellence', currently a buzzword in medical education policy documents, is characterized by 'a commitment to exceed ordinary standards'. Here, a return to classical Greece will help us to further define 'excellence' and also sharpen our understanding of 'virtue'. This, in turn, will lead to a better understanding, and appreciation, of 'empathy'.

In describing the relationship between rhetoric and athletics in ancient Greece, Debra Hawhee (2004: 17) describes a tradition of naming specific virtues, such as courage, but also of describing an overall 'virtuosity' (*aretē*). Hawhee describes Greek athletic competition as a form of 'rhetorical practice and pedagogy' in which competitors persuaded, or won over, the audience through their bodily prowess or virtuosity. In early Greek athletics, winners were judged by their ability to enter the field of play (*agōn*) as a warrior enters the battle, showing the virtues of courage, honourable engagement and physical prowess. However, as athletic contests matured, virtuosity was judged as excellent where it explicitly avoided moralizing, or piety. This subtle shift framed virtuosity as a highly focused or concentrated activity combining physical prowess (skill) with wisdom of the body (*mētis*) that is best translated as 'adaptability' and an art of timing or exploiting opportunity (*kairos*). This combination goes well beyond mere competence, turning sport into performance art. In the field of play that is the *agōn* of communication in medical practice, excellence might better be termed virtuosity, where virtuosity is a combination of skill (in reading, and responding to, cues), adaptability and the art of timing.

Let us explore this a little further with emphasis upon empathy. While technical virtuosity – for example as surgeon, diagnostician, psychiatrist – is easy to grasp, how might we frame virtuosity in the non-technical realms, such as communication and its subset of empathy? Arnold and Stern (2006: 21) describe empathy as a subset of 'humanism' along with respect, compassion, honour and integrity. Further, these virtues must be enacted (or performed) for them to have any meaning and this enactment is embodied in communication that is clinically informed and ethical. These authors distinguish empathy from compassion, where empathy is defined as a cognitive 'ability to understand another person's perspectives, inner experiences, and feelings without intensive emotional involvement' plus 'the capacity to communicate that understanding' (*ibid*.: 23–4). Compassion, in contrast, refers to the affective dimension of being 'moved by the suffering or distress of another and by the desire to relieve it'. As we shall see, when Homer describes what we might now call the skilful employment of empathy, he uses the term 'pity' that artfully collapses the modern technical (and arbitrary) distinction between cognitive and affective components.

Our shift from the virtue of the communicator to virtuosity in communication serves an important function – it links us back to classical thought in two senses. First, in Homeric Greek language (and then thinking) there is no equivalent of a modern sense of personal agency as intention (Padel 1992). Medical students come with the modernist cultural baggage of 'introspection', 'autonomy' and 'self-regulation' – descriptors that again would have had no meaning in Homeric Greek. The modern term 'empathy' implies something that comes from within oneself and is projected onto another, as the dictionary definition suggests. In Homeric Greek, there is no 'I' who is 'empathic'. Rather, pity is embodied in an action, or is a verb. Ruth Padel (1992, 1995), discussing images of suffering in ancient Greek literature, does what medical educators now encourage – she shows that a value or a virtue can only be understood in terms of a performance. It is not what the medical student thinks that matters, but how she acts.

In classical Greek, many verbs of thinking and emotion take a middle voice, for example 'to feel fear' – *phobeomai* – is neither active nor passive. Ruth Padel (1995: 23) suggests that the 'middle voice' verb in Homer is 'very close to passive, what is done to you by an outside agent'. Not 'I am disappointed', but 'disappointment is upon me' and this is known in the form of the resultant activity – disappointment as performance. If empathy, recast as pity, is considered as a verb rather than a personality trait, this unhooks us from 'character training' in medicine and undue reliance upon role modelling. Rather, we are now interested in how medical students act with patients. Returning to Homer makes us think of 'patient centredness' as a verb.

Second, while we have warned against cultivation of personality type in favour of consistently observable activities of patient centredness, a return to classical thought also helps us to reframe the virtuous personality in terms of identity. Let us return to the conceptual model of professionalism proposed by Arnold and Stern (2006: 22). As described above, a supporting pillar, or virtue, central to professional behaviour is humanism, which includes empathy and compassion. Humanism is defined as 'a sincere concern for and interest in humanity', without which, how could doctors treat a variety of patients with concern? We will not pursue here the difficulties presented by that weasel word 'sincere', connected as it is with probity or honesty. Rather, we are interested in the implications of 'humanism' and its relationship to identity.

Empathy has been both literalized and canonized particularly by Carl Rogers (2004) in the fields of humanistic psychology and person-centred psychotherapy. Rogers's holy trinity of therapeutic skills – empathy, congruence (genuineness or probity) and unconditional positive regard – has been drummed in to aspiring counsellors for half a century, with little critical attention. I (A.B.) recall that early in my psychotherapeutic training, I attended weekend-long 'empathy' workshops run by Rogers and his daughter Natalie. These focused on skills of attentive listening, discriminating between empathy, under-played empathy or sympathy ('would a cup of tea help?') and over-played empathy, identification or compathy ('you know, I had the same thing happen to me a couple of years ago, and...'). 'Compathy' is a neologism of the person-centred school. The end product of such training can be a caricature of the 'engaged professional' sitting attentively, nodding deliberately and reflecting ('tell me more...'). A symptom of this approach is the index in Roter and Hall (2006) – the primary text detailing research evidence on how doctors and patients communicate – having six entries for 'nodding', but none for 'pity'! (There are 13 for 'empathy').

Now, as long as humanistic 'person-centredness' is neither pious nor the exercise of political correctness, surely it offers a model for patient-centredness? Well, there are varieties of humanism and one can be humane without subscribing to modern humanism. Person-centredness readily aligns with narcissism – so characteristic of our age of celebrity status – that is a symptom to be cured and not a mode of curing. It is a short step from the inappropriate role modelling of celebrities, whether associated with eating disorders, body image, or being in recovery from multiple addictions, to the general health choices of impressionable adolescents. Cultivating the self is not necessarily a positive health choice. Further, putting the human at the centre of life can be said to have created an ecological crisis. We have become extraordinarily sensitive to our inner psychological states, yet wholly insensitive to the quality of our environment (Hillman and Ventura 1993).

In an effort to provide an alternative to the humanistic tradition's way of thinking about 'selfhood' and identity, Michel Foucault (2005) made a close study of late Greek and early Roman texts that describe a 'care of the self'. These texts do not address a core self that must then realize its potential (the view of Carl Rogers), but show how an ethical self can be developed, constructed, or produced. In the same way that athletes can attain virtuosity through practice and artful engagement, so persons can shape themselves aesthetically, or 'form' character. Such a background provides a new reading of medical education – not just as a technical training, but rather as an aesthetic self-forming, to shape a professional identity. Hawhee (2004: 93) equates this process with *phusiopoiesis*. First described by the pre-Socratic philosopher Democritus, *phusiopoiesis* is the '*creation* of a person's nature' (our emphasis) grounded in poetics or aesthetics, not in instrumental 'skill'.

Jerome Groopman (2007), David Stern (2006) and Shipra Ginsburg and Lorelei Lingard (2006) offer comment on professionalism that critiques the current technical–rational discourse constructing notions of 'empathy', while none of these authors mention *phusiopoiesis*, refer to Foucault's ground-breaking work on classical accounts of care of the self or engage with the topic historically. A seasoned American physician and practised communicator (a staff writer at *The New Yorker*), Jerome Groopman (2007: 17) suggests that how a doctor thinks (clinical reasoning and diagnosis) 'can first be discerned by how he speaks and how he listens'. Communication and diagnostic acumen are closely related – better doctors discover from the patient through close attention and build up a therapeutic relationship. It is still surprising to remind ourselves of the often-quoted statistic that doctors, on average, interrupt their patients 'within eighteen seconds of when they begin telling their story'. Less surprising perhaps, but still disconcerting, is the tendency for doctors to ask closed, rather than open, questions in the consultation.

Such remarks could be taken directly from one of the primers on self-fashioning that Foucault interrogates. Foucault (2005: 98–9) discusses texts by Philo of Alexandria (20 BCE–50 CE) and Epictetus (*c*.55–135 CE) that suggest those interested in care of the soul, as well as care of the body, could form a 'clinic' where you learn collectively how to do philosophy. We can readily translate this into contemporary medical education where aspiring doctors learn both how to treat the body and how to set up the circumstances that will offer a healing or therapeutic *relationship* with patients. Importantly, at the same time, the medical student is doing work on identity, or forming a style of life.

In Foucault's reading, Epictetus provides far more sophisticated advice on speaking and listening than most contemporary texts on the medical encounter (Foucault 2005: 339–40). For example, Epictetus warns about being captivated by the speaker and then not listening-through to what is underneath the surface talk. This recognizes that talk is acting rhetorically and certain persuasive elements must be challenged. Listening is also charged rhetorically. We can listen in various ways – hearing what we want to hear (rhetorical listening), missing the point (not listening well), or listening well (offering benefit both to speaker and listener), including knowing when to be silent. Speaking and listening are not instrumental but an art, requiring discrimination and diligent practice.

This links us to Stern's (2006: 7) suggestion that communicating well can be seen in terms of 'connoisseurship' (a term borrowed from the educationalist Elliot Eisner), as 'the ability to make fine-grained discriminations among complex and subtle qualities;' and to Ginsburg and Lingard's (2006) warning that communication within professionalism is not about what is a 'right' approach but what is *appropriate for context*. Again, judgement, or discrimination, an aesthetic quality, precedes the functional aspect of communicating. Ginsburg and Lingard switch emphasis from the teaching and learning of communication skills, or a body of knowledge concerning professionalism, to what people actually do in practice, emphasizing prior appreciation of rhetoric (how communication is used deliberately or unconsciously to persuade) and reflection (how do I justify my actions in retrospect, and how will this prepare me for future activity?). The latter resonates with Stern's (2006: 7) suggestion that, while connoisseurship is the 'input' for professional relationship with patients, there must be an output and this is 'critique', or 'public report' – a reflexive form of educational assessment and accountability. This leads us to suggest that structured reflection on real clinical encounters is a better way of learning communication than artificial (simulated) encounters in the skills laboratory or communication suite.

Finally, to reinforce our point about the difficulties of modern humanism's association with personalism and the cult of the individual, Fred Hafferty (2006: 294–6) notes that 'altruism' is a term that seems to be disappearing as the new lexicon of 'professionalism' takes hold. This also returns us to virtues closely associated with pity. Altruism is the opposite of egoism. Modern empathy does not require altruism – indeed, psychological introspection as a basis to cognitive empathy would seem to resist altruism by definition. However, pity and altruism are bedfellows.

Pity in Homer

Homer's use of 'pity' in the *Iliad* offers a striking reminder of the value of critically reviewing the status of words such as 'empathy' that have become part of the unexamined fabric of communication skills teaching. We examine scenes in the *Iliad* that elicit pity in the characters and the audience, offering a mix of the entirely familiar (a soldier saying farewell to his wife and child) and the bizarre (another soldier-hero fighting a river); of gentleness and savagery; of the homely and the foreign. Attempting to project our selves into the mindset of Homer's audience broadens our understanding of how words and actions are intimately linked. Again, it also reminds us that meanings are contingent on the age and peoples that form them.

At the end of Book 6 of the *Iliad*, there occurs a famous scene in which Andromache, the wife of Hector, pleads with him to stay within the city walls and not take the attack to the enemy (all translations are by Robert Marshall):

> Hector smiled, looking at his son in silence.
> But Andromache stood beside him, her tears flowing.
> She put her hand in his and called him and spoke to him.
> 'My lord, your passion will destroy you, and you take no pity
> On our little child, nor me, ill-fated, your widow
> Soon to be.'
>
> (Homer, *Iliad*, Book 6, lines 404–9)

And then at the end of this long speech:

> Hector, indeed you are father to me and dear mother
> And brother and strong husband.
> Come now, take pity and stay here on the rampart
> That you may not leave your child an orphan and your wife a widow.
>
> (*Ibid.*, lines 429–32)

Hector replies that he would feel shame to avoid the fighting and goes on:

> For I know this well in my mind and in my heart,
> That the day will come when holy Ilium (Troy) will perish,
> And Priam, and the people of Priam of the strong ash spear.
> But it is not so much the pain of the Trojans yet to come
> That troubles me, nor Hecuba herself, nor Priam the king,
> Nor of my brothers, who shall drop in the dust,
> Many and valorous, under the hands of men who hate them,
> As the thought of you, when some bronze-armoured Achaean
> Takes you off in tears, robbing your days of freedom...
> But may a mound of earth cover my dead body before I

Hear your cries and know they drag you captive.

(Ibid., lines 447–65)

This is followed by an iconic scene loved by the ancients where Hector stretches out his arms to his son but the baby shrinks away from him, scared by the horse's hair plume on his helmet. Hector laughs and removes his helmet, takes his son and invokes:

> Zeus, and you other immortals, may this boy, my son,
> Be as I am, pre-eminent in war among the Trojans,
> Great in strength, as I am, and rule over Troy with strength;
> And some day may they say: 'This man is better by far than his father'
> *(Ibid.,* lines 466–79)

He hands the child back to his mother, who takes him 'weeping and smiling at once'. (Now there is a good case study for building a therapeutic relationship – how would you feel towards the mother?) Her husband, 'noticing this, took pity on her' and says: 'no man will kill him unless it is fated, but no man may avoid his fate'. And then, in very simple language:

> So saying, glorious Hector took his plumed helmet;
> And his beloved wife returned home
> Turning often to look back [εντροπαλιζομενη].
> *(Ibid.,* lines 482–96)

'εντροπαλιζομενη' is an unusual word, otherwise used only of one warrior being pursued by another. And that ends the scene between them. She will not see her husband alive again, although this episode occurs early in the *Iliad.* We, the audience, know that. We are already familiar with the story and that is the point. Experienced doctors make good clinical judgements with relative ease because they access stored 'scripts' from previous, similar, encounters. This principle stands for communication exchanges also. But 'scripts' are also at hand in literature and perhaps the most common argument for the value of studying literature for practising medicine is that stories prepare you for patients' plots and characters; and genres, such as tragedy, offer archetypal 'scripts' (Kleinman 1988). Exposed to such scripts as the parting of Hector and Andromache, pity is, as it were, hard-wired.

The arc of tragedy

Homer's audience, indeed any later Greek or Roman audience, would have known the Troy story intimately; known therefore that it is scripted that Hector will die at the hands of Achilles and that Troy will fall. For them, and for us, knowing that Hector's words accurately foretell the fate of Andromache and that the baby will be hurled from the walls of Troy deepens the poignancy of the scene above. Such foreknowledge by the audience is characteristic of Greek tragedy (of which Homer was regarded as the father). Generally speaking, we prefer not to know how things will turn out. The pity of the ancient audience is greater because they know what will happen to Hector and his family – the arc of the tragedy. It is a feeling familiar to those caring for patients – the pity for someone of whose fate we have an understanding broader than, or certainly different from, theirs, given by the work doctors do. Entering the mind of the other, which we take to be an essential characteristic of empathy, is precisely excluded by the above definition of 'pity' because the other, the patient, does not always know his or her fate and this is complicated by the fact that the doctor knows the potential arc of the course of an illness that the patient suffers.

Hector's foreboding of the fall of Troy is correct. But Homer's *Iliad* ends before the fall of Troy, with Hector's death. He is killed by Achilles in revenge for Hector's slaying of Patroclus, the beloved friend of Achilles. Achilles defiles the body by dragging it around the walls of Troy and denying it burial. The climactic ending is the secret visit of Priam, the Trojan king, to the Greek camp to beg for the return of his son's body for burial. He starts by reminding Achilles of Achilles' own father, Peleus, and comparing Peleus' fate with his, Priam's, own:

> Reverence the gods, Achilles, and take pity on me
> Remembering your father, yet I am still more pitiful.
> I have endured what no man else on earth has endured before.
> I have brought to my lips the hand of the man who killed my son.
> (Homer, *Iliad*, Book 24, lines 486–506)

The Greek word *eleos*, used in this dialogue, can mean both 'pity' and 'mercy'. *Kyrie eleison* means 'Lord, have mercy on us', but also 'Lord, pity us'. In examining how wars are memorialized, Tatum (2004) hesitates between the uses of pity or compassion to describe the feeling of Achilles for the old man. He appeals to 'modern usage' to draw a distinction between the two words that we suspect does not exist for most contemporaries.

Since the death of Patroclus, Achilles has behaved like a savage, slaughtering the enemy in vast numbers even when they are disarmed and beg for mercy; he has sacrificed Trojan princes at the funeral pyre of Patroclus. Since his quarrel with Agamemnon at the beginning of the *Iliad*, Achilles' refusal to take part in the war has been morally suspect. With his later actions, he moved beyond the pale of acceptable morality. The above scene with Priam restores his humanity. He takes Priam by the hand and, knowing that his own death will come soon, tells Priam that suffering is the lot of man, that Zeus keeps two jars at his feet, evils in one and blessings in the other, which he distributes randomly to humans. In this speech, says Macleod (1985), 'there is endurance and sadness, but no bitterness, no railing or cringing'. And, 'This is also the fullest and deepest expression in words of Achilles' pity for the suppliant; for pity, as Homer and the Greeks represent it, is a shared human weakness. And it is pity which is at the heart of Homer's conception of poetry'. The body is restored and receives burial.

Such was the spirit of compassion infusing this last book of the *Iliad* that some late commentators argued it could not belong to the original version. One powerful argument for its integrity is the apparently unconnected scene between Hector and Andromache described above. It contrasts Hector, a man with a wife and child, the main defender of his city, who undertakes a task to which he feels ethically bound, with the solitary, selfish Achilles, driven only by wrath and a desire for revenge (Macleod 1985; Schein 1984).

There are also deliberate echoes in this scene that take us back to the very beginning of the *Iliad*, when Agamemnon harshly rebuffs the pleas of another father, and initiates events that lead to the deaths of Patroclus and Hector. The epic turns a great circle until a quarrel that started in Book 1 with a suppliant to a king, is resolved with a king who is now the suppliant. Both protagonists at the beginning (Agamemnon and Chryses) will survive the war; those at the end (Achilles and Priam) will die. Achilles is a better man than Agamemnon because he can regain his humanity and do what is right. The body is restored to Priam, who takes it back to Troy for cremation and burial. The pity of the audience is elicited for a final time by the lamentations of the three women most important to Hector during life – his wife Andomache, his mother Hecuba and Helen. It is striking that almost the last words of the epic are left to Helen. In a sense, she had nothing to do with him (as relative, wife or lover), but she is ultimately responsible for his death, because she left her husband to elope with Paris and brought the Greeks in pursuit to Troy. Hector and Priam are the only two of the city's inhabitants who have treated her with kindness and without reproach since she left her home. It leaves the epic on a note of ambiguity. We are left looking backwards and forwards to the wrongs done in the past and the many deaths to come in the future. Helen, the cause of the war, is one of the few to survive it.

Conclusions: empathy ancient and modern

Through a 'return to Homer' we have problematized the modern notion of 'empathy', a pervasive term in medical communication. By questioning what we see as a false division between the cognitive act of empathy and the affective state of compassion and by recovering a more poignant, ancient use of the now abused (and sometimes abusive) term 'pity', we have attempted to show how the Classics can enrich contemporary medicine as one face of the medical humanities. Indeed, at Peninsula Medical School we have developed a special study unit for fourth-year students entitled 'Homer and Communication in Medicine'.

Further, we have hinted at how knowledge of an epic story such as the *Iliad*, from the point of view of its tragic content, may provide a 'script' that prepares us for a deeper appreciation of the suffering of patients. The latter is an axiom of the literature and medicine school. In problematizing 'empathy' we have necessarily demanded complexity and ambiguity in an era where many medical educationists concerned with 'professionalism' have demanded simplification, clarity, instrumentalism, empiricism and measure. We have called for a return of empathy to its aesthetic ground as a challenge to the reductionist approaches characterized by instrumentalism, where empathy can be read metaphorically rather than literally. Finally, we have argued for a reading of empathy as a verb rather than a noun, so that empathy is context-specific, as act or performance, rather than personality condition. However, doctors who distinguish themselves through the quality of their communication and 'fellow feeling' may be seen as cultivating a style of life or work, as an aesthetic self-forming, a shaping of identity. If medicine is a kind of performance art then it is better nourished by the deeper structure of pity than the surface operations of empathy. Scripts are also better learned in the real field of play (the *agōn*) than in rehearsal in the artificial communication suite.

'Empathy' returned to an aesthetic ground in 'pity' does, and should, defy definition. However, socialized within an empirical, scientific tradition, most medical students, educators and researchers prefer clear concepts and well-defined boundaries. They will rejoice at the work of Hojat and colleagues (Hojat *et al.* 2002a, 2002b, 2002c) in utilizing a scale to measure empathy, discussed earlier, which assumes that one first knows what is being measured. This reflects a modern mindset that tells us we understand by anatomizing, rationalizing and articulating. It is an instrumental mindset that may, paradoxically, be the opposite of the empathic mindset that it both examines and teaches.

Examination of the *Iliad*, a foundation stone of Western thought, reassures us with scenes like those recounted above, with which we can identify easily. Yet we should learn from Homer that such identification is facile. For example, it is commonly assumed that women are more 'empathic' than men, and Hojat and colleagues confirm this as a significant difference in scores between male and female medical students (Hojat *et al.* 2002c). Yet Homer elaborates his view of pity and compassion largely through male characters. It can be argued that the sharp contrast between their heroic aggression and savageness and their familial tenderness makes the quality of pity more subtle, evanescent and complex. We have already argued that listeners to Homer's stories in the oral tradition may have been sensitized to pity, as the story unfolds in a characteristic manner. Yet Hojat and colleagues (2004), in a further chapter in their extensive research programme on empathy in medicine, suggest that medical students are desensitized, or lose empathy, as they move through medical school (yet see more patients). This is often explained as a necessary development of defence against the sheer volume of distressing circumstances that the doctor will meet. But previous chapters have outlined a more sophisticated model based on the production of insensibility in students as politics and aesthetics intersect in medical education. But these studies by Hojat and colleagues come with a health warning – the data are based on measurement of 'empathy' – again, an 'object' that may be constructed by its measurement.

If we take the core of the meaning of empathy as engaging with, and understanding, the feelings and mind of another, it may seem unsurprising that there was no word to describe this over two millennia ago. More importantly, the notion of cognitively entering the mind of another would have been incomprehensible to ancient Greece – at least for humans (Padel 1992, 1995). The Gods, or natural forces, may do this through dreams and do so in the *Iliad*. We should pay more attention to the metaphors we use in describing empathy. What do we mean by 'entering' the mind of another, or 'resonating with' it? We automatically locate the mind within the brain. Where Homer located it would have depended on what precisely was being described. Thoughts were located in the lungs (*phrenes*), the diaphragm (*thumos*), or the liver (*thymos*) and did not arise there but entered these organs as responses to events (Padel 1992); consciousness was more nebulous – an airy substance located in blood or breath. Emotions were more complex still, located in the chest, heart, liver, or breath (Onians 1988). But is this any cruder or more primitive than locating 'mind' in brain, especially in an age of 'distributed cognition'? The complexities of language, of course, will subvert such locations through metaphor – recall Titchener's embodiment of mind in locating empathy in the 'mind's muscle' – a way of saying that we are *moved* by things.

Recall the two events recounted earlier – the sacrifice of the princes and throwing Hector's baby son from the walls of Troy (the latter episode not in the *Iliad* but known to the audience and haunting the scene with Andromache described above). The *Iliad* is full of savagery – the killing of enemies by painful and grotesque means; boasting over the corpse; refusing to spare the life of a helpless foe. It is a small step to label those who do savage deeds as 'savages', or 'primitives'. Yet our own killing is savage, but done by others, usually at a distance, usually unseen. In the film *Troy*, Hollywood rewrites classical mythology to avoid unpleasantness and sweeten a pill too bitter for modern audiences. In the scene between Hector and Andromache, Hector shows her a secret way out of Troy and at the end of the film we see her and the baby escaping. Hollywood does not want to know about its heroines led off to concubinage and babies hurled from city walls. Yet such events still happen. Even if empathy could be taught, would it be fair to our students? Would not classes in narcissism and self-interest be of greater benefit? There has been no evolution, no progress in our moral sensitivity. That is why the stories of Greece and Rome resonate with us and can inform our ethical practice, while pity, sympathy, empathy and compassion have been examined formally in medical education for only half a century (Wilmer 1968).

5   Towards a medical aesthetics

Creativity and imagination in medical education

Weasel words

In the previous chapter, I problematized the weasel word 'empathy'; in this chapter, I do the same for 'creativity'. An air of optimism accompanied the early introduction of the medical humanities into medical education, as we saw from Chapters 2 and 3, but along with this came a certain naivety (much easier to see retrospectively of course!). For example, many applauded the potential of the medical humanities to introduce 'creativity' into medical education where 'creativity' was automatically linked with the arts. This ignored the fact that the arts can also be bland and inoffensive, or creative but highly offensive such as the arts in the service of totalitarian, masculinist politics – for example, F.T. Marinetti's fascist Futurism (Marinetti 1909). Marinetti applauded the energy and vitality of modernism and its fascination with sleek machinery such as the sports car, but through metaphors in which the frail, weak, dislocated or disabled were mocked, displaying the basest aspects of the fascist mentality – arrogance and superiority. Worse, Adolf's Hitler's pictures offer a good example of a fascist who also produced bland and inoffensive paintings (actually offensive because they are so bland!). Further, the descriptor 'creative' is bandied about without critical reflection on its various meanings. Indeed, as a weasel word, creativity conceals more than it reveals and rolls so readily off the tongue. So, let us take a more critical look at 'creativity' in the context of the introduction of the medical humanities into medical education.

Think improvisation!

Andrei Aleinikov (1989) coined the term 'creative pedagogy' to distinguish education concerned with creativity from education concerned with critical thinking. Aleinikov was concerned that critique can fall short of action, where a creative pedagogy in any disciplinary field seeks the indelible mark of recognizable innovation or invention. Such creative pedagogy has yet to bleed in to medical and healthcare education. This does not mean that there are not innovations in clinical education but there is, as yet, no organized subdiscipline that deals with 'creative clinical education'. Indeed, there appears to be no desire to struggle conceptually with the term 'creativity' that is treated as unproblematic, as if we were discussing the 'larynx' or a 'Mediterranean diet'.

Formal discussion of creativity in medical education is only two decades old. Handfield-Jones and colleagues (Handfield-Jones *et al.* 1993: 3) signalled the importance of creativity in medical education, but offered no discussion or conceptualization of 'creativity' itself, offering rather a catalogue of 'innovative techniques in clinical teaching' that is now depressingly familiar: 'experiential learning, role-playing, competition and games, stimulus materials, brainstorming and sub-grouping'. Pedagogy generally has come a long way in the decades since this article, refining its critical and conceptual approaches considerably. For example, 'experiential' learning was poorly defined in Handfield-Jones and colleagues' article – now we might conceptualize experiential learning as three differing states: learning *through* experience or doing (what Handfield-Jones and others offered as a limited view of experiential learning), learning *from* experience (reflection on action and reflexivity or values relativization), and learning *to* experience. It is learning to experience that is the focus of this chapter – how do we expand our horizons in real time to engage and realize creative endeavour?

Medical Education's (2002) special edition on the arts and humanities, including Shee Lippell's (Lippell 2002) 'Creativity and medical education' does not get us any closer to what is meant by 'creativity' either, where the term is used more as a mantra – an invocation rather than an explanation. A special 'Medicine and Creativity' issue of *The Lancet* (2006) offered some absorbing accounts of creativity in practice, such as what the arts can offer medicine. However, as the editorial suggested, the issue declined to define 'creativity' per se, but resorted to a proxy definition in terms of the 'diversity of contributions' to the special issue, again leaving the thorny issue of defining 'creativity' untouched.

Ness (2011: 1201) describes 'A pilot program to teach innovative thinking to health science students at the University of Texas', but this instrumentalizes 'creativity', turning problem stating into problem solving, neatly avoiding the issue of defining what it is that, in Ness's word, you are 'training' (can creativity be 'trained'; are 'creativity training programs' possible?). Salmon and Young (2011: 217) certainly do not think that 'training' is an adequate descriptor for learning communication skills in medicine and call for a more creative way of framing 'communication'. First, they suggest, communication is bigger than a 'skill'. Communication skills might be creatively reframed as 'skilled communication', where 'communication is inherently creative' and 'communication needs to be taught and evaluated holistically'. The authors suggest that: 'For communication teaching to be pedagogically and clinically valid in supporting the inherent creativity of clinical communication, it will need to draw from education theory and practice that have been developed in explicitly creative disciplines'. All very well, but this still leaves 'creativity' as ill defined.

Niamh Kelly (2012: 1476) draws on Ken Robinson's TED lecture (Robinson 2006), where Robinson argues that schools-based education produces good workers rather than creative thinkers. Kelly suggests that this also applies to medical education. She defines creativity in medicine as the engagement of the human imagination, where 'Medical education is... instituting programmatic changes that incorporate the sensibilities of the arts and humanities into medical school curricula.' Well, this is a big assumption and perhaps more wish fulfilment than reality, much as I value its optimism. What is missing from Kelly's enthusiastic support of creativity in medical education through the media of the medical humanities is critical engagement with the descriptors 'creativity' and 'imagination'.

Creativity, says Kelly, has 'hallmark features of imaginative thinking linked with the spirit of inquiry' and 'allows us to be in touch with *ourselves*' (Kelly 2012: 1476). I am not quite sure what she means by this, but I am comfortable with the sentiment. Her suggestion is that we should openly discuss with each other, both within medicine and medical education communities, what creative endeavours are currently gripping us. Such 'water cooler' and 'coffee room' conversations may 'serve to answer the question what would make creativity part of the medical vernacular, become commonplace – the rule rather than the exception?'

Danielle Ofri is a physician and author of perhaps the best book written on the relationship between medical practice and emotional states – *What Doctors Feel* (Ofri 2013). Ofri writes that creativity is stifled at medical school, where 'rote recitation inhibits the ability to think beyond diagnostic straightjackets' so that:

> Medical school can seem like an ongoing exercise of committing lists to memory, the only creativity being the mnemonics for memorizing branches of the facial nerve or diseases with anion-gap metabolic acidosis. When students present cases, there is a sense of roteness. A patient with chest pain, for example, becomes, 'Rule-out M.I. (myocardial infarction). Get an EKG, serial troponin levels, stress test, cardiology consult...
>
> (Ofri undated)

Ofri then offers a compelling case for thinking creatively from experience of clinical practice:

> I saw four patients with diabetes over the course of a morning. One was a young man whose glucose, weight and early-onset heart disease resist control, despite jogging 10 miles a day and eating like a rabbit. Another was an elderly woman with fragile bones, congestive heart failure and a medication list longer than my arm. A third was a middle-aged man

unable to compromise a single French fry in his diet. And the fourth was a middle-aged woman whose depression snowplows all of her other salutary efforts. Other than insulin dysregulation, these patients have nothing in common. Yet our medical approach is expected to be 'standardized'.

(Ibid.)

The Association of American Medical Colleges (AAMC) has a programme 'Teaching 'Creativity' in a Medical Education Scholars Program', first advertised in 2013 (see www.mededportal.org/icollaborative/resource/728), in which they place 'creativity' in inverted commas, as if it were a problematic or magical term, a black box. The programme promises to 'identify theories in creativity' but the website posts no indications of such theories. Let us stick closely to this term 'creativity' and hunt it down, or, as we shall see, expose its multiple facets, camping for a while in the field of creativity theory.

The general field of pedagogy and the particular discipline of psychology have wrestled with 'creativity' for longer and more intensively than clinical education. Erica McWilliam (2007), asking if 'creativity is teachable?', notes that Richard Greene's review of 552 articles published in 1996–2007 on creativity – mainly based in psychology – reveals 42 distinct models and seven higher-order types of models. McWilliam notes a trend, influenced by efficiency models in education, of unhooking creativity from 'artiness' and 'individual genius' and connecting it with both economic productivity and collaboration, trends that are discussed in more detail below.

Paul Haidet (2007) sniffs creativity in medicine in suggesting that doctors act like jazz musicians during encounters with patients, where collaborative improvisation is a key part of the job. Haidet too is suspicious of the 'creative genius' tag (for too long medicine has been in awe of the heroic individual, the conqueror), but also of the creative as linked to economic capital rather than the art or craft of medical practice per se. Learning from modern jazz improvisation, Haidet suggests that building space into communication with patients, developing a unique professional voice and 'achieving ensemble', or dialogue, are essential parts of both jazz improvisation and medical practice. While protocols derived from evidence are increasingly used to shape practice, this does not prepare you for the unique case – the single patient – presenting the unexpected. Immersion in the patient's experience also means following the patient closely, just as members of jazz groups follow each other's improvised solos, knowing how and when to back that solo and when to kick in with a solo of one's own. Improvised solos build on a basic vocabulary – chord sequences for example – but work around that structure to develop new expressions and meanings. Importantly, Haidet notes that potential improvisation is stifled by strict adherence to protocols.

This returns us to Adolf Hitler, who, upon invading Poland and Czechoslovakia, banned jazz and made jazz musicians play militaristic marching music (Skvorecky 1994). Anybody who knows jazz will appreciate that this is anathema to a jazz musician as you must play on the beat and cannot improvise or bend notes into 'blue notes' (slightly off key or sour). Jazz musicians hate to be tied down by protocols such as playing 'straight' from sheet music unless this is scored from previously improvised solos. Jazz too was associated with blacks, Jews and Gypsies as a corrupt music.

In Oliver Sacks's best-known work – *The Man Who Mistook His Wife for a Hat* – he describes a patient, 'Ray', who suffered from a severe case of Tourette's syndrome, where intermittent and unpredictable tics, grunts and grimaces would be peppered with expletives (Sacks 2011). Ray asked Sacks for help to control the alarming symptoms that were ruling his life. Sacks prescribed Haloperidol (Haldol), an antipsychotic drug. This had a dramatic effect in controlling Ray's symptoms, but a disastrous side effect. Ray was a jazz drummer and on the medication he simply failed to improvise, to play off and around the beat. Like the unintended consequence of medical education – described in Chapter 3 – to produce insensibility rather than sensibility, so Haldol stifled Ray's creative touch. Ray wanted his aesthetic mojo back. Sacks was sensitive enough to see how much the jazz life meant to Ray, so he suggested taking the Haldol on weekdays and ditching it on weekends when he played the most. This offered a smart solution and Ray regained his mojo – his jazz mind and feel – when he most needed it, late into Saturday nights. During weekdays the tics were muzzled and muted.

Medical education must educate for improvisers, who, like Ray, can play around and off the beat, getting underneath it and creating space around it. Yet medical education tends to standardize, in ways that, often inadvertently, produce practitioners who can only play from the song sheet. This kind of education stifles, rather than expands, sensibilities of students. In the language that I use throughout, medical education can anaesthetize or dull the senses rather than aestheticize or sharpen the senses. Again, medical education is then necessarily political as well as aesthetic and ethical, or shapes a political imagination, where the distribution of sensibility is an issue of the exercise of power in the hands of medical education faculty, especially clinical teachers, who in turn can be seen to be muzzled – like Ray's tics, grunts and expletives – by higher powers such as governing Councils and political masters. Clinical teachers do not of course go out of their way to make life dull for their students, but they can easily dull the imaginations of their students through falling into habitual patterns of teaching that do not encourage curiosity and innovation. In this sense, the historical and cultural frames into which they are absorbed already structure clinical teachers.

Where such teaching is institutionalized, within a traditional hierarchical and authority-led framework of medicine, students are not encouraged to exercise sensibility where they are, as novices, equivalent to the poor or underprivileged in a society. They do not have equal rights or access to social capital (until they have been properly socialized and gain legitimate entry into medical culture, with a formed identity). In this sense, students paradoxically occupy the same position as patients, deprived of certain rights in a politically weighted encounter privileging the experienced doctor or clinical educator. In employing the arts and humanities in diluted forms and as handmaidens to medicine in the early blooming of the medical humanities in medical education, so, again, medical dominance and inappropriate medicalizing of patients' experiences were not challenged. The arts interventions remained bland – uncritical and inoffensive, depoliticized and anaesthetized, occupying the same marginalized role as students, patients and 'other' healthcare practitioners on the clinical team. As medicine democratizes, partly as a result of more radical medical humanities interventions, so the arts and humanities can be empowered to play a critical role in medical practice.

A classic tactic of authoritarian structures in societies is to control both the forms of art that can be talked about, educated and publicly shown and the emotional regimes that accompany such art. For example, Soviet State Art after the 1917 Revolution is linked to public regimes of pride and identification. Again, Hitler banned 'degenerate' modern art that questioned and disturbed and replaced it with bland State Art invoking sentimentality and identification with nationalist myths. As noted above, Fascist Italian artists such as Marinetti employed hyper-energetic, masculinist and aggressive imagery tying together humans and machines in a vision that combined futuristic efficiency, masculine desire and ethnic cleansing. Jazz improvisation is a metaphor for breaking down – or democratizing – strict hierarchies (such as musical conventions). A creative medical education will 'think improvisation'.

Towards a medical aesthetics

While we have established medical ethics as an essential part of the curriculum in medical education, medical aesthetics remain peripheral. Yet medical aesthetics may make the difference between the merely competent practitioner and the exquisite practitioner who is a connoisseur of her craft. Medical aesthetics should not be confused with 'aesthetic medicine' that is often used as a descriptor for plastic surgery. Rather, medical aesthetics could be seen as a parallel interdiscipline to accompany medical ethics in the curriculum. Medical practice is (in)famously hard-headed, pragmatic and anti-intellectual and also anti-aesthetic. This sounds like the militaristic marching music discussed earlier, beloved of what 1950s jazz buffs – 'hipsters' – called 'squares'. Can we, as the jazz drummer and Civil Rights activist Max Roach suggested, 'Let Freedom Ring!' in medical education, bringing a hipster mentality? While there are many creative individuals in medicine and surgery, many medical students will eventually work as middle-of-the-road 'jobbing' doctors and not as innovators. But can we at least provide the conditions of possibility, through an inspiring medical education, to allow creativity to flourish, or for doctors to form an 'aesthetic' identity of connoisseurs?

As noted earlier, Michel Foucault (2005) argues that the making of the 'self', or identity construction through social process, such as entry into a community of practice (like medicine) can be conceived as an aesthetic process – one of self-forming or self-making, beyond mere crafting of skills. Aesthetic self-forming of identity is key to educating quality doctors who will make their mark, for here is the specialist who also comes to shape his or her specialty through innovation. And here is the specialist who specializes in creative approaches to relationship with colleagues and patients. In this chapter, the issue of creativity is approached systematically, to reveal a plurality of approaches. Identity construction of doctors through self-forming within specialities (including the speciality of generalism as a general, family or community practitioner) can also be seen as the specialty interest of the medical humanities in medical education, for it is here that forms of creativity are foregrounded as educational aims.

We have seen that medical aesthetics and politics cannot be separated. It is a common mistake across the medical humanities mixed community to imagine that drawing on arts and humanities perspectives in medical education is somehow free from power implications. This was a naïve position adopted by the first wave of those interested in establishing the medical humanities within the medicine curriculum, where the medical humanities were framed as light relief from the heavy constraints of the science-based curriculum, as a diversion or entertainment, or a non-critical 'friend'. Any educational approach that claims to be reflective (thoughtful) and reflexive (consciously critically engaged and able to relativize values that drive perspectives and actions) would move on from such a naïve position and argue for the value of the medical humanities in terms of reflective and reflexive educational practice and critical engagement with political (power) and aesthetic (form) issues. Those interested particularly in the radical and subversive arts (such as political performance art) will argue that 'thinking medicine' is already heavily invested with aesthetics and politics, and must be reflected upon.

Reflecting on 'creativity'

A recent edited collection – *Keeping Reflection Fresh* (Peterkin and Brett-Maclean forthcoming) – reminds us that educational practices such as Donald Schön's (1991) reflection-on-action and reflection-in-action need to be reimagined for each new age of learning such as the current transition into the deep information age geared around social media – lampooned brilliantly in *The Circle* by Dave Eggers (2013).

In 1999, I published an article that critiqued simplistic readings of Schön's model of reflective practice and warned against 'reflective practice' becoming a mantra (Bleakley 1999a), often invoked but rarely authentically practiced. I suggested that Schön's model should be progressed and reconceptualized, and provided a philosophical framework for this task. While reflective practice is now well embedded in health education (Johns 2009) its adoption has been slower in medical education (Mamede and Schmidt 2004), with the paper or electronic portfolio of professional practice as its main assessment medium (Ingrassia 2013). While the notions of reflection-on-action (how good was my consultation? Did I work well with colleagues today? Was that an ethically sound decision?) and reflection-in-action or monitoring practice as you go along (what should I do now? Is my manner too brusque?) are well established, something that I pointed out in my 1999 article and critique was that reflection-*as*-action is undervalued, sometimes not even recognized as an educational necessity. What do I mean by reflection-*as*-action?

Reflection-on-action can be rephrased as learning from experience, or reflecting on what one has done and subsequently adapting. This centrally includes the idea of 'reflexivity' or values relativization (Bleakley forthcoming). In reflecting on what one has done, it is useful to review the values that drive behaviour. This is essential for ethically- and morally-sensitive practice. Reflection-in-action can be rephrased as learning through experience, or doing. Skills learning leading to mastery requires hours of practice, but practice is improved through mindful attention as one practices – this is pedagogic orthodoxy. Reflection-in-action is temporally in the event. Reflection-on-action is temporally after the event. Reflection-as-action, however, temporally precedes the event, or prepares us for the event.

Here, all activity is by definition soaked in potential or possibility and is 'expansive' (Engeström 2008). This kind of activity can be described as learning to experience, or better, learning to re-experience. It accepts that learning is not primarily about reproduction of the known, but production or innovation. This is the process of bringing imagination and creativity to bear on ordinary learning to make it extraordinary – as a process of sensitizing – and it is best achieved through the media of the arts and humanities. This is the work of the medical humanities in medical education, where the arts and humanities are mobilized as media through which learning medicine is tangibly enhanced or made creative. But 'creativity', as I have said above, is a weasel word, concealing more than it reveals. Before simply accepting that we should introduce creativity into medical education through the medical humanities – as core and integrated curriculum provision – we should tease out what 'creativity' may mean. The remainder of this chapter critically interrogates 'creativity'.

Philosophies of lack versus philosophies of abundance

A conventional medical education is characterized by pragmatism and minimalism. Doctors teach students to focus on what works and what can be said succinctly. A by-product of this philosophy is instrumentalism – treating the person as 'patient' and further reducing the patient to 'symptom' and 'case'. A typical case presentation during a ward-based teaching round then consists of highly stylized, succinct presentations by students and junior doctors that are briskly treated by senior doctors as much for their style as for their diagnostic accuracy.

Here (necessarily abbreviated) is how the American College of Physicians suggests that you write up a case report abstract:

> Introduction: ... begin with a short introduction ... Case Description: ... follow the basic rules of medical communication; describe in sequence the history, physical examination, investigative studies, and the patient's progress and outcome. The trick is to be complete without obscuring the essence of the case with irrelevant details. Discussion: ... the best case report abstracts are those that make a small number of teaching points (even just one) in clear and succinct language.
>
> (American College of Physicians undated)

Such practice follows the form of a philosophy of lack rather than abundance, disguised as 'efficiency': be 'short', 'sequence', avoid 'irrelevant details', use 'clear and succinct' language – in other words, bleach out all narrative interests and certainly transform the patient's story into a 'report' or a non-story. This kind of explicitly functional presentation effectively processes the living and breathing human. Again, there is no desire for a tangible story, narrative tension, character or metaphorical content. The sharp end of this process is the drug formulary that gives an instrumental account of the drug and its expected effects and side effects, but in no instance offers a personalized case study. An interesting medical humanities session is to discuss a drug formulary with a class of medical students and contrast this with a series of YouTube video clips of people talking about their relationships to prescription drugs, especially in the field of mental health. Chapter 8 fully expands this point.

The first task of the medical humanities in medical education may be to acknowledge the value of an abundant imagination rather than simply a stripped back, minimalist style of clinical reasoning and communication with patients and colleagues. Medicine (surgery in particular) is famously pragmatic or hard-nosed, where certainty is valued over ambiguity and the patient's complex 'chief concern' is reduced to the doctor's version of the 'chief complaint' in which the patient is in danger of being objectified and reduced to an algorithm. Medicine is, however, driven by uncertainty or ambiguity and simultaneously saturated and riven with metaphor and aphorism (Levine and Bleakley 2012; Bleakley and Marshall 2012b); medicine is further an ur-example of complexity science and art at work (Bleakley and Cleland forthcoming).

Gilles Deleuze and Felix Guattari famously wrote an anti-Freudian (or revisionist Freudian) psychoanalytic text in which they begin with a philosophy of abundance rather than lack (Deleuze and Guattari 2004a, 2004b). While Freud described a world in which an unknown dynamic drives life (the unconscious) and we are forever trying to compensate for what we did not get in childhood, Deleuze and Guattari suggest that life is already abundant, rich and complex. The difficulty for modern people is to both appreciate and not be overwhelmed by this abundance rather than habitually translating this into lack. For Deleuze and Guattari, desire is a product of attempting to manage abundance, where for Freud desire is compensation for lack, for what one does not have or cannot reach. Abundance presents particularly in art through the Baroque and in ornamentation, trajectories that run against the grain of medicine's preferred style of reduction and stripped back minimalism.

I follow Deleuze and Guattari in suggesting that imagination and creativity offer a welcome, given abundance and attempts at reduction are ways of defending against such – admittedly overpowering – abundant fruits. While I 'type' different approaches to creativity below, this is for ease of comprehension and not because I want to translate the nonlinear complex field of creative life into a linear, albeit complicated, model. One kind of creativity is indeed a mechanical imagination where things can be put together in an ordered way, but this does not encompass the entire complex and dynamic field of the 'creative'.

My way into this inquiry is to first critically address the issue of what we mean by 'creativity'. In what sense may a medical education be called imaginative and creative? My aim here is to dismantle the notion that the 'creativity' invoked by the introduction of the medical humanities is somehow necessarily disruptive to scientific and logical thought, an aberration of practice, or an unnecessary adornment to practice that can readily be discarded and will not be missed. Rather, creativity in practices introduced by a medical humanities component or dimension to medicine should be seen as essential and necessary and productive rather than disruptive. Established medical educational practices such as use of problem-based, small group learning methods, the objective structured clinical examination (OSCE) as a form of practice assessment, use of standardized actor-patients in learning communication, learning anatomy without cadaver dissection, and learning a variety of invasive clinical skills in simulated settings were once radical innovations dependent upon creative activity.

The discussion of kinds of creativity below can also act as a helpful road map in accounting for innovations in medical education – their types, sources and aims. How will innovation occur in the future and will the presence of the medical humanities facilitate creative change? I am particularly keen that medical educators use this map consciously to inform curriculum planning and implementation that explicitly seeks transformational knowledge production rather than reproduction.

Constructions of creativity

Creativity is typically described in terms of (i) a product, (ii) a process or (iii) a creative individual (Mooney 1963; Taylor 1998; Lubart 1999). Mark Runco's trilogy of books on creativity challenges this division, introducing the importance of context or environment for creativity, suggesting that the field is now so extensive and diverse that earlier categorizations have been transcended (Runco 1996, 2006, 2011). In considering 'context' we might ask what does 'creativity' mean, for example, in a healthcare environment rather than, say, an engineering environment? Runco notes that studies of creativity have now extended beyond their disciplinary origins in psychology to embrace the cognitive sciences as they interact with cultural studies. However, the framework of product, process and individual, supplemented by context, remains a useful one.

Product approaches

Hennessy and Amabile (1988: 14) claim that 'most creativity researchers rely on a product definition' – something that can be judged as a creative outcome; but product approaches to creativity can be constraining and paradoxically counterproductive. In medical education, the simulation suite is often considered to be one of the most creative products in the last half century – a purpose built space defining an end-product activity. Drawing on the technological innovations of simulators designed for training airline pilots, medical educators in anaesthetics and surgery in particular have developed simulated environments in which both technical and non-technical (communication and teamwork) skills can be rehearsed and learned safely. This may include the use of high-tech manikins such as SimMan for 'crash' scenario training. As such simulations have become increasingly sophisticated, so they have paradoxically begun to cut off from reality where their supporters have become somewhat evangelical about simulation in learning (Bligh and Bleakley 2006). This has introduced an unintended counter-creative element in which learning is sterile as transfer becomes compromised. Where simulation sets out to provide a creative environment for learning, it may then actively work against patient safety by developing a false confidence in learning that resists transfer. This can happen across the domains of doing, thinking, feeling and intuiting.

As the work of Roger Kneebone and colleagues has shown, creativity in learning through simulation is not just centred around product but also process and context, reinforcing Runco's view above that studies of creativity must embrace context (Kneebone and Baillie 2008; Kneebone *et al.* 2010). Kneebone (Rees-Lee and Kneebone in press), for example, shows how surgeons can benefit from working alongside expert tailors to appreciate the process of creative craftwork requiring exquisite hand and eye co-ordination, shifting focus away from creative product. Rees-Lee and

Kneebone (in press) refer to this as expert bespoke tailoring providing a metaphor for surgical practice. Yet tailoring is more than a metaphor for surgical skills – it has obvious concrete parallels with surgical culture in the use of stiches, but also in the complexity of its craft which moves beyond mere competence, as Rees-Lee and Kneebone point out, into a complex interweaving of thinking, doing, feeling and intuiting as a creative process. Further, the apprenticeship of tailoring affords an identity construction through legitimate entry (at first peripheral and then central, as expertise develops) into a community of practice (Lave and Wenger 1991). Gaining an identity through entry into a 'closed' culture such as surgery is a complex and creative process in its own right, especially if this identity is partly formed through constructive active resistance to the norms of that culture – for example as a woman in a traditionally male world (explored particularly well by the surgeon Gabriel Weston in her 2013 novel *Dirty Work*, referred to in Chapter 4).

The potentially sterile learning encountered in the simulation suite can be made fertile and more creative through injection of a dose of reality, requiring process as well as product creative thinking. The process of learning itself is sensitive to context – where learning takes place. Learning to suture a wound in a busy Accident and Emergency environment with a drunk or aggressive patient, a frightened child, or a woman simulating that her bruising and wounds were caused by a fall when she has actually been physically abused by her partner, is clearly quite different from learning in a sterile simulation laboratory. Roger Kneebone and colleagues at Imperial College, University of London, in collaboration with St Mary's Hospital, have developed perhaps the most expressive and creative educational response to the limitations of learning in simulated environments, while not abandoning simulation and its safety features, but rather combining simulation with real clinical environments or perceptually pertinent features of that environment. This work has produced some of the most exciting 'medical humanities' research in postgraduate medical education, combining this with public engagement opportunities (supported by the Wellcome Trust).

For example, through a BBC Radio 3 programme titled *The Scalpel and the Bow* (see www.rcm.ac.uk/cps/bow), Kneebone and the Royal College of Music Professor of Performance Science Aaron Williamson discussed the use of interactive, simulated performance environments in educating both surgeons and musicians to perform under pressure. This includes outward-facing performance including team process and inward-facing aspects such as cognitive abstraction during performance. Collaborations between surgeons and jazz musicians can be productive in reframing what 'improvisation' might mean for a surgeon facing an unexpected situation, where a set of skills have to be reframed drawing on the cognitive and emotional capital of 'resourcefulness' (Kneebone 2013a).

A TEDMEDLive lecture by Kneebone (2013b) describes the use of a relatively cheap simulated environment – a portable, 'blow up' operating theatre – that can be used for medical and surgical education and for public engagement in a variety of ways. Where surgeons, for example, have a narrow field of focus in their work, the portable operating theatre can provide a space in which the table as the primary 'circle of focus' can be simulated with precision, where further circles of focus need only be roughly simulated – such as the peripheries of the operating theatre (for example, using a low-tech model of anaesthetic equipment, but with a 'live' anaesthetist present). High-tech silicone models of internal organs and simulated spilling and squirting blood provide realism as surgeons practice their craft. Conditions can readily be manipulated to provide, for example, an unexpected incident. Further, operating theatre teamwork can be practiced where roles can be swapped or performances varied. Finally, the public can be engaged in being shown how to perform techniques or in role playing members of the operating theatre team – especially good for engaging young minds and imaginations. In short, Kneebone has expanded our notions of what creativity in medical and surgical education can mean, focusing less on product and more on process and context – not simply the 'what?' of learning or outcome, but the 'how?' and importantly, the 'why?'.

Process approaches

Torrance (1988: 43) defines creativity as:

> the process of sensing difficulties, problems, gaps in information, missing elements, something askew; making guesses and formulating hypotheses about these deficiencies; evaluating and testing these guesses and hypotheses; possibly revising and retesting them; and finally communicating the results.

This 'in process' view places greater emphasis upon the dynamic of the creative event than upon its outcome that may be, as suggested above, the communication of the quality of the process rather than the showing of a tangible product.

Creative individual approaches

Torrance (1988: 47) also speculates upon 'what kind of person one must be to engage in the process (of creativity) successfully'. The history of medical education reflects the history of medicine that can be characterized as the valorizing of the heroic individual (Bleakley *et al.* 2011), reflected in medicine's passion for 'strong leadership' often linked to grooming for management roles. For example, greater emphasis is now being placed on grooming leaders as managers within the CanMEDS competencies framework in Canadian medical education. The rhetoric surrounding discussion of leadership roles is striking, almost imperial:

Visionary, change agent, influencer... these are the qualities associated with great leaders. And increasingly, these are the same abilities expected of medical specialists in order to provide high quality patient care in today's health care environment. To help residents and physicians prepare for their role as health care leaders, one of the proposed changes in the CanMEDS 2015 project is to increase the emphasis on leadership competencies in the CanMEDS Framework.

(Royal College of Physicians and Surgeons of Canada 2013)

Standard medical education texts still continue to refer to notions such as the 'adult learner' that are based on a philosophy of autonomy and heroic individualism, gendered male (Kaufman and Mann 2014). While such views are being eclipsed by sociocultural learning theories that stress collaboration (Bleakley 2006a) and small group collaborative learning models such as problem-based learning are now standard, autonomy and competition are still encouraged as standard 'lifelong learning' practices and medical schools persist in awarding a range and series of prizes for 'best students' in various categories. The creative individual is still revered within medical culture and this is reflected in medical education. The cult of the individual is reflected in the predominance of portraits of dead, white males who occupy the walls and halls of many medical school boardrooms, rather than, say, historically remarkable clinical or research teams, or significant women.

When David Irby (1978) wrote in the late 1970s about the attributes of great clinical teachers, you could smell the values of American frontier mentality – the unique, heroic individual fired by the Protestant spirit – rather than the more socialist view that creative endeavour is a result of collaboration and teamwork. Irby – a psychologist and therefore possibly biased towards study of the individual – did not, for example, seek out the attributes of great teaching teams (Bleakley 2014: part II). Such reverence for the inspired individual apart from his or her context is still pervasive in medical education and drives a reward culture based on personal achievements such as publication citations. Again, this cult of the personal and personality ignores networks, webs, systems, collaborations and identities based on multiples and social and cultural affiliations rather than character traits.

Conversations between product, process and persons

Barron (1988: 80), who wrote the first *Encyclopaedia Britannica* article on creativity in 1963, suggested that creativity is about bringing 'something new into existence purposefully' and that this 'something new' is 'usually a product resulting from a process initiated by a person', thus bringing us full circle or bringing person, product and process into conversation. Bearing this in mind, we might then in medical education design pedagogies in which process and product are purposefully crafted to be 'creative' and medical educationists themselves are recruited purposefully because they are identified as creative or inspired individuals – this, with the hope of producing creative doctors.

This, however, leaves us with two major obstacles. First, we have yet to decide on what we mean by 'creative'. And second, we have forgotten that 'creativity' does not occur in a vacuum, but within historical, cultural and sociomaterial contexts. How creativity within medicine unfolds can only be appreciated through considering contexts such as the technological. What is possible creatively is necessarily shaped by material contexts that in turn are products of networks of persons, artefacts and ideas. This is readily illustrated by the development of the scalpel where transitions from previously available metals have resulted in lighter, sharper and more durable carbon steel instruments (Bleakley *et al.* 2011).

As indicated above, a more recent interest in creativity research has moved away from characteristics of the creative individual to the potentially enhancing influence of context on sociomaterial process. While the establishment of creative learning environments is a central concern of higher education (Bleakley 2014: ch. 16), a prior question concerns the legitimation issue – why is one kind of environment considered 'creative' and another not? Lubart (1999: 339) again draws our attention to context, where 'creativity does not happen in a vacuum. When we examine a creative person, creative product, or creative process, we often ignore the environmental milieu'. Csikszentmihalyi (1999) notes the importance of context in terms of a legitimating audience – who, for example, in medical education decides what shall be a creative intervention? Increasingly, this is assigned to learners rather than teachers. The notion of legitimation raises another, fundamental question: to what extent is creativity socially constructed, where the methods by which creativity is delineated, defined and measured come to construct the object of their inquiry (Gergen 2001; Bleakley 2003)? For example, the study of creativity has surely been disciplined by modern psychology, where psychology delineates creativity as a primary domain of cognition (Hillman 1972a). The seminal psychological studies of creativity, the edited collections of Sternberg (1988, 1999), assume a constitutive phenomenon or object of inquiry open to psychological investigation and reflection and do not consider that the phenomenon under investigation may be constituted by those same psychological methods of inquiry.

James Hillman (1972a: 42–7) offers a fifth approach to creativity beyond process, product, personality and enriching environment – that of a phenomenology and typology of plural 'creativities'. Hillman describes six notions of creativity: differentiation, novelty, ferment, instrumental problem solving, eminence and renewal, considered to be 'archetypal' or universal forms. I suggest that such typologies are neither stable nor universal but subject to historical shifts and cultural variations and reconfigurations. However, I follow Hillman in seeing the value of differentiating kinds of creativity within a pluralistic world-view, a view that in its own right can be seen as a model of the creative. Kinds of creativity, as I outline below, may then be seen as a product of cultural discourse that is neither invariant nor pre-existent but in continuous emergence and flux as a complex conversation.

Over half a century of formal research into creativity has not resulted in consensus of opinion, demonstrating that the object of inquiry is unstable. Rather, there is dissension concerning definition, or flat refusal of definition as attempting to capture what is ultimately beyond definition (Bohm 1998). Where definitions of creativity are attempted, these are often expressed as definitive and inevitably reveal unaccounted for exclusions or 'surplus'. For example Sternberg and Lubart (1999: 3) define creativity as 'the ability to produce work that is both novel (original, unexpected) and appropriate (useful, adaptive concerning task restraints)'. The key notions here are 'newness' and 'usefulness' in relation to 'adaptation'. Such definitions construct creativity through exclusion, where what is not creative is useless or impractical. This would exclude most art that is not constrained by utilitarian concerns. Indeed, much art sets out to challenge the notion of utility itself, most famously parodying utility in Marcel Duchamp's showing of everyday objects such as a bottle rack or a urinal in a gallery context. Utilitarian approaches frame creativity as work, excluding activities such as play and daydreaming, the exercise of which may be the very psychological basis upon which a tolerance of ambiguity is developed, a key value complex in patient-centred medicine. Utilitarian theories of creativity may tell us more about the mindset of utilitarians than it does about the objects of their inquiry.

Creativity has been defined as a 'form of intelligence' that can be 'developed and trained like any other mode of thinking' (Gulbenkian Foundation 1982). This, again, tells us a great deal about the developmental and social engineering mindset of the authors, from which point of view a particular model of creativity is developed – one that sounds more like disciplining animals than developing a climate for democratic flowering of passionate ideas and practices. Further, the definition compounds the problem of reification, as creativity enters the minefield of operational, circular definitions – just like 'intelligence', 'creativity' becomes that which a creativity test measures. In contrast, a plurality of discourses concerning creativity acts to produce a variety of objects embodying differing values with equal ontological status, realized through differing educational practices. To further illustrate this historical and cultural contingency of discourses of creativity, we can turn to dictionary definitions (*Shorter Oxford English Dictionary*).

'Creativity' is a neologism, appearing in dictionaries only relatively recently. 'Creative' first appears in the English language in 1678, derived from the Latin *creativus*, referring to 'creation'. Its main synonym in this definition is 'originative'. However, in 1803, at the peak of Enlightenment rationalism and scientific inquiry, 'productive' was also introduced as a main synonym of 'creative'. Where 'productive' takes over from 'originative', we can see an historical and cultural shift in imagination of 'creativity' from creation myths (origination) to human (mainly mechanical) invention as 'productivity'. Put these two value complexes together and we see the backdrop for the definition provided by Sternberg and Lubert (1999) that refers creativity to both origination/innovation (the mindset of 'newness' or point of origin in developmental thinking) and production/labour/usefulness (the mindset of utility and application).

It is the latter that has become a dominant discourse (McWilliam 2007) where the capital of creativity is that which can boost the economy or provide for 'growth'. Creativity capital is then not distributed – according to a pluralistic view of differing kinds of creativity – in a democratic manner: for example encouraging medical students to experiment with different ways of thinking stimulated by a varied, interdisciplinary medical humanities curriculum. Rather, as with sensibility capital discussed in earlier chapters, creativity capital is defined and regulated by the institution of medical culture that in turn is shaped by a political economy that privileges the 'creative' as what is useful and boosts the economy. This closes down the potential democratic sharing of creativity capital in which a plural model of the creative is commonly decided among stakeholders including learners (students), colleagues (health care professionals) and consumers (patients).

The 10 kinds of creativity described below may help in informing different medical education strategies tailored to context. Links between the types of creativity described and teaching, learning and curriculum design are sketched. From the argument presented here, one would be sceptical of 'teaching' creativity, preferring rather to allow various kinds of creativity to emerge as fit for purpose or appropriate for context.

A typology of creativities

1   *Creativity as an ordering process*

As described above, the Latin root of the word 'creative' refers to 'origins', traditionally formulated through a culture's creation myths. Study of such myths may help us to understand how certain discourses concerning creativity come to be privileged. The Old Testament's Book of Genesis offers two competing creation myths – the seven days of creation of the world *ex nihilo* and the Garden of Eden, in which the world is already given as complete. The former describes order out of chaos and the creation of something from nothing. This models a process of creativity that is a progressive forming or differentiation, the operation of a logos principle involving movement from the simple to the complicated and invoking structures, boundaries, method, principles and classifications. This linear unfolding defines a traditional, developmental narrative and describes an analytic approach to diagnostic reasoning (type 2 reasoning) based on protocols such as decision trees. Such a notion of creativity defends against ideas of chaos and disorder and refuses overall pattern and metaphor for linked detail or metonymy. This approach can be stereotyped as masculine, where difference and plurality are absorbed into a governing principle of progress and then ordered hierarchically as taxonomy rather than typology.

Medical education has followed medicine in privileging the complicated over the complex (Bleakley and Cleland forthcoming). The complicated is made up of linear components that fit together like a jigsaw where the whole is the sum of its linked parts. The complex, however, is a dynamic system in which the whole exceeds the sum of the parts and is characterized by non-linearity (Capra and Luisi 2014). The complicated does not invite tolerance of ambiguity as its effects can be solved like an engineering problem. The complex, however, requires high tolerance for ambiguity. Dynamic, complex adaptive systems offer high potential for innovation through transformation, but also exist close to chaos. The medical humanities in medical education can offer a way to educate for tolerance of ambiguity in encouraging nonlinear thinking.

Medical education is currently struggling with how to accommodate holistic thinking in both science and clinical teaching and learning. It is 15 years ago at the time of writing that Pauli and colleagues set out a manifesto for shaping a future medical education through holistic and complexity thinking, arguing that medical science must shift from linear to nonlinear approaches and that medical education must follow (Pauli *et al.* 2000). Medical education has yet to grasp this nettle.

Introducing the medical humanities into medical education has often been a struggle, where the primary point of resistance is from basic and applied scientists – the teachers that medical students have most contact with in the traditional pre-clinical years. As the majority of medical students in graduate entry programmes will have studied a science major such as biology, medical students are socialized into biological science communities of practice before they engage with clinical communities of practice and a 'science' identity is often already established. The introduction of the medical humanities, requiring an appreciation of the forms and methods of the arts, humanities and social sciences, is usually attempted in the face of this already established identity construction and cultural socialization of medical students. There is, however, another route through which the medical humanities can be introduced – this is to explore with students and science faculty the intrinsic beauty and wonder, the aesthetics, of science and science practices in medical settings.

Complexity science, with its interest in pattern, form, emergence, process and transformation is already rich in aesthetic content and offers a powerful route into understanding why the medical humanities are important in medicine (Bleakley 2010; Bleakley and Cleland forthcoming). A starting point is again that science is fundamentally about appreciation, wonder and beauty; and that the scientific method has to be embedded in the possibility of forms of creativity that move beyond the linear, such as inspiration (see 7 below) and serendipity (see 8 below).

However, there is beauty too in logic and linear building, as an ordering process. Once the connection is made between stripped back forms of diagnosis and case presentations and minimalist aesthetic, for example, then a revelation occurs – there is a clear aesthetic to standard medical practices such as case presentations, but without this realization the forms remain sterile. With the realization, the forms can consciously be developed aesthetically as they are in minimalism, focusing on stripping back to bare essences, pure lines and clean forms. However, minimalism must be appreciated as an embedded form of complexity, where simplicity of form is not the same as simplicity of experience.

2   Creativity as rhythm and cycle

While the seven days creation story opens Genesis, it was a myth recorded some 400 years after the Garden of Eden story into which it seamlessly runs in the King James text. The Eden myth may have been recorded around 800 BC (Fokkelman 1987) and offers a different creation story and then a different construction of creativity to the ordering, anti-chaos myth of 'In the beginning God created the heaven and the earth. And the earth was without form, and void'. In the Eden myth, there is no creation of something out of nothing, but rather a tending of an already given whole, a 'garden' that is then open to appreciation and wonder prior to explanation. Such tending implies following a cycle, a rhythm, stressing timing, patience, opportunity and renewal that is stereotypically 'feminine'. This contrasts with striving onwards and upwards, as in the masculine, linear 'creativity as ordering' process (type 1 above). Further, the revelation of a given pattern illustrates type 1 diagnostic reasoning or pattern recognition, the typical way in which expert doctors reason.

The Garden of Eden myth is one of 'tradition' (creativity as conservation), characteristically opposed to progress. Once the fruit of the Tree of Knowledge of good and evil is eaten, innocence is forever blighted by experience as tradition gives way to progress, symbolized by banishment from Eden. Now we may be able to better appreciate the state of medical education, caught between the conflicting origin myths presented at the beginning of Genesis. On one hand, medical education wishes to develop beyond the constraints of its parent culture of positivist medicine through the introduction of the more radical thinking from contemporary pedagogies brought largely by educationists, social scientists and arts and humanities scholars – such as curriculum reconceptualization, postmodernisms, feminisms, queer theory, cultural studies, literary criticism, reflexivity, phenomenology, constructionist research approaches, Marxist-inspired sociomaterial learning theories and so forth. On the other hand, medical education is still grounded firmly in the conventions and traditions of positivist medicine, received with the bitter mother's milk of a tough-minded medical apprenticeship guided initially by anatomists and then by hardened, sometimes cynical, clinicians deep in the grooves of local cultural habits and resistant to change or innovation.

But this state of affairs is also, to pick up the critical theme running throughout this book, an issue related to the distribution of sensibility. In the Garden of Eden, sensibility capital is owned by a transcendent Being and withheld from Adam and Eve who remain innocent or unreflective about their condition of nakedness and pure existence – offering a kind of unexamined slavery. This is anathema to modern educationists, where learners should be offered the conditions for outgrowing their teachers. The parallel in medical education is the worst kind of master–apprenticeship relationship, in which resistance or dissensus is discouraged and experts hold sensibility and sensitivity capital. In the seven days of creation myth, a developmental process unfolds in which conditions are set up for humans to take control of their own destiny – or, sensibility capital is rapidly distributed, as its uses are formally educated (having been handed the keys to the car, do not expect a chauffeur to drive you around).

The serpent that tempts Eve to bite on the apple of the Tree of Knowledge is surely knowledge or wisdom itself allowing us to break out of the confines of habit, or turn learning from a state of innocence (a traditional, unquestioning apprenticeship) into learning from experience (questioning, questing and innovation). Returning to tradition and breaking the mould are two sides of the same coin of medical education each with its own creative possibilities and perhaps best termed, paradoxically, a 'radical traditionalism'. For some, however, tradition is an anchor that has become a hindrance, where the ship never leaves the harbour. Educational adventurers in contrast always have an eye on the horizon.

3   Creativity as originality and spontaneity

This type of creativity offers an idealized view of the child as 'naturally' creative and assumes that this condition can be recapitulated in adulthood. Play and spontaneity are seen as essential ingredients of innovation. This view is central to the argument rehearsed in earlier chapters made by the psychoanalyst Donald Winnicott (1971) and echoed by the literary scholar and philosopher Martha Nussbaum (2010) and the writer Mark Slouka (2010) that the humanities are central to educating for empathy. The argument, simply put, is that children go through a stage in which active play and fantasy play are central to learning how to position oneself in relation to others, in a proto-democracy. Where children are deprived of play or play-spaces, such positioning is not learned and those children can fall into habits of trusting hierarchies as forms of safety, developing authoritarian tendencies that are repeated in adulthood. However, a second chance for learning through play is presented in adulthood and this is appreciation of the Other and of difference through humanities such as fiction and drama. Indeed, as already noted, evidence shows that those who regularly read fiction have a more developed sense of democracy (Mar *et al.* 2010).

Arno Kumagai alerted me to recent work by David Comer Kidd and Emanuele Castano (2013: 377) that widens restrictive notions of 'empathy' to a more inclusive 'theory of mind' (ToM). Children must develop a wide-ranging cognitive (understanding the states of mind of others) and affective (tuning in to others' emotional states) sense of what is happening with others in social situations in order to effectively interact. Inability to do so leads to interpersonal deficits. Under controlled experimental conditions, Kidd and Castano show that reading literary fiction 'temporarily enhances' ToM, and the authors suggest 'ToM may be influenced by engagement with works of art'. Importantly, 'literary' fiction is different from pulp fiction, or romances and thrillers, through the use of linguistic tropes that make readers think otherwise, or engage actively rather than passively with the text. Such texts do not primarily entertain but educate through defamiliarization (discussed later at length). In brief, readers have to fill in gaps, invent and elaborate as well as be left, sometimes, puzzled and confused in the face of 'serious' fiction. The parallel in medical education, as discussed in Chapter 7, is the patient's narrative – complex, half-formed, laced with unsettling details, riddled with the 'unsaid' and so forth – that the doctor must 'read'.

Here is what Mark Slouka suggests:

> The case for the humanities is not hard to make, though it can be diffi-cult...not to sound either defensive or naïve. The humanities, done right, are the crucible in which our evolving notions of what it means to be fully human are put to the test; they teach us, incrementally, endlessly, not what to do, but how to be. ... The humanities, in short, are a superb delivery mechanism for what we might call democratic values.
>
> (Slouka 2010: 168)

The humanities too, says Slouka, are 'inescapably, political' because 'they complicate our vision, pull our most cherished notions out by the roots, flay our pieties. Because they grow uncertainty' (*ibid.*). They also educate for 'tolerance'. See how Slouka is caught between our two major creation myths – on the one hand extolling the virtues of moving beyond the confines of our teachers and conventions, but on the other, doing the humanities 'right' – suggesting that there is a tradition, a way, an initiation into the fold.

The physicist and complexity theorist David Bohm (1998: 1) opens his book on creativity with reference to 'originality', but goes on to include another dimension (*ibid.*: 6): 'perception of a new basic order', suggesting that this goes beyond 'childlike' spontaneity (see type 6 below). Bohm describes holistic reordering of form as a creative process that is in nature before it is in humans. It is the spontaneous production of new orders through certain intrinsic organizing principles, a transformational process, where the whole is greater than the sum of its parts. Here, I prefigure type 6 below: creativity as problem stating, where either the creative person intuitively grasps a totality of process, or a context emerges that makes us see the world anew. Bohm's view, while beginning in 'originality', can also be seen to encompass the holistic comprehension that exemplifies creativity as overall pattern, rhythm and cycle, echoing type 2 above. It shifts the idea of creativity from the spontaneity of the child to immanence in nature (type 6 below).

Nickerson (1999: 392–3) reviews a number of definitions of creativity all of which refer to 'novelty' or 'surprise'. However, simply producing some new idea or object is not necessarily creative, as the product may be trivial or harmful, Further, innovations in teaching and learning in medical education may be individually driven and unsupported by colleagues or institutional contexts, producing an unexpected burden for the innovator. Hence, many proponents of the novelty view of creativity, such as Nickerson, will add a rider: creativity must also be useful, appropriate, or have social value, referring us to type 5 below.

In the world of higher education, it has been argued that creativity has no place in the discourse of training for 'competence' (Leigh 1997: 5) that has now infected medical education to the point of obsession, despite thorough critiques (Hodges and Lingard 2012). However, a seminar devoted to that question produced a consensus view that creativity does have a place in an apprenticeship and training culture and offered a working definition: 'the production of something new whether it be totally original or a combination of existing components different from anything tried before in that context' (Leigh 1997: 5). Fennell (1997: 7), in response to Leigh's article, agrees that 'the distinguishing feature of creativity is a degree of "newness"' without replication or reformulation. Returning to creativity as spontaneity, the creative act is then constituted as an optimistic move into the unknown. From the perspective of creativity as an ordering principle (type 1 above), such playful spontaneity is self-indulgent, readily losing its focus in avoidance of application and labour and may then slip from playfulness into irrationality.

4   Creativity as the irrational

It is common in the arts, but uncommon in the sciences, to associate creativity with transgression and impulse, although, for example, Enlightenment science, especially chemistry, is littered with what may be seen from a contemporary perspective as transgressive and unethical, even foolhardy, experimentation (Uglow 2002; Kim 2004). The sciences may be characterized as seeking to reduce uncertainty through cumulative knowledge acquired by controlled experiment, where the arts explicit set out to cultivate ambiguity. The Romantic movement in particular is characterized by an interest in breaking free from order and regulation. From the 'day world' perspective the irrational is seen as dangerous, courting lunacy or destruction. From the 'nightworld' perspective of Romanticism, creativity is necessary experimentation: the suspension of intellect and expression of the instinctive and animal side of life, rejoicing in ferment, the primitive and the raw.

Harnessed as a political force, this is the breaking of an old order in revolution. Its social side is intoxication. Its extreme is annihilation: destruction as a creative act. Orr (2000) notes the novelist J.G. Ballard's contention 'that creativity needs chaos', or what the poet Baudelaire called 'derangement of the senses'. As noted above, the history of chemistry in particular is littered with examples of a paradoxical mix of creativity as an ordering principle (type 1 above) and as experimentation in the realm of the irrational. For example, in 1799, the chemist Humphry Davy (who also aspired to be a publicly recognized poet and shared a temporary but deep friendship with Samuel Taylor Coleridge) rigorously experimented upon himself over a period of three months with inhalation of nitrous oxide or 'laughing gas', meticulously recording the effects.

Davy notes inhalation of up to six to nine quarts from a green silk bag, three of four times a day for a week or more at a time, resting to record any ill effects and then returning to the same intensity of inhalation. Davy also encouraged others to inhale (including the poets Coleridge and Robert Southey and the inventor of the thesaurus, Peter Roget), studying their behaviour while they were intoxicated. Throughout this period Davy wrote poetry and prose, as well as keeping scientific notes based on rigorous observations related to dosage, timing and effects of the intoxicant (Knight 1992). Was this a rational study of the irrational, or a sympathetic study of the senses through derangement of the senses?

5   Creativity as problem solving

This type has affinity with creativity as progress (type 1 above), where creativity must demonstrate productivity. Aligning itself with the Protestant work ethic, creativity as problem solving is 99 per cent perspiration and 1 per cent inspiration. Usefulness, appropriateness, relevance and application are key notions in this discourse of instrumentalism. There is no 'breakthrough' without the sweat of preparation. Proponents of 'inspiration' (type 7 below) will argue that perspiration itself is not creative, but merely preparatory for revelation. However, the literary scholar Jonathan Livingston Lowes has carried out a painstaking case study that argues firmly for 'application' as creative practice in its own right. First published in 1927, Lowes's study of the genesis of Coleridge's poems 'The Rime of the Ancient Mariner' and 'Kubla Khan' demonstrates that the poet's inspiration may have been impossible without the perspiration (Lowes 1978). Lowes painstakingly catalogues, over 400 pages of narrative and a further 200 pages of bibliography and notes, the origins of every important image in these two poems as directed related to Coleridge's own literal or physical experiences, particularly through travel, reading and conversation with friends. This challenges the inspirational mystique of the creative process, shifting it to a more technical transformative process as a rearrangement of the known, that may provide the conditions for a shift in learning, aligning this construction with type 6 below – problem-stating as reordering of form in complex structures.

Lowes (*ibid*.: 391) also draws on a 'recycling' model of creativity (type 2 above) in a discussion of the creative act. He bemoans the convention that privileges 'originality' as a creative, for creative 'is one of those hypnotic words that are prone to cast a spell upon the understanding and dissolve our thinking into a haze'. There is, suggests Lowes, not some transcendent imaginative force at work – a 'shaping spirit' that 'sits aloof' in his own words – but, rather, there may be a simpler 'moulding of old matter into imperishably new forms'. The 'new' is then the recycled but refreshed or reinvigorated old. Imagination and creativity work 'through the exercise, in the main, of normal and intelligible powers'. No need for inhalation of nitrous oxide here as a shift in consciousness. Rather, the creative potential is already there in what we know. It is a matter of refining and redefining the known.

Lowes thus democratizes creativity. It is not the power of the individual genius but a birthright, a 'commonality': 'Creative genius' writes Lowes (*ibid*.: 394) 'works through processes which are common to our kind, but these processes are superlatively enhanced'. Here, Lowes refers to the influence of an enhancing context, or the provision of an educational intervention (Lubart 1999). This argument challenges the primacy of the individual creative genius (Howe 1999) and also focuses upon a creative process that is publicly accessible (Torrance 1988). Creativity then becomes a particular concern of a socially responsible higher education committed to widening access and promoting difference and equality of opportunity.

How, then, does one realize the potential for such enhancement where creativity is within the grasp of each of us? Lowes's own work offers the template. He demonstrates through *The Road to Xanadu* his own model of the 'well' in operation with the 'will'. The 'well' is a dedicated form of gathering and coagulation of life experience, through media such as notebooks. The 'will' is the reordering of this – often chaotic – material, as the exercise of a 'consciously constructive agency' (Lowes 1978: 367) such as expression through a formal genre of essay or visual form. In contemporary medical education, the portfolio, as a medium for reflection and assessment evidencing personal and academic learning and achievement, can be seen to offer a bridge between the 'will' and the 'well'. Productive movement between 'well' and 'will' defines the creative process. The challenge here for translating Lowes's model into a process for learning in medical education is how to offer a range of media for representation of learning that can be transparently and sympathetically assessed and compared for equivalence.

Howe's (1999) extensive study of biographies of publicly recognized creative people, while focusing on person rather than process, product or context, concludes that creativity is largely application. His account is peppered with words and phrases such as 'hard work', 'application', 'practice', 'sustained work', 'diligence', 'perseverance' and 'attentiveness'. From the point of view of creativity as inspiration (type 7 below), the 'application' model returns us to a familiar value complex – that of the Protestant work ethic with its pieties and puritan joylessness that resists or excludes the child-like (type 3 above) and the irrational (type 4 above) as legitimate sources for creative life. Further, where creativity rests in instrumental practices and functional forms, then craftwork is restored to the realm of the creative, challenging the modern separation of arts from crafts that offers genius to the artist but refuses this for the artisan.

6   Creativity as problem stating

Where type 5 above may stress simplicity in functionality, the problem stating construct is based on the creative as complex. Applying Stuart Kauffman's (1995) model of complexity to biology, Brian Goodwin (1995) suggests that biodiversity, as an effect of evolution, may be viewed as a process of maintaining maximum complexity 'this side' of chaos. This metaphor describes one kind of creative moment. Maximum complexity at the edge of chaos characterizes not only weather systems but also improvised solos, baroque ornamentation and a good deal of medicine. Problem solving approaches (type 5 above) are readily aligned with creativity as an ordering principle (type 1 above) where a linear approach pieces together components to arrive at a solution, however complicated. This has often been the basis to problem-based learning approaches in medical education.

However, the reality of much medical practice, in messy and complex situations, is that problem solving cannot be achieved. Ambiguity and uncertainty must be suffered (see Chapter 9) in more open-ended processes of problem stating. It is better perhaps to think of patient-based learning (PBL) methods as PPBL – person- and population-based learning, in which problem-stating under conditions of uncertainty is just as important as problem-solving under conditions of certainty. In learning, as we have seen, Donald Schön (1991) describes the 'swampy lowlands' of practice as more familiar territory than the technical-rational high ground. Creativity here is exercised as expert problem stating, including 'problematizing' or not taking initial and easy formulations for granted but interrogating them critically. Such approaches challenge the model of a spiral curriculum where the simple leads to the more complex. Rather, curricula may be reformulated in William Pinar's (2012) term as 'complicated conversations', that I would recast as a mixture of 'complicated' and 'complex' conversations. Here, teachers do not act as facilitators of learning, as in classic PBL, but as democratically sensitive participants in a conversation, wearing their expertise lightly.

7   Creativity as inspiration

The Romantic view of creativity accepts the value of the irrational (type 4 above), but is also centrally concerned with the artistic vision described as a response to being touched by the Muse (Graves 1961). Here, inspiration is a product of living in imagination, cultivating metaphor rather than literalism. This type of creativity is clearly in conflict with the problem solving type (5 above) that stresses perspiration over inspiration and the developmental view (type 1 above) that privileges progressive forming. Critics of the developmental view point out that Mozart wrote seven symphonies by the age of 10 and 14 symphonies by the age of 15. Mendelssohn produced his greatest music in his youth, while later in life he was far more industrious but had lost his flair. Humphry Davy too showed increasing industry and application in the second half of life but a deep decline in inspiration (Knight 1992).

The primer for the inspiration perspective is the poet Robert Graves's *The White Goddess* (1961) that offers an idiosyncratic historical view of the place of the Muse in poetic life, where the Muse is always female. For Graves, as for William Butler Yeats before him, the Muse is a literal inspirational assistant (or a series of assistants in Graves's case, often lovers). Paradoxically, the woman Muse occupies a secondary, passive 'medium' position to the primary vocal creativity of the man, thus excluding her possible creativity, where the active production of the male poet is what is broadcast and remembered. Homer too invokes the Muse as the opening lines to both the *Iliad* and the *Odyssey*.

8   Creativity as 'making strange' and 'indirection'

The poet Samuel Taylor Coleridge (see type 5 above) applauded the creative spontaneity of the child (see type 3 above) but was aware that adult creativity must move beyond what is 'childish' while continuing to cherish the 'child like'. The psychoanalyst Donald Winnicott also recognized the value of this same approach in calling for an 'adult play' as a mode of creativity, seeing the value of the arts as not only providing such adult play but creating conditions for tolerating and valuing the expressions of others as an education into democracy. In 1817, Coleridge wrote in *Biographia Literaria* that one could 'carry on the feelings of childhood into the powers of manhood', where such feelings could 'combine the child's sense of wonder and novelty with the appearances which every day for perhaps forty years had rendered familiar'. This, suggested Coleridge, 'is the character and privilege of genius' (Coleridge 1956). Rendering the familiar unfamiliar need not however involve dialogue between a child-self and an adult-self. There are many ways in which one can be dislocated creatively through making the familiar strange.

A standard approach to educating for a humane medicine is to focus on educating empathy for patients and colleagues through media such as literature, film and drama. Margaret Edson's play *Wit*, discussed earlier, is a good example of a commonly used piece of conventional drama evoking identification and catharsis. But there are other ways to promote, or provoke, reflection about the 'other'. Given that 'empathy' is a contested notion as we saw in the previous chapter, are there other ways to educate the sensibilities and sensitivities of medical students that challenge the 'empathic route' while still maintaining that identification with the suffering of patients is central to caring medicine? An obvious starting point is to consider what medical students might learn from wholly unfamiliar persons (and situations) they initially consider disgusting, alien, or even abject – out of empathy's reach.

Danielle Ofri tells a story entitled 'The Doctor Can't See You Now', a recollection of an incident from her first placement in the Emergency Department as a first year medical student. At 3 a.m. her bleeper went off for the first time, asking her to attend to a patient. A nurse pointed in the direction of 'a disheveled black woman...clearly homeless, with shaggy, matted hair and dirt encrusted clothing' (Ofri 2013: 8–9). As Ofri approached her, 'a pungent odor enveloped me, the fetid smell of an unwashed body and moldering clothes'. Worse, she spotted a cockroach scurrying about in the folds of the woman's sweater. Feeling that she was about to retch, Ofri backed out, retreating to the safety of the triage desk, where she could only look in pity at the woman and curse herself for not having the courage to do the job that she was asked to do. A nurse's assistant then appeared and helped the woman to her feet, talking to her, holding her close and helping her towards the shower room, where she could clean up. Ofri 'sat hidden behind the desk, awed and humbled' and then 'I sank back into my chair, realizing how much I needed to learn about medicine' (*ibid.*). Something is going on here beyond mechanical 'empathy' to encompass deep concern and justice – identification with wider humanity. No classroom course on 'communication skills', 'professionalism' and 'empathy training' is going to touch this realm. Only experience of the kind Ofri describes will help. But we do need conceptual frameworks to better understand these complex social interactions.

Arno Kumagai and Delese Wear (2014) describe a form of creativity in medical education that shifts us out of the familiar sphere of instrumental, 'lukewarm' compassion and empathy into the less familiar world of Bertolt Brecht's dramatic method as a pedagogical technique. Brecht challenged the traditional notion of drama evoking empathy (identification with characters) to produce drama of ideas, through which the audience would aspire to critical thought and social action. His scripts placed the audience in a zone of deep unfamiliarity, forcing them to see the familiar with fresh eyes, or to make the familiar strange – Brecht's 'alienation effect'. This process has subsequently been pushed to its limits by performance artists such as Bob Flanagan, Stelarc, Ron Athey and Orlan, discussed earlier, whose self-inflicted bodily wounding and morphing demands a thinking otherwise of an audience about what we mean by 'normal', 'health', 'wellbeing' and 'illness'. Like Charlie Chaplin, whom Brecht admired and later befriended, the playwright wanted the audience to see the world through the eyes of the underdog and to learn the disruptive techniques of resistance (Rancière's 'dissensus') that would upset the status quo. Such techniques, as Kumagai and Wear note, can be traced in modernism to the work of the Russian Formalist art critic Viktor Shklovsky, who coined the term 'defamiliarization' in 1917. Defamiliarization can readily be employed in medical education, especially in encouraging students to make their own, original art works, as a means of gaining a range of perspectives on patients (Kumagai 2012).

Kumagai (*ibid.*) describes how, in the Family Centered Experience (FCE) programme at the University of Michigan Medical School, first- and second-year students are matched with volunteers from the community with serious or chronic illness. Patients visit the homes of these volunteers and come to understand the contexts of their lives in relation to their illnesses. Making sense of these experiences can be achieved through 'thinking otherwise', using the media of original art such as painting, sculpture, collage, film and photography, where students represent issues learned through the programme in a process of defamiliarization of habitual ways of thinking and perceiving. This is a process that I have also been involved with at Peninsula Medical School, UK, for over a decade. Here, all 4th year students participate in a longitudinal programme that allows them to integrate experiences with patients through a variety of visual art, music, drama and writing opportunities, facilitated by experts in those fields. Students then present finished work to each other and to a wider audience of clinicians and the public, as with the Michigan initiative. Such work is also formally assessed, using criteria drawn from arts and humanities education.

Kumagai provides a sophisticated conceptual rationale for educating students into thinking otherwise. First, engagement with the media of the arts allows for tacit knowledge to be exercised where students 'know more than they can tell', moving away from the constraints of demonstrating instrumental competencies. Such tacit knowing allows students to tap into their patients' worlds in important ways, providing an alternative metaphor for knowing beyond 'empathy'. Second, is another way of knowing described by the philosopher Hans-Georg Gadamer as a fusion of horizons, a dialectical method. Rather than me adapting to your worldview, or you adapting to mine, we might consider how our horizons can meet to offer a prospective dialogue, to which we both can adapt and that is essentially 'open'. This horizon is necessarily communal and fluid.

Just as Brecht's theatre uses unfamiliar perspectives to unsettle the audience, so Jacques Derrida (1968) coined the term *différance* to describe how language can be used to defamiliarize. *Différance* means both 'to defer' and 'to differ'. Let us take Danielle Ofri's situation described above as a first year medical student faced with a situation in which her emotions (disgust and physical repulsion) were at odds with her moral conscience (I took an oath to study medicine in order to help all people, without discrimination). In recognition of the differing social status between her and the homeless black woman, she differed; and in her act of retreating to the triage desk, she deferred. But the deferral is not necessarily a retreat – rather, as with Ofri, it can act as a sanctuary to afford the sweet and sour moment of recognition of difference that allows for our value system to be suddenly, critically and deeply interrogated: often in a state of shame where things are brought sharply into focus and keenly felt. This, suggests Derrida, is what language does to us all the time, or has the potential to do if we allow language its free play. Our tight value systems can suddenly be split open into many possibilities as we are suspended in a moment of *différance* that offers a potential for defamiliarization and a 'seeing otherwise'. We usually refer to this as a 'dilemma' and of course its chief content is ambiguity or uncertainty.

Although Ofri was serendipitously relieved of her professional duty by the human act of kindness shown by the assistant nurse, it was precisely this moment of modelling by another that shifted Ofri's values from distanced professional concern to close personal concern. Derrida shows that, in the play of language as in the play of social activity, defamiliarization both differs (considering something in different, usually more complex, terms) and defers (alters perceptions).

Derrida (1968) suggests that *différance* is a position in language that resists 'closure' or remains open to possibilities and likens it to the 'middle voice' of Homeric Greek language, discussed in the previous chapter, paradoxically resting between the active and the passive. This voice does not locate 'truth' in either self or other but suggests that there is a third position, constantly deferred, that is a horizon of shared possibilities, a common voice 'to come'. Derrida's later work (Derrida *et al.* 2004) described democracy this way, as a project that is far from complete, preferring the descriptor 'democracy to come' (an horizon of shared possibility and responsibility) rather than a democracy achieved (Bleakley 2014).

In personal correspondence, Arno Kumagai writes that 'making strange' through exposure to a new medium of expression, is 'to have a disruptive influence on perception and taken-for-granted ideas that is ultimately generative of new ways of seeing, new possibilities of being in medicine and in the world'. Kumagai notes that the turn from a descriptive 'first wave' of the medical humanities to an engaged and critical 'second wave' is in itself a reflexive act – a way of making the medical humanities strange to its practitioners and exponents as if they were seeing it for the first time. Certainly such turns in cultures can be alienating for those hankering after the old ways. But such turns usually indicate movement from a handmaiden or supportive role to an actively critical engagement. In the slow progress of social justice, the Western and Northern post-industrial world prides itself on developing equality between men and women (although we might recall that women were not granted the right to vote in Switzerland until 1971, and in Liechtenstein – the richest country in the world, by measure of gross domestic product per capita – in 1984), on children's rights and on racial and ethnic tolerance, yet medicine is – relatively – historically fresh to ideas of gender equality, patient inclusion, collaborative interprofessional team-work and widening access to a medical education.

Kumagai (2012) critically notes where many medical humanities initia-tives fall short. Such initiatives are usually described as taking medical students beyond self-centredness and personal reflection into activity that encompasses the 'horizon' of the 'other'. This is the usual project of 'empa-thy'. However, this can be taken further. As indicated above, drawing on the philosopher Gadamer's work, Kumagai notes that accommodating the hori-zon of the self to the horizon of the other can still lead to subordination of one view to another, inviting a third position that is a 'fusion of horizons'. Art, suggests Kumagai (2013), offers a key horizon, where 'thinking other-wise' is invited as we transcend our individual or institutional, limited, horizons. Agitated reflection ensues that can move us out of our restricted views to a place of discomfort and sublimity described by Martin Heidegger as the 'mystery of being'. This place can be imagined as the 'common well' that is the deep transformative potential for all humans but normally having restricted access through social injustices. Such injustices, in turn, can be framed as the poor handling of humanity's 'common wealth' such as sensi-bility capital, dictated by various structures of power.

In the following chapter, I note Catherine Belling's (2011) concern that encouraging medical students and doctors to be reflective about patients in the affective domain – raising feelings – is complex, because what a doctor feels is also tied up with what she 'should' feel in exercising professionalism. In using 'indirection' – by focusing upon works of art as a medium, or 'third thing' after the practitioner and her patient, through which feelings can be reflected upon – Belling points out that more authentic reflection may ensue. Arts media provide, in Kumagai's sense, a third place or fusing of horizons, where reflection is not so 'full frontal' or direct but can be indirect or subtle, yet experience and consequent action are mediated profoundly. Use of more sophisticated techniques such as indirection point of course to expertise, indeed connoisseurship, in pedagogy within medical education and remind us that faculty development remains a sticking point in creative initiatives in medical education involving the medical humanities.

At Peninsula Medical School and in other contexts, indirection has been used as a teaching device for both students and faculty through what we have called 'art ward rounds'. Here, an expert (practicing artist, critic, art historian) takes a group of clinically oriented people (students, clinicians) to a new clinic – that of the art gallery or museum, where the 'patients' are the art exhibits. Instead of analysing the lives and personalities of the artists who made the work, the 'art round' diagnoses cultural dis-ease through symptoms shown in the art works themselves, returning to Nietzsche's view of artists as 'diagnosticians of culture'. For example, in a recent 'art round' with medical students, an early David Hockney painting showed clear reference to his homosexuality and the necessarily furtive means by which he contacted other gay men for sex. Hockney painted several pictures during the early 1960s with this theme, when homosexuality was still underground and outlawed formally in Britain. The students were encouraged to discuss how this painting diagnosed an illness in society – that of intolerance towards same-sex attraction, affection and love and then how such societal prejudice, as an illness, could be treated. Recall that Hockney was painting under extreme prejudicial conditions in which homosexuality was considered by the establishment as an illness to be cured.

9   Creativity as serendipity

'Serendipity' entered the English language in 1754, after Walpole's *The Three Princes of Serendip*, who 'were always making discoveries, by accidents and sagacity, of things they were not in quest of' ('Serendip' was the former name of Sri Lanka). Serendipity as creativity could be seen as a subset of type 7 above, where fortunate chance seems to arise more often (or is noticed) where there is 'preparedness' – openness to imaginative possibility. Synchronicities, planned fortune, fortuitous accidents and fruitful detours seem to develop against a backdrop of tolerance of ambiguity and acceptance of the possibility of inspiration arriving out of the blue. The fifth of William Empson's prototypical 'seven types of ambiguity' used to effect in literature – discussed at length in Chapter 9 – is 'a fortunate confusion, as when the author is discovering his idea in the act of writing' (Empson 1991: vi).

While trial and error can be forced into an ordering process (type 1 above) it can also amble along a crooked and then forking path, or loop back on itself, to stumble across the unexpected. Dan Noel (1986) has investigated Walpole's coining of the term and suggests that he was punning on 'serenity' and 'dip' (seren-dip-ity). The active process of creation in serendipity may be literally to dip into a text in a calm fashion and see what comes up, by chance. This is quite different from both frantic search and pedantic research. Many will have experienced this serendipitous method, opposed to a systematic literature search using search terms, as they plunge head first into the Internet through a search engine such as Google and simply follow the links that turn up, hoping for fortuitous and fruitful connections.

As Umberto Eco (1999) suggests in *Serendipities*, apparent mistakes can be fortuitous, or produce interesting side effects. Certain 'lunacies', such as

Columbus setting out to 'discover' the Indies by sailing westward, prove to be serendipitous. Accidental by-products are commonly reported in science, arts and humanities research, but this type of creativity may be neglected in medical education in an era of obsessively detailed learning outcomes and curriculum descriptors. Serendipity has perhaps become the unconscious or tacit dimension to such limiting pedagogical frameworks.

10   Creativity as resistance to the 'uncreative'

We have seen from earlier chapters the importance that resistance or dissensus plays in the possibility of redistributing sensibility capital, or altering the fabric of sensibility. Similar to political resistance, we can also be in a permanent state of alert to challenge what we see as the 'uncreative' in life. The poet John Keats described a parallel to this condition as living in 'negative capability': 'when a man is capable of being in uncertainties, mysteries and doubts without any irritable reaching after fact and reason' (in Claxton 2000: 49). This condition is also one of critique, or critical examination, refusing the habitual. Creativity is then a condition of paradox, as a general inhibitory state. The 'uncreative' – the mundane, literal, dull, mediocre, mechanical, trivial, habitual, predictable and routine – is actively denied or kept at bay. This may be seen as an 'inoculation' view of creativity, inoculating against the disease that is the ordinary. The conditions for creativity are then afforded by vigilance for the intrusion of the ordinary as a default position, rather than an explicit cultivation of the extraordinary.

Creativity is then multivoiced, plural and polymorphous. Should this sound fuzzy to more scientifically inclined medical educators, recall that in Chemistry, 'polymorphous' refers to crystallization of a compound in at least two distinct forms; and in biology, the serial occurrence of different forms or stages of an individual organism. Let us celebrate such multiple possibilities and actively support the many faces of a democratic medical education rather than fighting our corner for a favoured approach.

6   Close noticing

Observe, record, tabulate, communicate. Use your five senses. ... Learn to
see, learn to hear, learn to feel, learn to smell, and know that by practice
alone you can become expert. Medicine is learned by the bedside and not in
the classroom. Let not your conceptions of disease come from words heard
in the lecture room or read from the book. See, and then reason and
compare and control. But see first.

(Sir William Osler, quoted in Bryan 1997: 114)

Sensibility and sensitivity

'Sensibility' is defined in the *Shorter Oxford English Dictionary* (OED) as
'the specific function of the organs of sense' or, simply, quality of perception. In the seventeenth century, this plain description of general perceptual
attentiveness morphed into the particular – as 'emotional capacities'; and by
the eighteenth and early nineteenth centuries 'sensibility' was often associated with an educated or refined taste, but also the capacity to 'feel
compassion for suffering' of others, aligning it with empathy, discussed in
Chapter 4. Such refinement of taste is traced by Barker-Benfield (1992: xvii)
in British society in the eighteenth century, where it came to a head as
'manners'. Once, then, 'sensibility' referred to the commonly shared
mechanics of perception, its definition resting on 'essentially materialist
assumptions', but by the eighteenth century, sensibility referred to 'a particular kind of consciousness' invested with 'spiritual and moral values', in
short, sensibility had become class-based civility or 'refinement'. In Jacques
Rancierè's terms, discussed in Chapter 3, the sensible, the fabric of the sensible, or sensibility, had become a form of capital owned by the wealthy few,
wrested from its ground in the common and subject now to political
control, the boundaries of taste carefully policed.

'Sensitivity' – 'Having the function of sensation or sensuous perception'
(OED) – is considered to be synonymous with 'sensibility' but there is an
important qualitative difference, one of intensity, where such a perceptual
response is acute: 'feels quickly and acutely' (OED). This difference in
intensity aligns sensitivity much more with 'feeling' and emotional states

rather than sense perception in everyday usage. I will treat sensibility as the potential of the senses for close noticing and sensitivity as the potential for consideration of the feelings of others, noting that they work in concert.

In medicine, as in eighteenth-century British society, observation and close noticing and feelings for patients became organized socially as capital, through power and authority structures inherent to medical culture, policed by medical education, as argued in previous chapters. Such sensibility capital is distributed or withheld in fair and unfair ways, often unconsciously, both facilitating sensibility and producing insensibility in medical students, patients and other healthcare practitioners. My concern in this chapter is to:

1   Map out what is meant by the terrain of the sensible in medicine and healthcare.
2   Focus on the process of close noticing as the key clinical practice dealing with sensibility, exhibited in the physical examination and clinical judgement.
3   Analyse the processes by which sensibility capital is formed, held and distributed (or maldistributed) by those in power (senior clinical teachers). And how the relatively 'poor' and 'disenfranchised' (students and patients in particular) in medical culture can disrupt patterns of maldistribution of sensibility and production of insensibility through resistance.

This is a rather long and bumpy ride, and I apologize in advance for the bruising that it may cause in some.

Kinds of reasoning in the senses

Following Aristotle, Martha Nussbaum (2001: 290) notes that medicine is a 'stochastic' art – that is, an art with a high degree of uncertainty and random chance. Novices in medicine suffer greatly from such randomness because they have not yet learned how to focus on salient features of a situation that give a greater sense of certainty – for example learning how to recognize signs and symptoms in order to arrive at a diagnosis. As they gain expertise, they form cognitive schemata – generalized representations formed from many exposures to individual symptom types – that allow them to make clinical judgements according to pattern recognition ('I know this, I've seen many before'). Pattern recognition, or non-analytical reasoning, becomes a form of 'tacit knowledge' or an 'indwelling' of a phenomenon (Polanyi 1983; Engel 2008). This kind of reasoning is termed Type I or System I, as opposed to rational, logical and deductive forms of reasoning following rules, known as Type II or System II. It is widely accepted that in everyday cognition, as well as in expert judgements, both forms of reasoning work together as a dual system (Frankish 2010).

Studies of eye tracking by doctors using visual skills during diagnostic process also show two processes at work – global impression and focal search. Where novices and juniors use mainly focal search, experts rely more on a global impression, a holistic grasp of the image. Global impression is like System I (holistic and intuitive) clinical reasoning, where focal search is like System II (logical, analytical) reasoning (Norman *et al.* 2007). We might then 'hothouse' or accelerate the clinical reasoning capacities of novices through introducing deliberate, planned exposure to common visual stimuli – in other words, meet plenty of patients early in a medical education with emphasis upon expert guidance (scaffolding learning) through briefing and debriefing. Recall William Osler's wisdom at the head of this chapter: 'Medicine is learned by the bedside and not in the classroom. Let not your conceptions of disease come from words heard in the lecture room or read from the book. See, and then reason and compare and control. But see first' (Bryan 1997: 114).

The received wisdom is that medical students, in the absence of tacit knowledge held by experts, should use formal, logical, analytical methods such as hypothesis generation and forms of differential diagnoses to avoid misdiagnosis. Norman, Young and Brooks (2007) challenge such a sharp differentiation between novices and experts, suggesting that novices start using pattern recognition much earlier than was previously thought. However, novices tend to draw on a different pattern recognition process to experts. Experts use two types of pattern recognition – first, the prototype, where numerous examples of a pattern are averaged into a typical example that is matched against the new perception; second, the exemplar, where many exemplars of an object or pattern are held tacitly and scanned and matched against a new perception. While novices and experts use both strategies, novices tend to categorize according to single prototypes, where experts categorize according to multiple exemplars. This means that across a group of novices, a common prototype will be held, whereas across a group of experts, differing exemplars are drawn upon. This is why experts may disagree about a more ambiguous judgement. The shift from novice to expert is, of course, on a gradient and not set as an opposition.

These two types of perception – averaging and use of multiple exemplars – have their political counterparts in two kinds of democracy. The first, averaging, is movement towards a norm. The second, multiple exemplars, is based on respect for difference. Normative democracies tend to be skewed towards meritocracies or mild autocracies, in which those who best uphold the norms or give evidence of having succeeded to meet those norms (meritocracy) place pressure on others to conform (mild autocracy). Feminists in particular have pointed out that this form of democracy tends to be biased towards male, white, northern European–North American values, and is maintained not just through social forms (such as medical hierarchies) but also language use. Thinking 'difference' opens up a new field of democracy that is more radical, disturbing and unstable, but ultimately closer to genuine exercise of equality and equity.

To return to use of exemplars, individual cognitive architectures distributed across a group of experts, say a team of consultant dermatologists, radiologists or histopathologists, add up to significant material capital for working with patients. Experts will be working with visual symptoms at gross and microscopic levels and both naturally and virtually (in images such as X-rays or scans). But this shared cognition also provides a rich resource for collaboratively teaching medical students and junior colleagues. In the realm of perceptual clinical judgements, or use of the senses and close noticing, this collective wisdom can again be termed 'sensibility capital' organized as a fabric of the sensible. Following from Chapter 3, we can ask: (i) 'how is such capital acquired and used?' (an aesthetic question concerning the education and use of the senses and the gaining of identity as a connoisseur in a specialty); and (ii) 'how is such capital shared among others who do not hold this capital but are ready to acquire it as students or patients?' (a political question concerning the use of authority and power in deciding how capital shall be distributed).

Five main factors in current medical education frustrate the fair distribution of sensibility capital across experts and novices such as medical students or the patients treated by those expert doctors:

1   Experts cannot readily access knowledge and strategies that are tacit in order to explore these with novices. Mechanisms of introspection and reflection themselves have to be learned by experts in order to mine tacit knowledge and make it explicit. We do, however, have a hundred years of psychoanalytic tradition to draw on to offer a model of how the unconscious can be made conscious.

2   Experts are reluctant to encourage novices to use pattern recognition in the absence of experience because this may lead to misdiagnoses. However, experts do not judge well how more advanced medical students for example have already gained pattern recognition ability in some areas of medicine. Further, novices are likely to over-diagnose without the checks of pattern recognition against analytical forms of reasoning.

3   Medical education still does not offer early and consistent exposure of medical students to patients, relying instead on teaching abstract protocols and logical decision processes such as 'paper' (virtual) case-based differential diagnosis.

4   Students do not have enough exposure to experts disagreeing among themselves about more complex judgements. This would expose biases in favour of serial exemplars rather than generalized, collapsed prototypes as the mechanism by which pattern recognition works. Just as better experts read their individual patients as one in a series of exemplars of 'chief complaints', yet still bear these individual patients' 'chief concerns' in mind (Schleifer and Vannatta 2013), so students could be educated through a release and sharing of such sensibility capital.

5   Clinical experts may lack the pedagogical expertise to scaffold learning in novices.

Where sensibility capital is withheld, or equitable sharing is frustrated, in each of the five examples above this produces and reproduces insensibility in novices as an unintended consequence of medical education. The shared or distributed cognition across a group of experts in a specialty is not a handicap to medical educators but a benefit – it shows students how serial exemplars based on real patients (the idiographic), rather than collapsed prototypes based on typical or generalised cases (the nomothetic), inform clinical judgements. As Immanuel Kant suggested, the idiographic typifies a descriptive humanities approach, where the nomothetic is typical of scientific reasoning. If expert judgement in medicine veers towards the idiographic (series of exemplars within a class of symptom) then we should be thinking much more about medicine as an art of judgement readily informed by humanities frameworks.

In distributing sensibility capital, senior doctors are bound by historically formed conventions. A democratic gesture involves sharing capital of sensibility through clinical education, collaborative teamwork and patient-centred practices. An autocratic gesture involves withholding capital of sensibility from other stakeholders to maintain an authority structure, or distributing capital in ways that demean or mock learners or restrict understanding and practice. Jacques Rancière (2010), as described in Chapter 3, calls this a 'policing' of sensibility. Any stakeholder is free to resist the dominant discourse, for example through seeking out more enlightened teachers, self-informing, joining pressure groups, and so forth – that Rancière calls 'dissensus'. Michel Foucault (2002) called this the exercise of 'capillary power' as a form of resistance against sovereign power, in which subtle acts of resistance accumulate to flow against the grain of the dominant power structure. Homi Bhabha (2004), in the context of describing forms of resistance among colonized people, notes that these acts of resistance – as 'mimicry' and 'sly civility' – can be subtle coded performances recognized by the oppressed but by-passing the perceptions of the oppressor.

In Margaret Edson's play *W;t*, discussed in the Introduction, there is a scene in which Vivian Bearing, an English literature professor and expert in John Donne's poetry, who is dying from advanced ovarian cancer, is the 'object' of a Grand Round. As the senior and junior doctors gather around her bed and objectively and coldly discuss her condition rather than address her, she engages in a parallel, mocking interior monologue:

> 'Grand Rounds'. The term is theirs. Not 'Grand' in the traditional sense of sweeping or magnificent. Not 'rounds' as in a musical canon, or a *round* of applause (though either would be refreshing at this point). Here, 'Rounds' seems to signify darting *around* the main issue ... which I suppose would be the struggle for life ... *my* life ...
>
> (Edson 1999: 36)

Here is a scenario that illustrates the maldistribution of sensibility and the production of insensibility in a working surgical team undergoing a crisis that leads to a serious consequence – the unnecessary death of a patient. In 'Just a Routine Operation' you can watch a YouTube video account by an airline pilot, Martin Bromiley, of how his wife Elaine died in March 2005 under tragic circumstances (Laerdal Medical 2011). Elaine was undergoing a routine operation but the anaesthetic team had difficulties in fitting a laryngeal mask and then establishing an airway after the anaesthetic had been administered. Normally, after several attempts at intubation and noticing that oxygenation levels were falling, the operation would have been cancelled and the patient allowed to recover naturally from the anaesthesia. On this occasion, the anaesthetic team, composed of senior doctors and aided by a consultant surgeon, got locked into attempting to intubate Emily long after vital signs showed that she was lacking oxygen. A team of nurses came into the room and immediately diagnosed the problem, leaving a tracheostomy set for the doctors to use for introducing an emergency airway. The presence of the set was ignored as intubation was pursued.

One of the nurses saw immediately that Elaine was turning blue and booked a bed in the intensive care unit. The doctors told her that everything was under control and the bed was cancelled. Emily died as a consequence of the doctors' collective error. The sensibility capital they held as a team of experts was extremely high, but was not mobilized as they got locked into a 'heads down' situation without seeing the wider picture. The nurses exercised their sensibility capital through commonly noticing deterioration in vital signs, but this failed to be distributed as the doctors ignored its value. The doctors meanwhile continued to produce insensibility across the entire team as the nurses were persuaded out of the legitimacy of their sensibility capital through the exercise of hierarchy – they were basically ignored and felt that they could not speak up. The team was literally an-aesthetized or starved of sensibility – and of sense making – through historically determined power structures that were not adequately resisted by the nurses.

An extreme model of this scenario of the interaction between the politics and aesthetics of resistance is developed in Peter Weiss's (2005) novel *The Aesthetics of Resistance*. Only the first part of this three-part masterpiece has been translated into English. It is set in Berlin in 1937 and centres on teenage working class students who, guided by their parents, are undercover resistance fighters against the Nazi regime. Their political resistance is shaped aesthetically, literally through visits to museums and art galleries where certain works of art provide stimulation for shaping political forms and through close reading of literature. In other words, Weiss links sensibility (aesthetics) directly to politics (power). The teenagers recognize that the function of art through the ages has not been simply to represent and uphold dominant forms (Church-inspired, State-inspired or Patron-inspired art), but to challenge dominant ways of thinking. Most importantly, exposure to art teaches these adolescents forms of close noticing. It is only through such acute perception that resistance can be formulated not as a direct political confrontation but as a slow erosion of dominant and oppressive forms.

Medicine would couch this scenario in terms of militaristic metaphors, where the enemy is disease and the cure is a slow process of formulating exactly how the disease operates biochemically, physiologically and psychologically. Only then can resistance form itself into an effective movement, just as the immune system adapts through series of exposures and mimicry.

Arts-educated observation

Caroline Wellberry and Rebecca McAteer (forthcoming) note that observational skills learned through medical education have been honed by a supplement of arts-based observation interventions in many medical schools – usually visits to art galleries or museums where curators or art historians help students to notice more closely. I return, critically, to the developing literature in this field later in this chapter. I have already noted paradoxes in medical education that may result in unintended insensibility and the most obvious of these is that the diagnostic gaze is highly controlled and specified. It is not the ordinary gaze of persons upon the world. Honing this gaze visually, or through other senses, is in turn confounded by the fact that the environments in which the gaze is exercised – clinics, hospitals, consulting rooms, operating theatres – are often perceptually anaesthetizing environments. They are often either poorly lit or flooded with artificial light, overheated or too cold and with depressing low ceilings. There are of course exceptions, where hospital design explicitly sets out to sensitize (Bleakley *et al.* 2011).

Education of sensibility to recover what specialization may have driven out – the ordinary perceptions in human encounters that allow for sensitivity to the Other – is a priority for medical education. Wellberry and McAteer, both doctors, suggest that beyond education in arts-based observation, nature writing serves as a model for educating close observation. This may appeal to medical students as natural history overlaps so clearly with receiving a patient's history. Further, close reading of texts can encourage close reading of the patient as text, a point elaborated by Bleakley, Bligh and Browne (2011). Finally, medical students must be able to say what they see in terms of public narrative and 'the ability to craft this speech as public narrative' (Wellberry and McAteer forthcoming) is surely at the heart of a humane, patient-centred practice. Importantly, Wellberry and McAteer see the honing of sensibility as opening a door for resistance – where medical students and doctors can turn their newly honed gazes upon the institution of medicine itself, not just critically but constructively, in formulating appropriate interventions.

The art of medicine can be thought of as a connoisseurship of symptoms. Doctors must learn to closely observe, whether reading physical symptoms direct from the body or images, such as X-rays and scans. This is driven of course by a morbid curiosity – not because doctors like to see suffering but because they want to track down precisely what is causing the suffering. Close sensing is of course what artists of all varieties do – whether looking in visual art, listening in music, or attuning kinaesthetic senses in dance and performance. Doctors need to extend close sensing to smell also (Ursitti 2008), for example to the fruity smell of a diabetic's ketone build-up, or worse, coma. Where sensitivity or empathy is absolutely central to humane care, then sensibility or close noticing precedes this. It makes sense that medical students should learn close noticing from experts in clinical contexts and this can be intensified through working with artists to educate the senses.

Where 'technology has given us an extended eye' (Ursitti 2008: 2), is this merely extending the clinical gaze, or further objectifying patients, as 'hands-on' medicine becomes a distant memory? Nobody has fought harder within clinical education to remind us of the importance of educating the senses for close noticing than the senior physician and successful author Abraham Verghese, currently based at Stanford University medical school in California. As we have seen, Verghese is a champion of hands-on 'bedside skills' such as auscultation, palpation and percussion. He is also a champion of the preservation of the languages of tropes – resemblances, similes and metaphors – that support diagnostic acumen or expertise (Chen 2009; Verghese 2009).

Across a series of talks and through his non-fictional and fictional writing, including his bestselling novel *Cutting for Stone* (2009), Verghese has tirelessly reminded medical educators and the general public of the value of medical students learning to become connoisseurs within their chosen profession – to value the art and craft of their work (see for example Verghese 1992, 2007). Indeed, this brings an important identity construction as medical students learn the rituals of the physical examination as an expert performance. Patients literally bare their bodies and metaphorically bare their souls for doctors and in return doctors should provide a professional performance in a collaborative cultural ritual of transformation. If the doctor sells the patient short, the ritual is incomplete and the full identity construction is never achieved for the doctor or the patient. Verghese, in an interview for *The New York Times* (Chen 2009), notes that 'It's so easy for the doctor to just slide into a room and not think … But for the patient it is high drama and hugely symbolic.'

While proxy testing and imaging have of course offered great advances for medicine, they also afford the symptom of over-diagnosis (Welch *et al.* 2011) and potential objectification of the patient that ruptures the ritual exchange described above that is the classic bedside encounter. In the interview mentioned above (Chen 2009), Verghese says: 'The busy practitioner struggles with time pressures … But hurrying through makes us just hurry through. We order a lot of tests because we think we are saving time or because we are uncertain. If you spend more time listening to a patient or being more thoughtful, you end up saving time'. This returns us to Wellberry and McAteer's point that a good model for close noticing is natural history, where patient and intense observation is key to knowing what is going on. Patient and patience are related etymologically.

In Verghese's *Cutting for Stone* there are a number of examples of why a medical education is about educating sensibility for close noticing. One character's description of the symptoms of typhoid fever alerts us to 'See how her (the patient's) eyes keep roving as if she's waiting for something? A grave sign. And look at the way she picks at the bedclothes – that's called carphology, and those little muscle twitches are *subsultus tendinum*'. Through one of his characters, Verghese gives a brilliant mini-lecture on resemblances in medical diagnosis – descriptive names for different physical signs, expanded later in this chapter:

> Yes! A treasure trove of words! That's what you find in medicine. Take the food metaphors we use to describe disease: the nutmeg liver, the sago spleen, the anchovy sauce sputum, or currant jelly stools. Why, if you consider just fruits alone you have the strawberry tongue of scarlet fever, which the next day becomes the raspberry tongue. Or how about the strawberry angioma, the watermelon stomach, the apple core lesion of cancer, the peau d'orange appearance of breast cancer... and that's just the fruits! Don't get me started on the nonvegetarian stuff!
>
> (Verghese 2009: 223)

This is the stuff to get poets and visual artists salivating. Yet we must remind ourselves that this is an aesthetics of suffering, of symptom. Fascinated as we are, a 'bamboo spine' (Figure 6.1) spells out a debilitating condition – ankylosing spondylitis, a form of arthritis associated with long-term inflammation of the joints in the spine; and an 'apple core lesion' (Figure 6.2) – cancer of the colon. Medical students then have to apply a moral imagination and an ethical dimension to the aesthetics and politics of the distribution of sensibility through medical education. The sensibility that is being educated is one of acute awareness of potential suffering. Yet we must remind ourselves that artists are connoisseurs and diagnosticians of the suffering of culture – Edvard Munch's 'The Scream' or Francis Bacon's screaming and distorted figures are our common wealth, common social capital, ways in which each of us may ponder the realities of suffering.

Having set out a conceptual framework for challenging current forms of the maldistribution of sensibility through medical and healthcare education, I will now turn to why it is important to shape close noticing in clinicians.

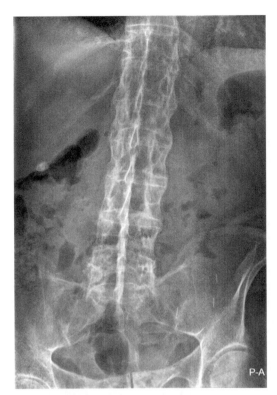

Figure 6.1 Bamboo spine
(ankylosing
spondylitis)
Source: Stevenfruitsmaak

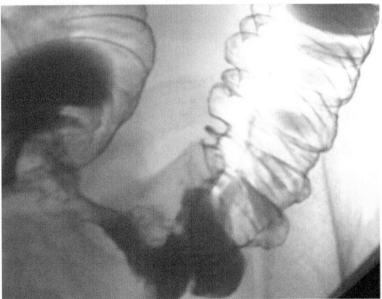

Figure 6.2 Apple core lesion (colonic carcinoma)
Source: Dr Richard Farrow

Making sense of diagnosis

Consider this description of a clinical practitioner at work:

> Around midnight he started getting a bit more pale...and his lung
> sounds were ok. They had a few crackles but nothing really significant
> ...by about 2am he was looking quite a bit worse and very wet...So I
> got blood gas and the pH was 7.2...I finished giving the bicarb about
> a half hour previously and I looked at the baby and he looked much
> worse than he had before...His mouth was just open slightly. He was
> gasping to try to breathe. He just looked awful, looked absolutely terri-
> ble...So I gave the Lasix (*Furosemide*, a diuretic), but at that point the
> baby was looking so bad that I didn't even wait for the Lasix to take
> effect before I went ahead and did another blood gas.
>
> (Benner *et al.* 2009: 117)

Albeit rather dated, this account beautifully illustrates the perceptual basis
to healthcare. The decisions made to treat this ill baby were based on a close
noticing of qualities, primarily visual ('getting a bit more pale', 'looking
quite a bit worse'). But also, sensitivity is involved ('He just looked awful,
looked absolutely terrible'). Ways of 'looking', embedded within a moral
practice of concern and care, are central to diagnostic acumen and may be
best educated through clinicians working in tandem with those whose
primary work is also 'looking', such as visual artists and art historians. The
latter, of course, 'care' mainly for material objects. It is their aesthetic
concern that underpins beautiful architecture, elegant instruments, engaging film and television, popular culture and so forth, as 'diagnosticians of
culture' in Nietzsche's phrase (Smith 2005). My point is that morality
informs an aesthetic.

Where the situation of physicians teaching students in clinical settings
affords relevance, the addition of artists affords meaningfulness. Ingredients
for a successful core medical humanities provision are twofold:

- education of sensibilities and sensitivities set in live clinical contexts;
  and
- with physicians, artists, humanities scholars, patients, and students
  working democratically to improve patient care.

The practitioner looking at the sick baby above is a nurse. Nurses are often
defined in terms of lack in relation to the work of physicians within a hierarchy. This example of sensitive close noticing is purposefully chosen to
raise three issues. First, to question casual and exclusive use of the common
descriptor 'the medical humanities'; second, to ground the artistry of clinical practice in the senses, in aesthetic work; and third, to address the issue
of democratizing clinical practice. The first issue can be dealt with briefly.

Although this book concentrates on medicine and therefore continues use of the term 'medical humanities', as explored in the Introduction and Chapters 1 and 2, this can be seen as exclusive and undemocratic in an era of collaborative, patient-centred, interprofessional teamwork. The generic term 'health (or healthcare) humanities' is explicitly inclusive, where 'humanities' is taken to include the arts and the humanities-leaning social sciences. The second issue – grounding practice artistry in the senses – also involves making a case for the shared praxis of the health humanities, to democratize the previously exclusive domain of the 'medical gaze'.

The medical/health humanities can be summarized as the humanity (sensitivity) and artistry (sensibility) of medicine and healthcare. How this is educated depends, again, upon a structured collaboration between clinicians, artists, humanities scholars, students, patients and the public. Sensitivity encompasses ethical care, where sensibility is *aesthetic labour*, such as the expressive close noticing of the nurse in the example above. 'Medical aesthetics' complements the established field of 'medical ethics'.

I have emphasized (possibly over-emphasized) the value of a model that treats sensibility as capital, but of course the aesthetic labour of medical students, patients and healthcare colleagues is intimately tied in with sensibility capital. If, for example, a medical student goes out of her way to incorporate a more innovative approach to her medicine informed by the medical humanities that she has engaged with through the curriculum, senior clinical educators should not exploit this labour through, say, belittling it as 'soft and fluffy'. She should be rewarded appropriately for that labour.

As indicated in the opening to this chapter, we must unhook ourselves from the legacy of aesthetics as 'high art' and that aesthetics is confined to 'pleasure'. The root of aesthetics is the ancient Greek *aisthanomai* – meaning perception by means of the senses, or 'sense impression'. Aesthetics is to do with *quality* of life as experienced through the senses. This includes not just the pleasurable, but also the perplexing, the disgusting, the sublime, the perverse and the abject. For Nietzsche (1984), ill health paradoxically provides the conditions of sensitivity needed to become an acute diagnostician of culture, thus problematizing the notion of the 'health' humanities. Education of the senses in terms of 'lay' connoisseurship (close noticing), or 'professional' connoisseurship (pattern recognition and close diagnosis in expertise), is an educated bodily event. The arts and humanities create ambiguity, to destabilize and challenge unproductive habits such as abusive exercise of legitimate authority, so that creative ways of living can emerge. This, again, is a basis to democracy.

But there is a prerequisite for both citizenship and professionals working in democratic team settings – persons must be sensitized, aestheticized to notice closely and not dulled, or an-aesthetized. Without the evidence of the senses, debate cannot ensue about the logic of practices. Further, tolerance of uncertainty and ambiguity is central to performing that debate.

Intolerance of ambiguity is the central character trait of the authoritarian personality type resistant to democracy (Adorno *et al.* 1950) as discussed in earlier chapters. An 'aesthetics of resistance' (Weiss 2005) is needed to counter such authoritarianism, also noted earlier.

Let us return to the nurse above, making qualitative judgements based on sense impressions, or doing aesthetic work. In 1859, Florence Nightingale (in Quain 1883: 1038) wrote that close noticing is 'The *sine qua non* of being a nurse', where 'attending to...one's own senses...should tell the nurse how the patient is'. This is the aesthetic labour of healthcare. Again, who would wish for an an-aesthetic healthcare service? This would be dull, uninspired, ugly, unimaginative, flat, ungracious, clumsy, insensitive, tiresome and numbing. Aesthetic work is elegant, inspiring, beautiful, imaginative, animated, dignified, graceful, sensitive, distinctive and passionate. In the context of art history, Rudolf Arnheim (1969: 206) describes a sophisticated kind of looking as 'intelligent vision', but reminds us that this 'cannot be confined to the art studio'. Arnheim suggests that such intelligent vision can succeed in other disciplines 'only if the visual sense is not blunted'. We must, in Arnheim's phrase, 'think with the senses' and think acutely. As the art historian James Elkins suggests, 'Most sciences...have specific visual competencies', and these present 'ways of seeing waiting to be explored' (Elkins 2003: 87).

Polanyi and Prosch (1975: 31) argue that education of the senses is essential for good science, where 'no science can predict observed facts except by relying with confidence upon an art: the art of establishing by the trained delicacy of eye, ear, and touch a correspondence between the explicit predictions of science and the actual experience of our senses to which these predictions shall apply'. Bardes, Gillers and Herman (2001: 1157) note that 'clinical diagnosis involves the observation, description, and interpretation of visual information', where such skills 'are also the special province of the visual arts'. The arts, it seems, offer essential capital for distribution across to the culture of medicine in educating for close noticing. But does this work? What does the evidence tell us from studies in the field and can that evidence be trusted?

Can exposure to the arts hone observation?

Evidence suggests that observational capability in medicine and healthcare can be significantly improved through tutored looking at pictures in art galleries, where close noticing or attention to detail is cultivated. The use of the visual arts for educating the senses has entered medical education relatively recently but has made an impact, as Wellberry and McAteer note above. Previously, the arts appeared in the guise of arts therapies or arts in health, where the medium, such as painting, offered the therapeutic intervention and not the quality of the artwork. In utilizing art to teach close noticing, the quality of the work is paramount, but of course the students themselves usually do not engage in any art-making activities. Rather, they are learning connoisseurship, through the media of curating, criticism or art history. There is a considerable literature and tried-and-tested set of practices in this area of 'how to look', in particular James Elkins's (2008) *How to Use Your Eyes*.

Usually, the focus is on developing, first, better observational capability and, second, interpretive capabilities; but also the power of the visual arts to elicit an emotional response in the observer is recognized. Bringing these three components together is the goal of numerous contemporary art-and-medicine classes that, again, often take place in museums and may be led by museum educators, curators and art historians. For example, Florence Gelo at Drexel University College of Medicine describes how she brings doctors in a Family Medicine residency training programme to Philadelphia art museums and encourages them to describe to each other their emotional responses to a painting, to notice details and to interpret (see http://litmed.med.nyu.edu/Annotation?action=view&annid=12975).

Andrew Jacques and colleagues (Jacques *et al.* 2012) at Ohio State University College of Medicine have teamed up with Columbus Museum of Art to develop a two hours' long programme for medical students in which art is observed critically and collaboratively. A critical thinking strategy – 'observe, describe, interpret, prove' (ODIP) – is used, and it can be transferred back for example to use on a ward round where close observation of patients is necessary.

Such work is only a decade old at the time of writing and hence only in the first flush of its possibilities. The vast majority of such work has been initiated and piloted in North American medical schools as elective programmes for early years, usually first year, medical students. The problem with this constituency is that first year students are less likely to be critical of such programmes as they are not yet fully socialized into medical school culture; and they do not have very much in the way of preliminary clinical experience with patients to act as a background against which to make sense of the close observation techniques that they are learning.

In 2001, Ruric Anderson and colleagues from the Department of Medicine at the Medical College of Wisconsin called for a reformulation of how physical diagnosis is taught in the light of growing evidence that showed a decline in emphasis placed upon teaching physical skills and in students' ability to learn such approaches where intensive support and expertise was lacking (Anderson *et al.* 2001). They suggested that greater emphasis should be placed on teaching students to look closely in the physical examination. In the same year, Bardes and colleagues at Weil Cornell Medical College, New York, described an educational collaboration between an art museum and a medical school where students were taught how to observe, describe and interpret portraits and then transferred this back into clinical settings by examining photographs of patients' faces (Bardes *et al.* 2001). This increased students' ability to read emotional expression on the face.

A study at Yale University in 2001 suggested that an arts-based intervention – systematic looking at representational paintings – could improve the observational skills of students (Dolev *et al.* 2001). This was more rigorous than Bardes and colleagues' study: 146 first-year medical students took pre- and post-test scores on dermatology photographs; 81 students looked at paintings and discussed them, while the other 65 students did not receive this intervention. The post-intervention scores showed a 10 per cent increase in positive recognition scores for the experimental group who had discussed the paintings, suggesting that this had a significant influence upon their ability to look more closely at the clinical test material.

In 2002, Rodenhauser, Strickland and Gambala (2004) carried out a survey of arts-related activities beyond the literary across North American medical schools. They noted that while literary activities were introduced to medical schools in the 1970s and 1980s as part of the first wave of medical humanities interest, arts activities were not introduced until much later, but took off more rapidly. A 2002 survey of all North American medical schools with a 65 per cent response rate showed that over half of the schools responding involved the arts in the curriculum, to include visual arts, performing arts and music, on top of an established literature provision. These were, however, mainly elective provision, typically involving less than 20 students and were rarely part of formal assessment or curriculum evaluation. While this interest is encouraging, it is a long way from the ideal of a core and integrated medical humanities curriculum discussed in Chapters 1 and 2.

A cognitive psychologist, Abigail Housen (2002) and a visual art educator, Philip Yenawine (1997), developed a set of techniques called 'visual thinking strategies' that employed 'thinking aloud' collaborative and critically dialogical conversations where you describe what you are seeing in the company of others, as a composite picture is built up. Reilly, Ring and Duke (2005) describe the use of a visual thinking strategy in residents' medical education using a 'think aloud' techniques based on viewing three well-known medically themed paintings – Sir Luke Fildes's 'The Doctor', Robert Pope's 'Mr S Is Told He Will Die' and Rembrandt's 'The Anatomy Lecture of Dr Nicolaes Tulp'. The authors do not say how many learners were involved or how they were recruited and the outcomes are reported only in terms of participants' satisfaction. The value of the research is that, in borrowing from visual thinking strategies, the methods of investigating close looking in medicine were extended. In 2011, at the University of Texas Health Science Center, San Antonio, Klugman, Peel and Beckmann-Mendez (2011) set up 90-minute-long art rounds with both medical and nursing students using visual thinking strategies as the method. A pre- and post-test on 32 students showed significant increases in observation skills, tolerance for ambiguity and even the desire to learn communication skills.

Shapiro, Rucker and Beck (2006: 2623) noted that: 'medical educators have periodically experimented with using arts-based training to hone observational acuity'. Well, at this point – 2006 – there were very few published accounts, as we have seen. The authors set out 'to better understand the similarities and differences between arts-based and clinical teaching approaches to convey observation and pattern recognition skills'. In a matched cohorts comparison of just 38 third-year medical students, the authors found that tailored clinical activity to improve pattern recognition and hone observation does indeed improve these abilities in students. The clinical activity group benefitted most from learning about pattern recognition, possibly because of relevance of the material. However, an arts-based approach adds value, where 'students also developed skills in emotional recognition, cultivation of empathy, identification of story and narrative, and awareness of multiple perspectives'.

The largely functional approaches to close noticing were now extended, to include affective responses that clearly have an influence upon how one 'looks' or gazes in clinical practice. Despite what doctors may claim about professional behaviour, there is a difference between a physical examination performed on somebody who disgusts you as opposed to a patient for whom you feel attraction or respect. Elizabeth Gaufberg, a physician and educator and Ray Williams, a director of education at a university art museum, have developed an educational innovation in which they buck the trend of teaching close observation of visual material through tutored visits to art museums (Gaufberg and Williams 2011). In what they call 'The Personal Responses Tour', medical learners randomly select a question from a prepared set that invites an emotional response, for example to think of a memorable patient – such as one you found it difficult to empathize with – and then find a work of art that somehow resonates with that patient and dwell on the connections. The task lasts one and a half hours. Catherine Belling (2011) points out that encouraging doctors to be reflective about patients in the affective domain – raising feelings – is complex, because what a doctor feels is also tied up with what she 'should' feel in exercising professionalism. In using 'indirection' by focusing upon works of art as a medium – or 'third thing' after the practitioner and her patient – through which feelings can be reflected upon, Belling points out that more authentic reflection may ensue. Use of more sophisticated techniques such as indirection point of course to expertise, indeed connoisseurship, in pedagogy within medical education.

At the Department of Family Medicine, University of Cincinnati, Nancy Elder and colleagues utilized a medicine–art museum collaboration for second-year medical students attempting to compensate for the fact that 'teaching the skill of observation is often short-changed in medical education' (Elder *et al.* 2006). The 'Art of Observation' was an elective course with only 17 students. Education into 'looking' and 'seeing' provided by the museum was evaluated retrospectively – as students completed clinical rotations – through an online evaluation. Students claimed that the course had improved their clinical skills in observation and description. Again, the study is weakly designed, using a small, self-selected sample likely to be positive towards the experience from the outset and utilizing vague self-reports. This is easy prey for medical humanities sceptics.

Deborah Kirklin and colleagues at University College London medical school improved on the 2001 Yale study by Dolev and colleagues above by setting up a far more rigorous study in a clinical setting (Kirklin *et al.* 2007). They systematically evaluated the effects of an arts-based educational intervention on the development of observational skills in primary care of both doctors and nurses. The procedure tested was confidence in diagnosing and referring suspicious pigmented skin lesions. One group received an arts-based, 90-minute-long observational skill training (delivered by an artist), where the control group received practical training in the management of psoriasis. There was a significant difference in the quality of judgement between the two groups in favour of the arts-based intervention group. The intervention was fairly simple – the artist gave participants common objects such as a coconut, a piece of carpet, some bubble wrap, an orange and a piece of broccoli to handle unseen and then asked the participants to handle the same objects seen, describing tones, colours, shades and so forth in detail. All participants then described three photographs of dermatological symptoms. There are limitations to this study, such as the possible short-term only gains from the arts-based exercises. However, it is a telling and important reminder that education in 'looking' can become education in 'seeing' and the research design was far more sophisticated than previous inquiries in the field.

At McGill University, Canada, Boudreau, Cassell and Fuks (2008) eschewed the paradigm of experimental investigation into capability in clinical observation to ask a panel of experts just what constitutes expert close noticing in medicine. They distilled four pedagogical principles and eight core principles of clinical observation as a basis to developing a course in clinical observation for first year medical students. The main educational principle is that learning must occur in live clinical contexts, challenging the dominant emerging paradigm of learning in museums and transferring to clinical contexts. Of the eight core principles, perhaps the most important is that 'observation is distinct from inference' – importantly, students must describe what they see and not what they expect to see. Boudreau and colleagues' paper significantly moves theorizing of close noticing forward, where perceptual, cognitive and cultural elements are seen as inseparable. It also models one way in which sensibility capital can be distributed.

Naghshineh and colleagues set up a course for first- and second-year medical students at Harvard in 2004–5 called 'Training the Eye: Improving the Art of Physical Diagnosis' (Naghshineh *et al.* 2008). The authors responded to evidence that physical examination skills had declined among students because teaching these skills had declined. A course in 'visual literacy' was set up in which unbiased observation was linked to physiological and pathophysiological reasoning. A group of 24 students engaged in a course to improve observational capability or visual acumen through structured observation of artworks and a life drawing session, where instruction was provided into how to link this to patient care. Thirty-four students were used as a control group. The groups were tested pre- and post-intervention on ability to read patient photographs. There was a significant difference between the two groups, with those who had taken the visual art education course showing greater sophistication in reading clinical symptoms.

Samy Azer, based at the King Saud University College of Medicine in Saudi Arabia, shows that medical students better learn surface anatomy of the abdomen through drawing rather than merely describing verbally (Azer 2011). Other studies cited by Azer (*ibid.*) – have shown that students learn surface anatomy effectively through drawing on the skin. These visually oriented studies have a well-developed literature. This suggests that students should not simply be learning from artists and applying this to practice but should be doing art themselves. While arts-based observation education studies reported so far suggest benefits, they suffer from lack of hands-on experiential learning, craved by medical students.

The first issue in the body of research on close noticing discussed above is to separate out what is seen from what is inferred, or to investigate the relationship between the two. Visual thinking strategies provide a conceptual framework for understanding this and collaborative thinking aloud research provides an appropriate method for inquiry. A second move in extending research is to incorporate study of affective responses and not simply perception. A third move is to engage students in art-making themselves so that close noticing becomes a part of making an artefact, where sketchbooks can act as reflective diaries. This is established in core, compulsory medical humanities units in some medical schools such as the University of Exeter medical school and Plymouth University Peninsula School of Medicine, created out of the dissolution of Peninsula Medical School, UK, that developed the first core, compulsory undergraduate medical humanities curriculum in 2002 (Bleakley *et al.* 2006). Chapter 1 gives an outline of other UK medical schools that have developed significant medical humanities components.

A third, significant move in researching how the visual arts can be used to educate close noticing has been established at the University of Southern California Keck school of medicine, in collaboration with Los Angeles' Museum of Contemporary Art. Schaff, Isken and Tager (2011) noticed the tendency in medicine-art projects for teaching observation to use portraits or figurative art. At first glance, this makes sense, as medical students will be dealing with bodily symptoms and facial features in learning consultations and physical examinations. However, the authors cleverly thought that non-representational or abstract art might be just as important to study, as this includes a high level of ambiguity or uncertainty and tolerance of ambiguity is a key feature in medical practice. How might students be taught 'to observe describe and interpret complex information' from non-representational artworks? Here, they must learn to tolerate high levels of ambiguity and engage in collaborative thinking and appreciation. The step-wise process of close noticing, pattern recognition, matching to experience, engaging with multiple hypotheses and testing these, utilizing intuition and then comparing the outcomes of this process with the judgements of others in a collaborative process is learned from discussions about non-figurative art and translated to medicine.

Michael Baum, a distinguished surgical oncologist and Visiting Professor of Medical Humanities at University College, London, approaches paint-ings in a quite different way, teaching medical students through forensic examination of paintings, revealing that painters not only learned from dissection, but also from close study of the dead. A fifteenth-century paint-ing by Piero di Cosimo in the National Gallery, London, shows a dead woman, a Nymph, mourned by a Satyr. The mythological setting suggests that the woman has been killed accidently by a spear during a deer hunt. Close examination of the painting, however, shows, suggests Baum, that both hands 'are covered with deep lacerations. There is only one way she could have got those. She has been trying to fend off an attacker who has come at her, slashing in a frenzied manner with a knife or possibly a sword' (in McKie 2011). The woman's left hand is bent back in a way that suggests she has received a serious injury at points C3 and C4 on the cervical cord, causing nerve damage that would flex the fingers exactly as painted by di Cosimo. A diagnostic 'ward round' in the gallery could continue in this way – for example a self-portrait of Rembrandt shows that he was probably suffering from rosacea, reddening the facial tissues.

Such forensics on Old Masters seem somehow distanced from the contemporary world of the medical student and may seem arcane. Would students not equally enjoy and learn from study of Andres Serrano's large-scale photographs from the morgue (of which a selection can be viewed via the 'Works of art' link at www.artnet.com/awc/andres-serrano.html), or from Christine Borland's repersonalization of a woman's skeleton used for anatomy teaching in which she refleshed the object to recover the person – an Asian female (a piece called 'From Life'), discussed in Chapter 2 (Borland 2006)? Borland was surprised, indeed shocked, to find that, at the time, she could buy a human skeleton from a catalogue used by anatomy departments in medical schools. She worked with forensics experts to reconstruct the Asian woman or repersonalize her, also serving as a metaphor for the need to educate for a personalizing medicine rather than the dominant mode of de-personalizing through objectifying patients.

There is, then, a developing literature on teaching close observation to medical students, with certain models, particularly the medical school–art museum link becoming dominant in the field. But there is a long way to go in developing more sophisticated research and in challenging two sticking points in particular – most research is done with first year students and projects are at the periphery of the main medicine curriculum. A literature review by Perry and colleagues (Perry *et al.* 2011) found no evidence for significant and lasting effects on behaviour of arts-based interventions in medical schools, but this is probably because such interventions have not been well designed. A systematic programme of research is needed in which longitudinal interventions are made and evaluated.

Programmes based on looking at artwork in galleries and museums and then applying this to medicine are now ubiquitous. For example, Richard Pretorius and colleagues have documented such a course at Buffalo University, run since 2005 (Pretorius *et al.* undated). First-year students learn from studying paintings how observation can help through sensitizing to visual cues such as colour, shape and form. Jasani and Sacks (2012) at Robert Wood Johnson medical school, New Jersey, show that utilizing visual art can enhance the clinical observational skills of medical students. But, again, their sample was small (110 students) and the intervention short (three hours). The students were drawn from year 3, however, and so had some clinical experience. The students studied art images using visual thinking strategies and made diagnoses from photographs of patients. Pre- and post-test scores showed a difference in the kinds of language that students used to describe symptoms.

Where pre-test descriptions involved generic descriptive (non-specific) words such as 'normal' and 'healthy', post-test descriptors involved specific language such as 'Her left arm is flexed at the shoulder and elbow with the hand clenched in a fist'. Post-test language included reference to patients' emotional states and surroundings and included more speculative thinking (subjunctive mood rather than indicative language). Thus, not only were close observations heightened, but also interpretation and reflection increased, enriching observations. The authors note that this was a one-off study and may not have lasting effects.

There are, then, worrying concerns that arise from these studies. They do not innovate in the curriculum with enough force or central presence. Further, they are poorly conceptualized. Simply training for close observation is not the same as structurally challenging the nature of the clinical or diagnostic gaze – this is the bigger project of democratizing medicine. Further, it is important to ask what 'art' is being looked at in gallery and museum visits and does that matter? And who are the artists or curators who might be employed to work in arts-based educational activities with students? At the back of my questions is the niggling worry: does the 'art' itself matter? To artists, curators and art historians of course it matters. Yet the medical humanities culture blithely talks of using 'art' – particularly visual art – as if this were a generic category, without discrimination.

For example, in the Naghshineh *et al.* (2008) study mentioned above, students were asked to study Gauguin, Turner, Sargent, Munch, Picasso, Steen, Manet, Pollock and Monet mainly to look at abstract features such as pattern, colour, composition and form. Given that one of the criticisms of the use of art in medical humanities in medical education is that studies in museums may lack transfer to the bedside, would the same not apply to the art that is chosen here to represent principles? I have nothing against these artists, but what would be 'hot' for contemporary medical students may be to study contemporary performance artists asking questions about the status of the body, particularly the medicalized body, including the gendered body, the HIV positive body, the dysmorphic body, self-harming, the drugged body, the body in pain and so forth.

Such artists include Gina Pane, Orlan, Stelarc and Ron Athey; while visual artists such as Christine Borland, mentioned above, ask questions about medicine's depersonalization processes. Borland's (2006) body of work over more than two decades has consistently wrestled with issues that arise from the medical culture's view of the 'normal' body. Students may relate more easily to a comix/graphic artist such as Ian Williams (2014), who is also a general practitioner. Orlan (www.orlan.eu) does not deal with abstractions and principles of close noticing but with shaping the body through surgery to challenge gender stereotypes and to illustrate the 'theatre' or performative side of surgery. Ron Athey (www.ronathey.com) performs the body perceived as abject – the marginalized and stigmatized body. Ian Williams (www.graphicmedicine.com) confesses that your local GP is likely to be neurotic or carries symptoms, but is not allowed to expose or explore these. With the singular exception of Paul Macneill (2011), commentators have failed to inquire into why the arts employed generally in the medical humanities are 'benign and servile in relation to medicine'. As Macneill points out, treating the arts as a mere 'resource' rather than a vehicle for critique is both missing an opportunity and demeaning. As we have seen, Macneill calls, perhaps inappropriately, for a more 'muscular' approach to utilizing the arts in medical humanities.

Artists and doctors collaborate in 'thinking aloud'

Starting with the kinds of assumptions that Macneill prompts, some research had already been carried out well before Macneill's observations, linking close noticing and medicine. Alan Bleakley and colleagues (Bleakley 2004; Bleakley *et al.* 2003a, 2003b) describe a research project on 'ways of seeing' that attempts to anatomize and theorize sense perception within the domain of medical expertise, where visual artists and doctors are paired in 'thinking aloud' conversations. The method involved analysis of videotaped conversations between artists and physicians about profession-specific ways of looking and seeing, where artists visited clinics and physicians visited studios.

One element that emerged from this research was how expertise may either reach a comfortable plateau that becomes habitual, or may continue to develop as a generative connoisseurship. Experienced physicians said that comparing their work with that of experienced artists had challenged their comfort zones and rekindled their passion in the artistry of visual diagnosis. In Japanese, a distinction is made between 'ordinary seeing' and 'active seeing'. In English, this is equivalent to the distinction between mere 'looking' and active 'seeing'. 'Active seeing' in Japanese is used, for example, to describe a doctor looking at a patient. The same word (*miru*) also means 'to have sexual relations' and a 'stolen look'. This deeper kind of seeing is then eroticized – *passionate*, or life giving. Experts said that although they had developed considerable skill in close noticing, this often felt less than passionate and talking with artists has rekindled the desire to 'look again' with a fresh eye.

Can doctors then benefit from collaboration with artists in inquiry into clinical judgement practices and will this lead to a new identity construction? Bleakley and colleagues' methodology draws on traditions of collaborative action research, participative inquiry (Reason 1994) and appreciative inquiry (Cooperrider and Whitney 1999). Appreciative inquiry emphasises that while practice may already be good, continuous reflection, as an art in itself, can bring further enhancements. This approach also stresses passionate, heart-felt involvement with subject matter as a legitimate research stance, rather than cool detachment. The methodology is not grounded in emancipatory or personal growth agendas, but interested rather in identity constructions through resistance to regulative and normative discourses, following the trajectory of Michel Foucault's late work (Bernauer and Rasmussen 1994) where processes of 'aesthetic self-forming' are described.

The dominant discourse of technical medical judgement marginalizes aesthetic approaches to practice and constructs doctors as technicians. Where artists are familiar with forming images, doctors may form aesthetic identities through appreciation of clinical images, as a basis to expertise in a specialty. In this project, the artists' interventions have focused the doctors on the inherent aesthetic of the 'informational' images (Elkins 1999) they habitually meet with an objectifying medical gaze. The artists also model the value of generation, rather than reduction, of uncertainty.

The project was unusual in its interest in identity formation as a research outcome and added another twist to this approach where it shifted the focus of the doctor's identity away from personality towards how the doctor gives metaphorical personality to the presenting clinical image. Typically, a specialty such as pathology strives to reduce uncertainty at all costs, but in the process may lose the tolerance for ambiguity that is the hallmark of deliberate practice (Fish and Coles 1998). Where clinical judgement is restricted to, and by, technical procedure and protocol, and then loses its 'artistry' (Schön 1991), we can characterize this as being authoritarian towards the image. Less reflective 'image authoritarians' may be more prone to classic diagnostic errors, such as premature closure, by not seeking alternative or innovative explanations (Schmidt and Boshuizen 1993).

Research data were gathered in a number of ways and in differing forums:

- Public seminar and debate and conference presentations: these formal settings, documented through videotaping, audiotaping and notes, involved framing of typical episodes of clinical and aesthetic judgements in the visual domain, to which invited audiences of doctors and artists responded.
- 'Thinking aloud' work-based exchanges (artists to clinics and doctors to studios). These allowed practitioners to swap live practices and 'stories'. The deliberative and reflective processes were documented through extensive notes.
- Doctors talking to clinical images such as X-rays, pathology slides and photographs of skin conditions. These model typical clinical formulation responses and were audiotaped and transcribed.
- Minuted review and round table discussions progressing models and insights with the project convenor, a medical educator and psychologist. This was an iterative process.

Data were triangulated with a literature review and expert opinion culled from presentations within the local medical and medical education community. Data analysis followed grounded theory principles in coding, categorizing and model building. Five kinds of practice were noted:

1 *Habitual practice.* Experts may see what they habitually expect to see and not notice what is there, so that 'perceptual readiness' occludes fresh seeing. This calls for an outside challenge to 'describe what you see, not what you expect to see'.

2 *Saturated practice.* The expert eye may become tired through over exposure to everyday material and needs to be refreshed. This is linked with (1) above, and calls for an outside challenge to reframe the conventions of 'looking', 'seeing' and 'saying' within the specialty. Doctors may need to be reintroduced to the conventions of their looking through reframing involving the interventions of visual artists.

3 *Restricted practice.* Experts may fail to gain a balance between an evidence-based, technical approach, and idiosyncratic practice artistry. The latter allows for greater tolerance of ambiguity and for innovation. It promotes a more flexible diagnostic capability under conditions of complexity, uncertainty, ambiguity, uniqueness and ethical conflict. Practitioners who employ such artistry tend to be interested in the value of heuristics as well as scientific objectivity, but also are more likely to collaborate with others in reaching judgements.

4 *Aesthetic practice.* This is a logical extension of (3) above and calls for an explicit acceptance that the work of diagnosis needs an educated sensibility of discrimination between qualities. This is an aesthetic, not a technical, dimension, although it is informed by technical (scientific) knowledge. Key here is the forming of an aesthetic identity as a 'connoisseur'. Second, where such connoisseurship is of informational

images, the aesthetic dimension can be extended to such images, so that the traditional distinction between informational, non-expressive or non-art, images and 'art' images is collapsed. Third, experts judiciously draw on a range of visual heuristics that offer vivid similitudes and metaphors, referring the clinical image back to a natural referent (for example 'strawberry gallbladder' – see Figure 6.3). This tacit storehouse of images and metaphors prepares and enhances perception and then diagnostic acumen. Such a focus is characteristically avoided in traditional continuing education in the medical specialties.

5   *Ethical practice*. This is a logical extension of (4) above. Sensitivity to isolated matter of the body (an X-ray image, a pathology specimen, a photograph of a skin condition) is extended as a humanizing move to embed that abstracted clinical interest and judgement back into the lives (and deaths) of patients. Such active movement between isolated sign, symptom and bodily matter or image and the phenomenological realities of patients is an active component in the forming of a doctor's identity as an ethical practitioner. This would offer a challenge to the traditional diagnostic gaze that dehumanizes or objectifies.

Democratizing the medical gaze in medicine

Close noticing, as argued above, is not simply naïve looking, but is a historically, culturally and socially formed process that can be conceived as capital, owned by experts and distributed by them according to structural rules of power. The diagnostic looking, or 'gaze', of the doctor, has been widely studied and debated since its description by Michel Foucault (1989)

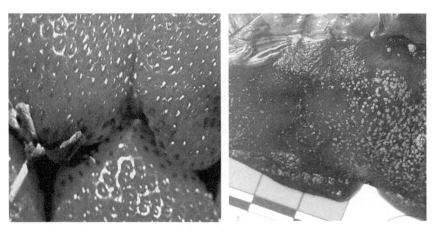

Figure 6.3 Strawberry gallbladder: fatty deposits in the gallbladder (right) resemble a ripe strawberry in appearance (left)

Source: Dr Joe Mathew/Dr Robert Marshall

as a gaze of power or authority as well as a scientific gaze. Bleakley, Bligh and Browne (2011) and Bleakley (2014) argue that the democratization of the medical gaze through the rise of interprofessional teamwork and patient-centred practices, serves to distribute the capital of the gaze among a wider group of stakeholders.

Further, the basis upon which the medical gaze is learned, that of dissection, is obviously dissolved in medical schools that do not include dissection as part of the process of learning anatomy, such as Peninsula Medical School, UK and its subsequent Plymouth University and Exeter University schools (McLachlan *et al.* 2004; McLachlan and de Bere 2004). Grant (2014) notes that some Canadian and North American medical schools are considering learning anatomy through limited dissection such as prosections. But the argument concerning distribution of the medical gaze has not yet entered this debate that is still centred mainly on functional availability of cadavers rather than a more sophisticated pedagogical debate about what is the best way to learn anatomy, rather than the most effective initiation rite for medical students, or how to bring those students into intimate contact with death (Bishop 2011).

The work of Bleakley and colleagues described above explicitly sets out to challenge the dominance of the medical gaze through democratization, by introducing an equal debating voice – that of the artist. The medical gaze or 'perception', the key performance element described in Michel Foucault's (1989) account of the birth of the clinic (modern diagnostic medicine in the teaching hospital), rests on an idiosyncratic, socialized connection between 'seeing' and 'saying'. The act of looking deep into bodies through literal dissection is linked with an exclusive diagnostic vocabulary that affords an imperialism of the gaze. What the doctor says is 'true' (knowledge is power) and this is reinforced by it being said in the doctor's exclusive professional domain, the clinic (authority), to reinforce identities (that of the doctor and that of the patient). The 'gaze' is then not confined to literal sense-based diagnosis, but offers a metaphor for professional solidarity, making sense of medicine as a cultural discourse.

Sensibility capital in medicine, then, is actually a complex web of forces and not simple a repository of knowledge and skills. At the heart of this web is the identity construction of the doctor as specialist, whose connoisseurship is perceived by others especially laypersons, as magical. This of course can inflate doctors' importance – the focus of a raft of anthropological and literary studies. For a recent confessional account of how one famous neurosurgeon has wrestled with the issue of self-importance, see Henry Marsh's (2014) *Do No Harm: Stories of Life, Death and Brain Surgery.*

Aesthetic ways of knowing in healthcare

Every clinical educationalist is surely familiar with the ground-breaking work of Donald Schön (1991) on the 'artistry' of professional practice and

Barbara Carper (1978) on aesthetic knowing in nursing. Neither of these approaches has been formally progressed for its reference to aesthetic concerns, but has often been reduced to a frame for instrumental skills or educational technologies. An exception to this is the work of Della Fish and Colin Coles (Fish and Coles 1998) on progressing Schön's view of practical knowing (itself derived from the pragmatism of John Dewey). They translate professional 'artistry' as 'deliberative critical appreciation' of one's own practice, but explicitly ground this in ethics (moral inquiry) rather than aesthetics.

Schön's (1991) work on the development of judgement in the professions through reflective practice resulted in a description of the 'artistry' of professional practice. But Schön did not progress this idea through grounding in formal work on aesthetics (Bleakley 1999a). Subsequent work on reflective practice as personal or procedural knowing in healthcare (Freshwater and Johns 2005; Kember 2001), while referring to both Schön's notion of 'artistry' and to Carper's aesthetic way of knowing, has also not formally progressed the idea of practice artistry through grounding in aesthetic theory drawn from philosophy, cultural studies, art history and psychology. For example, work on visual intelligence and the visual mind shows a healthy interdisciplinary collaboration between scientists, social scientists, artists and art historians (Arnheim 1969; Jones and Galison 1998; Elkins 2003), but has hardly touched clinical education.

In a nursing education context, Carper (1978: 23) describes four 'fundamental patterns of knowing' informing healthcare practice: empirics or scientific knowledge; personal or self-knowledge; ethics or moral knowledge; and aesthetics, which she refers to as 'the art' of nursing. Carper refers to 'the esthetic perception of significant human experiences' (*ibid.*), appropriately formulating aesthetics as the integration of sense impressions and acts of appreciation. However, while the four ways must overlap in practice, Carper separates ethics, or moral knowing, from aesthetics, where moral knowing is 'the capacity to make choices within concrete situations involving particular moral judgements'. Moral judgement can, however, be grounded in aesthetic appreciation, where discrimination between qualities, close noticing and perceptual engagement with an Other precedes and forms the ethical act. This synthesis results in an aesthetic and ethical self-forming, or an identity construction as a sensitive and appreciative practitioner and a connoisseur of clinical symptoms (Bleakley 2004).

Jane Cioffi (2000a: 266; see also Cioffi 2000b, 2002), in a study of nurses' experiences in deciding to call for emergency assistance for patients, shows the importance of close sensory noticing of signs and symptoms: 'You can tell by looking at someone...you pick up on the little things...no warmth, bit cool'. One nurse says in the study of a patient: 'The colour is not right...could be greyish not quite greyish as that is too far...more sallow, pallid' (Cioffi 2000a: 266). Recall the nurses who made similar rapid perceptual judgements about Elaine Bromiley in the scenario described in Chapter

4, where the doctors, holding the primary sensibility capital, brushed off the nurses' advice, resulting in the death of the patient through mismanagement of an airway. Such connoisseurship, for that is what expert, close observation amounts to, has a long history. In Leviticus 13 from the Old Testament, written around 400 BCE, there is a section on 'how leprosy is to be recognized', where diagnosis is through sense-based reasoning or pattern recognition. Here, 'If the priest, looking at the place on the skin, finds that the hairs have turned white and the skin of the part affected seems shrunken compared with the rest of the skin around it, this is the scourge of leprosy'. Further, such pattern recognition is educated through use of a vocabulary of resemblances between symptom and natural referents. Rabbis, who were the healers, identified over 30 shades of white from natural referents, including 'wool', 'quicklime' and the 'skin of an egg'. Are there similar colour charts or vocabularies for medical students today?

As cognitive psychology research (Lakoff and Johnson 1980, 1999; Way 1994) indicates, the most complex expert decisions are grounded in thinking in metaphors, as schemata or coding constituting tacit knowing. In clinical reasoning in medicine, pattern recognition of a complex of symptoms can be explained as a match between the presenting patient and an 'illness script' that is a sophisticated encapsulation of knowledge as a network of metaphors and resemblances (Boshuizen and Schmidt 1995). Expert judgement is often referred to as 'intuitive' or based on 'gut feeling', descriptors which tend to make the process mysterious rather than transparent. Advances in cognitive psychology that model representations of knowledge serve, however, to partly demystify expert knowing. Reber's (1993) rigorous experimental psychology research demonstrates how people learn and store rules that they do not comprehend explicitly, but which help them to more expertly perform linguistic acts. People learn tacit transformational rules that they cannot explain but can nevertheless mobilise. Reber calls such learning 'implicit', the storage of knowledge 'tacit' and the site of storage 'the cognitive unconscious'.

Gaston Bachelard (1964, 1983, 1986) refers to the same site of knowledge representation as a 'poetic imagination' (see also Bleakley 1999b), offering an aesthetic descriptor. Such 'sites' in themselves are metaphors and their naming reveals a rhetorical strategy at work. Reber's technical description persuades us of the 'reality' of such a cognitive site of knowledge representation, where Bachelard's description appears more abstract and perhaps less convincing technically but more attractive aesthetically.

Abductive judgement

Charles Peirce (1931) described knowing in the senses as 'abduction' or abductive reasoning, to distinguish it from inductive and deductive reasoning (Schleifer and Vannatta 2013). Inductive reasoning involves working forward from evidence to set up a hypothesis. Deductive reasoning involves testing a hypothesis through gathering evidence. In Peirce's description, abductive reasoning is the very moment of the generation of the hypothesis itself: 'the operations by which theories…are given birth'. Hallyn (1993) argues that hypothesis generation in science is a form of poetic imagination that can be distinguished from inductive and deductive reasoning that are the logical elements of scientific thinking. Deduction refers to the consequences arising from accepting or rejecting a hypothesis through consideration of evidence. Induction refers to agreement or disagreement between reality and a hypothesis or theory that is evidence generation. Abduction refers to reasoning in, not beyond, the senses. Abduction is essential to the progress of science as it refers to the possible rather than the evident. The possible is the stuff of poetic imagination.

Hypothesis forming is then intuitive and poetic – a hypothesis has the status of a 'heuristic fiction', acting like a metaphor. Metaphors produce necessary ambiguity in thinking that feeds back to, and enriches, perception. Without ambiguity, we would become authoritarian in our thinking, refusing alternatives and failing to appreciate contradictions. In reducing ambiguity, science may claim rigour, but without ambiguity and its consequent poetics, science has no vigour.

We have seen that experts make clinical judgements based on pattern recognition. While this is instrumentalized as System I (or non-analytical) reasoning (Norman and Eva 2010), such judgements can be described as intuitive. They are based on tacit knowing and hence, by definition, cannot easily be made explicit. While expertise is gained through experience, the point of a structured education is to intensify such experience and get the best out of each patient encounter. The paradox for experts, as explained earlier, is that they cannot directly pass on to novices the fruits of their experience because they cannot readily frame tacit knowing in an explicit way. Novices must continue to use analytic rather than intuitive clinical reasoning, where they do not have the necessary experience upon which to reason in the senses, because the senses are not formed by appropriate tacit knowledge representation such as a set of metaphors or narratives.

Abraham Verghese describes such abductive reasoning, in this case based in the sense of smell, on a teaching ward round:

> Smells registered in a primitive part of the brain, the ancient limbic system. I liked to think that from there they echoed and led me to think 'typhoid' or 'rheumatic fever' without ever being able to explain why. [However,] I taught students to avoid the 'blink-of-an-eye' diagnosis… the snap judgement. But secretly, I trusted my primitive brain, trusted the animal snout.
>
> (Verghese 1999: 299)

Verghese echoes the fears of many clinical teachers, that students should avoid pattern recognition or Type I/System I reasoning. Norman and Eva

(2010) however encourage early support of System I (pattern recognition) reasoning as long as students are exposed to multiple examples. As we shall see, it is not simply exposure that facilitates recognition of symptoms, but the nature of the patterns themselves, as resemblances, where the more striking the resemblance (strawberry gallbladder, bamboo spine), the easier the recognition.

The 'snap judgement' in the senses is what the philosopher George Santayana calls 'animal faith'. Bleakley (1999b) terms this the 'animalizing imagination' – it is a reflective judgement in the senses that is the intuitive moment of formulating a hypothesis. James Hillman (1972b) describes animal faith as a reflection, but 'neither after nor even during the event... Rather *it is the manner in which an act is carried through*' (italics added). Hillman calls this 'style', effectively claiming an aesthetic home for pattern recognition, as any artist would suggest. But style goes wider than pattern recognition, into pattern formation as habits of the heart, or typical ways of responding. This has important resonance for the aesthetic of healthcare practice. It is not simply the technical accomplishment of the act, but also the style that matters, as the manner in which the act is carried through. An act of care must be caring, must engage the patient intentionally as 'cared for'. A judgement should have form as well as content.

Resemblances

In medicine there is a large vocabulary of resemblances that can act as heuristics or short cuts to diagnosis. A 'strawberry gallbladder' (where the gallbladder has excess fat) uncannily resembles a ripe strawberry (Figure 6.3); a 'nutmeg liver' (where the liver is engorged with blood) resembles a cut nutmeg; an 'apple core lesion' on an X-ray showing colonic carcinoma shows a characteristic apple core shape (Figure 6.2), and so forth. Experts do not like to encourage novices to resort to heuristics, preferring them to develop an analytical, differential diagnostic method in the absence of clinical experience. Experts themselves, however, regularly rely on pattern recognition as a short cut. Recall Verghese's account above – 'I taught students to avoid the "blink-of-an-eye" diagnosis...the snap judgement. But secretly, I trusted my primitive brain, trusted the animal snout.'

Of course, heuristics bring the danger of bias, and this is well documented for the professions in general (Kahneman *et al.* 1982) and nursing in particular (Palmer 2003; Thompson and Dowding 2002; Fonteyn and Fisher 1995). Fonteyn and Fisher (1995) argue that heuristics are particularly important in nursing judgements that they characterize as less focused upon 'diagnosis and hypothesis generation' and more upon the abilities to 'distinguish between relevant and irrelevant patient data...and to make decisions that assist in accomplishing the overall treatment plan for each patient'. But this description does not address the rapidly changing face of nursing where 'Nurses will increasingly be asked to diagnose disease'

(Thompson and Dowding 2002). Indeed, it does not account for the host of everyday unspoken sense-based judgements that nurses make about patients that have stronger or weaker diagnostic consequences. Emphasizing the potential biases and errors arising from the use of heuristics may be over-stated, or may be overshadowed by the larger spectre of the need to conform to evidence-based approaches. Shielding novices from engaging with pattern recognition early in their careers may deny the development of sense-based judgement acumen and certainly its acceleration or 'hothous-ing', for there is a further element to abductive reasoning that must now be discussed that is desirable to learn early in a healthcare career.

The poetic imagination

Abduction is reflective judgement in the senses. How can sense-based judge-ment be 'reflective'? Surely, what Verghese describes as the use of the 'animal snout' is by definition pre-reflective? Hillman's (1972) and Bleakley's (1999a) arguments for a reflective sensing that displays as style – the manner in which an act is carried out – were noted earlier. This collapses reflection into perception, where ethical deliberation is preceded and formed by aesthetic appreciation.

The quote earlier from Nightingale is still the orthodoxy a century later. We still tend to see sense-based observation and reflection as different epis-temological activities, whereas Nightingale suggested that 'Observation tells us the fact, reflection the meaning of the fact' (in McDonald 2009: 723). By separating sensation, perception and reflection, we miss the integrated or holistic nature of expert judgement. James Gibson's (1979) 'ecological' model of perception suggests that an individual is not a passive recipient of sense data. Rather, the environment 'affords' such data. The environment acts on the individual to shape perception and to 'capture' attention through pattern and form. Thus, repeated exposure to patients with similar presenting signs and symptoms 'affords' a perceptual depth in the expert healthcare practitioner, who more easily recognizes such patterns than the novice, because the environment has shaped her perception.

This shaping is represented, as argued earlier, as a condensed and tacit form: metaphor, image or script (narrative) that is stimulated upon further pattern recognition or matching. Thus, an active cycle of perception is set up between the affordance of an environment (such as the presence of patients) that comes to act as an 'attractor' for the senses and forms the senses and the senses themselves that are further formed or shaped from within through a poetic imagination, an active repository that constitutes tacit knowledge. Indeed, Gibson's (1966) model also assumes that the senses do not work independently, but as systems. Pattern recognition (as accommodation to the environment) allies with a heuristic (as assimilated rule) across the senses to form clinical judgement.

Abductive reasoning is, again, not simply a passive sense-based process, but an active perceptual process in which the senses are informed and prepared by a poetic imagination that is the embodied reflective component. An example of such preparation and heightening of the senses is wine appreciation (Brochet and Dubourdieu 2001). A naïve taster simply tastes the wine and may or may not experience a variety of sensations. When told that the Californian Viognier you are about to taste will be a subtle mix of dry peach with smoky pear and lemon, on drinking the wine one's taste is already educated leading to differentiation and appreciation. You are now on the road to connoisseurship. In the same way, and at a simple level of resemblance, the 'strawberry gallbladder' prepares and informs the senses so that perception is heightened or educated and the diseased gallbladder is diagnosed.

Gaston Bachelard (1964, 1983, 1986) wrote a series of texts showing how the poetic imagination can prepare and enhance the senses. By the poetic imagination Bachelard means a sensibility educated or formed by culture. The arts make the ordinary extraordinary and educate us to see in new ways, preparing the senses for deeper perceptions. If we return to the nurse who is already making subtle judgements concerning how the patient looks ('The colour is not right . . . could be greyish not quite greyish as that is too far . . . more sallow, pallid'), imagine how her senses may be further educated or heightened through influence from a poetic imagination of off-greys. The aesthetic of greys can be gained from natural referents such as the palette of greys in a thunderhead, or that offered by the winter weather of northern Europe. This is enhanced through, for example, poetry that reformulates these greys of the weather; or the use of the metal lead in the work of the visual artist Anselm Kiefer, offering a range of greys as a referent. Precise referents are then established as diagnostic guides in terms of how the patient 'looks'.

Gradually, the practitioner builds a storehouse of tacit referents as metaphors, images and narratives. This is repeated in the linguistic register as aphorisms or maxims (Levine and Bleakley 2012). This tacit knowledge is enhanced enormously through organization into a poetic imagination – rich metaphors, images and stories that are readily excited in the diagnostic moment of pattern recognition to work back on the senses, enhancing perception or bringing closer noticing through differentiation and appreciation.

There is a final part to this puzzle of turning how we 'look' (surface looking) into how we 'see' diagnostically (deeper perception). We must be engaged with the patient, passionate about the work. The process of diagnostic seeing is then eroticized or given extra intensity, charged with compassion. As mentioned earlier, in Japanese, a distinction is made between 'ordinary seeing' and 'active seeing' (Elkins 1999). 'Active seeing' (*miru*) is used to describe a doctor looking at a patient. The same word (*miru*) also means 'to have sex'. This deeper seeing is then passionate or life giving. The practitioner is fully engaged by the work. 'Erotic' is not of course read literally, but acts as a metaphor for passionate engagement. This reveals an ethical layer to the model of abductive reasoning developed here. The prior technical and aesthetic elements of a diagnostic judgement may be in place, but this is completed within an overall act of care that is the ethical gesture.

The visual rhetoric of clinical practice

This chapter argues then for a formal education of what Florence Nightingale described as the 'power of attending... to one's own senses' in clinical judgement. Establishing a formal aesthetics of practice in a curriculum requires advice from experts in the field of aesthetics. However, the field of healthcare practice research can do much to help itself in developing a poetics of practice. First, as described earlier, it can formally build on the leads provided by Schön's notion of practice 'artistry' and Carper's aesthetic way of knowing. We can resist reducing artistry to functional (efficient cause) effects such as the 'training' of communication 'skills'. This merely leads us back to the technical rational 'high ground' that Schön suggests is not the best place from which to approach uncertainty, ambiguity, uniqueness and value conflicts in practice. Given that important instances of clinical judgement cannot simply be approached by technical-rational means, it is important to keep alive the study of heuristics and sense-based judgement in clinical reasoning. However, in an age of evidence-based healthcare, such forms of judgement are not developed well in the literature in comparison with technical-rational approaches such as decision analysis.

At the same time as we attempt to reduce uncertainty through fine discrimination can we not also educate for tolerance of ambiguity so that we do not slip away from the diagnostic problem at hand to invoke technical-rational decision analysis modes too early in the process of judgement? In other words, can we save the art of bedside clinical judgement from the suffocating grip of analytical decision models? The hope is to preserve close, imaginative and committed care of the patient, where compassion and sense-based judgement are two sides of the same coin. This is not to devalue the worth of decision analysis methods. Rather, again it is a plea to not lose the art of clinical judgement to such methods.

An aesthetic healthcare is sensitive, elegant and appreciative and faces up to the sublime, the terror of illness. It is, however, perhaps easier to grasp an aesthetic healthcare by what it is not: an-anaesthetic. To anaesthetize is to dull. We do not want our practices to dull or be dulling, to be habitual, or to recycle tired conventions. While we have developed a sophisticated healthcare pragmatics and ethics, the aesthetic arena has been neglected. This chapter calls for the urgent development of a sub-discipline of healthcare aesthetics. The stochastic art of practice – referred to by Martha Nussbaum at the beginning of this chapter to describe medicine – is not a mystery and can be formally educated.

7 Can narrative medicine take the strain?

Essential, not desirable

In Chapter 6 I argued that close noticing is an integral part of clinical acumen and to frustrate its early education is a mistake. In the same way, understanding and using narrative capabilities are central to clinical education. Listening to 'stories' can be extended from the verbal to noting and reading temporal signs and symptoms on the spatial body, such as rashes, coughs and lung crackles; and readings through intermediaries such as tests and imaging. Educating these aspects of close reading and close noticing is central to the medical humanities and cannot be considered to be fringe or supplementary to a medical education, but must be seen as core and integrated. The frustration or denial of such a medical humanities-infused education leads to the production of insensibility and insensitivity in medical students rather than increasing the capital of sensibility and sensitivity that is key to improving the quality of clinical work.

What is a narrative?

To 'narrate' comes from the Latin *narrare* – 'to give an account of', 'to relate or recount', but also 'to know' (*Shorter Oxford English Dictionary*). The Russian Vladimir Propp first studied the formal structure of narratives in the 1920s, demonstrating that folk tales had a common plot structure and set of functions – such as encounters between heroes and villains. Structuralists (such as Claude Lévi-Strauss) later suggested that the common narrative forms identified by the formalists such as Propp indicated that language provides a universal set of rules through which cultures generate and transmit ideas. Language thus shapes cognition or the ways we think in commonly shared, rule-bound and systematic ways. However, experimental modernist writers such as James Joyce and William Faulkner expressly upset or subverted conventions of story such as plot and, while poststructuralists follow the structuralists in accepting that language shapes thought, they suggest that the search for universal rules of how such structuring happens is fruitless and that attention should be turned away from meta-narratives – archetypes and universal forms – to the differences shown in the proliferation of localized or 'small' narratives (*petit récits*) (Lyotard 1984).

The value of the shift from structuralist thinking to post-structuralist thinking is that it focuses us on the value and meaning of difference at a local level. Thus, we can instantly appreciate that common, public uses of language to talk about health and illness are quite different, for example, from the specialist language that medicine uses to describe symptoms and disease. This difference in language use causes a gap between patients' experiences and those of doctors, where meanings are lost in translation across the two communities (Marshall and Bleakley 2013). What is then important is to respect such difference through democratizing differing stories. This does not mean that we should ignore structuralism's lessons. Some 'big' stories are very helpful in making sense of individuals' everyday stories. For example, later on in this chapter I will show how understanding genres in story (such as the epic, tragic, comic and lyrical) can help us to better appreciate how medicine as a culture may be restructured in the project of democratizing medicine and doctoring.

A good example of the local case of how narratives may be structured is what Kathryn Montgomery Hunter called 'doctors' stories' (Hunter 1991b). Hunter (now Kathryn Montgomery) wrote the first book on 'narrative medicine', focusing primarily not on patients' stories (which later became the trend), but on how medical knowledge is structured narratively. Hunter famously claimed that medicine is not a science per se, but a 'science using' activity in which informing scientific knowledge is wound into a narrative practice. Just as patients tell stories, so doctors have their own conventions of turning those stories into medical stories, structured as 'cases'. Cases in turn are – because they are embedded in a cognitive process of diagnostic reasoning – embedded in a genre, that of the 'detective story', or 'sleuthing', so that the use of cues and clues is endemic to the structure of cases.

Hunter recognized that there is an incommensurable gap between patients' stories and doctors' stories. Yet, it is precisely this gap that may offer the opportunity for medicine to work at a technical level. However, this gap cannot grow too large, otherwise medical interventions become iatrogenic, or produce symptoms themselves. While doctors and their patients share a common humanity (and one of the central features of this is storytelling), in professional settings doctors understanding patients is a little like an anthropologist studying an 'other' culture. There is much room for misunderstanding and misinterpretation of the 'other' (the patient) by the anthropologist (the doctor). The first of these is objectification – patients becoming known and addressed by their symptoms only.

Kathryn Hunter (1991b: 27) suggested that doctors read the patient as 'text' (Bleakley *et al.* 2011). She borrowed this, as she acknowledges, from a 1904 essay by Sir William Osler, who says 'It is a safe rule to have no teaching without a patient for a text, and the best teaching is that taught by the patient himself' (in Bliss 1999: 238). Doctors must then become close, attentive readers. Yet where do they formally learn such capabilities? This has been left more to the vagaries of a haphazard apprenticeship rather than a carefully designed educational experience in which textual readings (say a bedside encounter) are formally analysed in a briefing and debriefing set-up, where issues such as text, subtext, intertext and context are discussed. Such a pedagogical context could involve a clinician working with a literature scholar – as Margaret Edson (1999) shows in her play *W;t*, the thought processes of the English literature scholar and the senior oncologist could readily be brought into fruitful conversation. For example, how the patient 'presents' (text) is not just confined to symptom but goes wider, to the patient's concerns (context). What is the patient not saying or revealing (subtext) and how is this accessed? How might the conversations between the textual worlds (what is said, left unsaid, and performed non-verbally) of the patient and healthcare teams be understood (intertexts)?

Hunter (1991b: 131) then concludes that 'the medical retelling of the patient's story' is a double-edged sword. It 'has potential for healing and for harm'. Contemporary anthropologists and ethnographers are in no doubt that, in relaying the stories of the 'other' culture, they do not seek truths, but the ability to tell a moral and satisfying story (Geertz 1973). So doctors must seek to translate back and forth between the worlds of their patients and the relatively closed world of medicine in ways that honour the patient. This is achieved in three ways: first, recognition of the gap between the patient's story and doctors' subsequent stories; second, constructing a mutual story carefully through close listening in the consultation and close noticing in the physical examination; and third, restoring the subsequent medical story to the patient in a way that is not simply understood but also appreciated. Just as we grant doctors permission for intimate examinations and intimate knowledge of our lives so, as patients, we should expect that such exchanges are not misappropriated or abused, but are reciprocated.

The clinical encounter then provides a rather unusual dynamic for story-telling exchanges. In the reciprocal narratives of the clinical encounter, a patient first tells a story to a doctor. This is framed within a set of quite hardened cultural conventions in which the patient submits to the doctor's perceived professional capacity, often expressed as a relationship of power and authority in favour of the doctor. Further, while the patient 'presents' the story of his or her 'chief concern', symptom(s) or condition, the doctor is geared up to 'take a history' through a formalized and habitual routine as a set of questions ('where does it hurt?', 'when was the last onset?', 'has there been any bleeding?'). Taking a psychiatric history too follows a conventional format. Despite the attempts of some medical schools to teach their students how to 'receive' a history, 'taking' a medical history remains a dominant convention again suggesting a power differential at work. Moreover, medical schools do not stress enough that a large proportion of an encounter with a patient will be psychological and not physical, especially in general practice (and obviously in psychiatry). Further, stories may be by proxy, or heavily contextualised, such as parents telling their children's stories in paediatrics; and they are non-verbal as well as verbal. Stories may be largely reminiscences (care of the elderly) and compromised or curtailed (cognitively challenged or intellectually disabled patients).

As the patient tells his or her story (there may also be an intermediary involved such as a translator, carer, or an adult reframing a child's account), the doctor gradually tells a story back to the patient as a first formulation of a diagnosis or differential diagnosis, with an aim to provide a final diagnosis and treatment plan. This may involve referral to a specialist, tests, prescribed drug regimes, lifestyle advice, referral to a counsellor, dietician, physiotherapist and so forth. We thus have a mesh, or a reciprocal relationship between the patient's 'lay' story and the doctor's story as a professional and ethical response, where roles of teller and listener interchange. Intimacy may enter the dialogue if the patient and doctor are familiar with each other such as a regular patient at a GP surgery, such that side-talk is introduced to 'oil' the communication and regulate emotional exchanges. The kinds of language that are used will depend on the level of intimacy. However, the doctor will use specialist language ('it's probably atherosclerosis, but only an angiogram will tell us') in his or her story, translating across to lay language where the patient asks for clarification or looks confused ('it's probably a clogging up of a blood vessel, but only testing for that will let us know').

The doctor, at a second level, may then engage in another storytelling or narrative sequence that is highly formalised – passing on the patient's 'case' to colleagues in a clinical education context. Here, the case narrative follows conventions such as high compression (brevity) and use of technical language. The 'case' – possibly presented at ground rounds for hospital settings and general practice meetings or psychiatric team meetings for community settings – turns the patient's 'chief concern' into the 'chief complaint', where there is focus only on symptom, diagnosis, treatment plan and prognosis. The chief complaint narrative may bleach out the chief concern narrative with which this sequence of stories started, medicalizing the patient and changing the narrative for convenience. It is the chief complaint narrative that is then formalised into the patient's notes (actually the doctors' and healthcare teams' notes) rather than the 'chief complaint' and the 'chief concern' forming a parallel pair of notes.

These narrative forms and levels – the patient's story, the doctor's response in the clinical encounter and the doctor's recounting in the highly conventionalized case presentation – have been widely studied in terms of embodying aspects of the traditional forms of narrative described by the formalists and structuralists, such as characters, plot and tropes (style, achieved through use of linguistic devices or figures of speech such as rhetoric, genres, metonymy and metaphor). I will describe and illustrate the uses of such tropes throughout this chapter.

A story or narrative is set within a historical, cultural and social context that determines how relationships between speakers, listeners and stories shall be structured. In preliterate societies, such as archaic Greece, the oral tradition of the stories that were later written down by Homer as the *Iliad* and *Odyssey* was highly structured. Storytellers relied on memory and audiences responded through knowledge of familiar structures and characters, although some improvisation was possible. A similar formulaic approach applies in the structured case presentation of medicine (Marshall and Bleakley 2011).

Novelists and poets, however, capture the far wider range of potential narrative presentations that are also familiar from idiosyncratic patient presentations in GP's surgeries, clinics, and emergency departments. For example, how does the author present a character and place the reader in relationship to that character in anticipation of an unfolding plot? In possibly the greatest American novel, *Moby Dick*, through the first sentence Herman Melville grabs the reader's attention in the most striking and unexpected way: 'Call me Ishmael'. Immediately, you, the reader, are drawn into an intimate and trusting relationship with the storyteller, who later introduces the chief protagonists. The three words of introduction offers no more than an exclamation point, a model of minimalism. How, for example, does your general practitioner greet you?

James Joyce's *Finnegan's Wake*, written over 17 years and first published in 1939, is widely regarded as the prototype for experimental writing and complex language play, yet it has the simplest of narrative forms – a circular loop. So the novel (actually a metonymic chain of word play) finishes as 'A way a lone a lost a last a loved a long the'. The first page of the novel begins 'riverrun, past Eve and Adam's, from swerve of shore to bend of bay, brings us by a commodious vicus of recirculation back to Howth Castel and Environs'. Thus, the 'recirculation', a river running (the Liffey), as the last line brings us back to read *Finnegan's Wake* anew: 'A way a lone a lost a last a loved a long the riverrun, past Eve and Adam's, from swerve of shore to bend of bay, brings us by a commodious vicus of recirculation back to Howth Castel and Environs'. We are situated by Joyce in a real place near Dublin, but in a timeless way (past Eve and Adam's) encapsulating a model for narrative as a timeless form, a circular loop. Recall – in Chapter 5 on types of creativity – the original Garden of Eden myth presenting a ready-made world for discovery within a time zone of the eternal return.

The doctor treating the patient may inhabit this Joycean trope of the Eternal Return, seeing medicine as an enclosed and self-referential culture to which she has gained access. The patient too enters this trope of the Eternal Return where the doctor has seen so many of these presentations before. The patient becomes a 'type', treated through pattern recognition or Type I clinical reasoning (Chapter 6). The doctor's clinical reasoning mindset is one of matching up the last line of the novel with the first to return to the familiarity of Howth Castle and Environs, the closed world of Dublin city that is an example of the archetype of all places – Eden or 'Eve and Adam's', Dublin standing for this patient's particular suffering of a bad dose of influenza that is a type or pattern or 'Eve and Adam's' instantly recognizable to all clinicians and where they feel at home. But what is not apparent is, first, the doctor's thinking process made plain to the patient; and second, the complexity of that doctor's thinking process made plain to herself, or the tacit dimension to her use of 'Intuition in Medicine' (Braude 2012). The patient, of course, has not read the medical version of *Finnegan's Wake*.

Hillel Braude (2012: 120) draws on the work of Alvan Feinstein to suggest that clinical reasoning has a tacit or intuitive dimension that is built up from experience of many, similar, patient encounters for particular disease and illness categories. In Chapter 6, we saw how such examples were grouped as a series of exemplars for experts rather than a prototype, the cognitive mechanism of novices, thus maintaining focus on the individual patient as a series (idiographic approach) rather than the typical, or averaged, patient of population studies (nomothetic).

Braude's approach avoids talking about 'narrative' or 'story', preferring to represent embodied and tacit medical knowledge in terms of Venn diagrams and 'precise clinical language derived from observation and not deductive inference', where 'clinical epistemology must develop a richly descriptive language that is both scientifically reproducible and thick enough to match the passion-filled domain of clinical medicine'. This approach challenges the common accusation that what medicine teaches through the cultivation and ritual of case presentations is reductive. Braude suggests that this is not the case – the 'reduction' is invisible as it refers to tacit or implicit knowledge accessed through 'intuition' and 'abductive reasoning' (see Chapter 6). There is nothing mystical about intuition – it is the process of calling forth embodied and tacit knowledge structures held in memory storage as a response to certain patterned cues. David Bohm (2002) modelled what he calls an 'implicate order' that can reproduce itself at the quantum level as well as the level of consciousness – a spot of ink is placed on glycerine in a revolving container and the glycerine is then wound. Eventually the ink becomes a fine thread and then disappears as an implicate order – fully wound in to the glycerine. The revolving container is then wound in the opposite direction and the ink spot is recovered.

A specialist may hold a well-developed tacit pattern knowledge of 'acute rheumatic fever' that can be represented as a Venn diagram of overlapping constituents (severe carditis or inflammation of the heart, carditis, chorea or involuntary movements, arthritis and arthralgia or joint pain). Overlaps between these conditions produce a local narrative of rich descriptions. However, medicine teaches medical students and junior doctors to present these thick and rich descriptions in minimal ways. This, as pointed out earlier, is akin to the visual and literary art forms of minimalism, in which the appearance of a stripped-back object or utterance does not mean that the thought behind it or the passions it may evoke are not rich and complex. Minimalism, like Kathryn Montgomery's appropriation of Holmesian sleuthing, is a favourite genre of medicine because it bypasses unnecessary elaboration. We 'get' the picture of James Joyce's *Finnegan's Wake* as an Eternal Return to a staging post, or familiar world (the environs of Dublin, the Garden of Eden, the hospital ward, the consulting room, the patient's presenting symptom as omphalos or centre of the world) without having to recite the whole, complex book. This does not mean, however, that we have not learned the contents of the book in our apprenticeship, through our encounters with patient's stories and their encounters with developing medical knowledge, now wound into the glycerine of our minds or stored tacitly as 'scripts'.

By contrast, imagine if medicine were practised in the manner that another great innovator in Modernist writing besides James Joyce, William Faulkner, wrote. This is the first paragraph of *Absalom, Absalom!*:

> From a little after two oclock until almost sundown of the long still hot weary dead September afternoon they sat in what Miss Coldfield still called the office because her father had called it that – a dim hot airless room with the blinds all closed and fastened for forty-three summers because when she was a girl someone had believed that light and moving air carried heat and that dark was always cooler, and which (as the sun shone fuller and fuller on that side of the house) became latticed with yellow slashes full of dust motes which Quentin thought of as being flecks of the dead old dried paint itself blown inwards from the scaling blinds as wind might have blown them.
>
> (Faulkner 1936)

In Joyce we have an epic sweep in the connection between the final and first lines. In Faulkner there is already tragedy in the air – keeping the light out, a feeling of chronic decay sustained as a single, interminable sentence that literally takes your breath away in the telling and attention to detail – both exhausting and exhaustive. Both Joyce and Faulkner capture what patients may bring to consultations with their doctors – time stretched to an eternity in chronic suffering. Yet doctors are trained to respond with the crisp, let's-get-to-the-point greeting of Melville's 'Call me Ishmael' and the tight universal myth of Joyce's Eternal Return through a set of tacit medical scripts, expressed as a to-the-point connection between symptoms and diagnosis. There is no time for the exhaustive detail Faulkner would want us to appreciate. And yet, surely this detail has to be acknowledged, because this is the world that the patient brings to the consultation. Further, this detail is actually the webbed architecture of a tacit medical diagnostic script.

Narrative, according to Schleifer and Vannatta (2013), has the following features: a sequence of events, an end, recognizable agents, and a witness who learns from experience or who is concerned about the end of the narrative. Narratives are both articulated and received. Time in a narrative is then often split between when the story happened and the telling of the story, which may be much later. Even children recognize 'ill-formed' narratives as 'stories' (*ibid.*: 95) suggesting that 'narrative knowledge' is a 'cognitive inheritance'.

Kathryn Montgomery Hunter's insight, now almost taken for granted, is that medicine is a tale of two stories – the patient's and the doctor's – characterized by differing approaches to uncertainty: 'Medicine, then, is a science-using, judgement-based practice committed to the knowledge and care of human illness and characterized by its varied and ingenious defences against uncertainty' (Hunter 1991b: 47), where patients' stories are laced with uncertainty. Doctors, then, need what Rita Charon (2006), an experienced doctor herself, came to call 'narrative competence' to engage these differing approaches to uncertainty and ambiguity. Charon (*ibid.*: vii) has tirelessly argued that doctors need to acquire more than a passing acquaintance with narrative in medicine, so that medicine is 'practiced with the narrative competence to recognize, absorb, interpret, and be moved by the stories of illness'.

Charon (2006: 155–74) inaugurated the educational practice of the 'parallel chart', where students write a chart of their experiences with patients, such as what the patient brought up for them in terms of associations or memories. The parallel chart is the first step towards students learning to hold two imaginations at once – the technical imagination of the doctor treating a patient and that of the flesh-and-blood feeling person who is attending to the needs of another fellow human being. This requires dual mastery of technical, medical narrative and everyday or lay story.

Paul Ricouer defines a lay story technically:

> a sequence of actions and experiences done or undergone by a certain number of people, whether real or imaginary. These people are presented either in situations that change or as reacting to such change. In turn, these changes reveal hidden aspects of the situation and the people involved, and engender a new predicament which calls for thought, action or both.
>
> (Ricoeur 1990: 150)

A story has a plot ('a sequence of actions and experiences'), usually with a crisis or turning point ('situations that change' to 'engender a new predicament which calls for thought, action or both'); and characters (a plot is 'done or undergone by a certain number of people, whether real or imaginary'). The gripping thing about stories is that after the crisis or turning point, very unpredictable things may happen (stories 'reveal hidden aspects of the situation and the people involved, and engender a new predicament'). Therefore, close listening to stories requires tolerance of ambiguity. While telling stories can be therapeutic (it can also be distressing and excessive or indulgent telling of particular stories can be symptomatic of mental illness), listening to stories can be therapeutic too. Medical students and doctors, however, have to listen to many stories professionally without necessarily being allowed to tell their own, intimately.

Again, medicine is a stressful occupation with the highest rates of suicide, suicidal ideation and drug and alcohol abuse across the professions (Dyrbye *et al.* 2008; British Medical Association 2012). A 2012 UK General Medical Council report detailed 1,384 doctors who had been assessed for health concerns over the past five years, including around half abusing alcohol and drugs and half with mental health problems. Female doctors are particularly prone to depression. The Practitioner Health Programme – a confidential service for sick doctors – recently had 554 referrals over five years, 85 per cent of which were mental health problems. Doctors are, however, resistant to seeking help. A recent NHS health survey questioned a sample of 2,500 doctors in Birmingham, UK, where only 13 per cent said that they would seek help for addiction or mental health problems, and 87 per cent said that they would self-medicate rather than seek help or advice. Another survey showed that 81 per cent of doctors fear being stigmatized should colleagues discover that they were suffering from mental health problems or addiction. Doctors, then, are 'at risk' and need supportive 'recovery' options, one of which is telling their stories to professional listeners.

Rita Charon in particular suggests that it is not enough for doctors to simply be aware that they practice narrative-based medicine. This would produce reflection of a kind but may not have impact upon practice. Rather, they must see narrative as part of the expertise they should obtain as professional, ethical practitioners. If practising 'non-technical' medicine – communication and teamwork – is as important as the technical or scientific practice, then doctors must gain 'narrative competence' and move on from basic reflection to a deeper reflexivity – inquiring into how their levels of narrative capability may be affecting their ability to offer responsive, creative and imaginative care. Practising storied medicine must be informed fully by principles of narrative and knowledge of the chief concerns of patients, just as practising safe and effective medicine must be informed by up to date science (including complexity science of populations) and expertise in presenting and managing the patient's chief complaint. Charon's choice of 'competence' is unfortunate in light of critical attention concerning the limitations of that term (Hodges and Lingard 2012), where 'narrative capability' may be a better descriptor. Competence literally means 'good enough'. Charon wants doctors and healthcare professionals to move beyond this, to show a deep engagement with story and its potential.

Charon (2006) thus details what doctors need to *know* and *value* about narrative in five key areas:

1   Temporality: our conception of time is given meaning through narrative. Clearly, this is of key importance to medicine in terms of our

mortality. Disease is largely a result of ageing and experience of temporality itself then becomes a neurosis (for which faith in an afterlife might be seen as a rationalization or a cure). Many of us become fixated upon death, that becomes an enemy rather than an ally, and feel that we are poorly prepared for our deaths.

2   Singularity: where science explores and explains the universal and the law-bound, medicine largely deals with the idiosyncratic individual, the singular. This is the paradox of medicine – where evidence-based medicine reduces the individual to the chief complaint, missing the chief concern, which is existentially of greater importance to the individual.

3   Causality and contingency: narratives gain their meaning from plots. Something happens, and something happens to somebody. But what gives narrative tension is that a twist occurs in the story. While medicine's main claim for expertise is diagnostic acumen, the hope is that every story is quite predictable. When these symptoms are seen, then this is the cause, and this is the cure or treatment plan. However, the plots of patient's lives within which their symptoms are embedded are not as straightforward as that, but contain the unexpected, the ambiguous, the twists and turns that make the plots of novels so compelling. Further, in consultations patients introduce stories at the middle, not the beginning and end, that are necessarily incomplete.

4   Intersubjectivity: plots generally unfold around characters and their relationships with and to each other. Medicine, too, is an intersubjective practice. Indeed, how well communication happens in clinical teams and between patient and doctor in the consultation is an integral part of medical treatment.

5   Ethicality: stories introduce morality where, as Charon indicates, the receiver of a story – often an intimate confession – owes something to the teller by virtue of now knowing the story. Such intimate knowing confers power upon the listener, but may strip the teller of power in a kind of naked revelation. Telling the doctor about symptoms may bring shame or embarrassment as well as vulnerability and fragility. These conditions may be compounded through poor listening, exposing an immorality in the doctor's behaviour. Medicine and healthcare are ethical practices increasingly being understood as narrative performances (Nelson 1997; Charon and Montello 2002). For example, medical students learn to act like doctors through scripted performances that are influenced by their teachers' role modelling. How then, do they work with a script that includes unprofessional behaviour? How do they respond to traditional methods of teaching by humiliation and 'pimping'? Finally, medical students often take classic bioethics cases, often used in teaching, as 'neutral', in the same way that they might treat clinical cases studies as technical information rather than a tightly packed narrative. Tod Chambers (1999) treats classic bioethics cases sometimes used in teaching as literary texts and reveals their rhetoric, revealing that

the way the case is written already biases the reader towards a particular interpretation, which in its own right can be read as unethical.

Charon (2006: 107) points to the 'clinical dividends' to be gained from education in narrative: 'development of the clinical imagination, deepening of empathy for patients, awareness of the ethical dimensions of clinical situations, and the development of the capacity for attention'. Building on the foundations provided by Kathryn Montgomery and Rita Charon, Ronald Schleifer and Jerry Vannatta have fully integrated narrative approaches into clinical practice and provided a stunning rationale that will act as a touchstone for narrative medicine for many years to come (Schleifer and Vannatta 2013). *The Chief Concern of Medicine* argues that doctors cannot realize the potential of narrative approaches to medicine without engaging with literature (*ibid.*). This would be like learning about symptoms without ever seeing a patient. Further, narrative medicine must have a well-developed epistemological framework for understanding why it works in practice. This means systematically approaching a complex field of narrative approaches and organizing it into categories and forms or 'schemas'. In this way, narrative medicine can be better taught. The book brings critical thinking into the medical humanities via emphasis upon narrative.

Of the schemas through which narrative knowing and treatment of patients may be organized, the most important is that which centres round the difference between the patient's 'chief concern' and 'chief complaint'. Doctors interested only in the chief complaint reduce person to symptom and context to medical text. Doctors must develop schematic understanding of their patients as well as scientific understanding. The former, the province of the arts, humanities and social sciences, is the introduction of subjectivity and intersubjectivity into medicine, which cannot be bracketed out.

Schemas provide both a 'parallel chart' and a counter to protocols in medicine. They are frameworks, but have qualitative focus and large flexibility. For example, a narrative schema would be fairly similar to the narrative competences demanded by Rita Charon, discussed briefly above. This would include the anatomy of a story – the main components, such as characters and plot – and what a story does, such as disrupt expectations and intensify interest. For example, medical students can be taught to 'attend to the surprising fact' – some anomaly in a narrative or text (the patient's story in relation to her presentation; what is left out of the story; how the story relates to previous accounts) that may not be immediately or self-evidently important often turns out to provide a clue. Other schemas include how medical students and doctors respond to metaphor and allusion rather than factual statement and understanding stories told from an 'other' cultural or values perspective.

Ronald Schleifer and Jerry Vannatta have gone out of their way to write a text that is not a textbook and they have succeeded. James Meza and

Daniel Passerman (2011) have written a textbook that captures the new paradigm of what Charon (in the foreword to their book) calls a 'stereo-scopic way of knowing in clinical medicine' (*ibid.*: ix) – thinking at the same time with narrative-based and evidence-based medicine. Meza and Passerman suggest that such stereoscopic thinking can be achieved through a philosophical framework of relativism, in which it is understood that 'facts' are historically, culturally and socially contingent.

Against narrative

Reading the world narratively is one approach among many that has gained particular significance within medical education. Narrative medicine is grounded in reading literature – novels, short stories and poetry – with medical themes (Greenhalgh and Hurwitz 1999), the basis of many 'litera-ture and medicine' courses. Besides mainstream narrative approaches to medicine and bioethics, such as interest in typologies of 'illness narratives' (Frank 1995), narrative is widely used in medical education research (Bleakley 2005); cross-cultural studies of illness and healing (Mattingly and Garro 2000); the study of clinical reasoning across health disciplines (Mattingly and Fleming 1994) and within medicine (Montgomery 2006; Groopman 2007); and in integrating psychotherapy and medicine (Broom 1997).

Further, narrative approaches to medicine have been studied in the context of telling fictional stories to public audiences through media such as film and television (especially medical soap operas) (Moody and Hallam 1998). Recently, there has been an explosion of interest in digital story-telling – using narrative online, for example in developing online communities who might employ stories in a confessional manner, or as an educational medium (Alexander 2011; Page and Thomas 2011). Typical of such narratives are 'survivor' stories, for example of mass trauma such as in the wake of conflict, as well as mental health, in which use of stories has been related to the development of resilience (Gonzales 2012). Stories, too, have moved with the times, so that there is now a growing interesting in 'graphic medicine' or comics and graphic art drawing on medical themes, such as Ian Williams's (2014) delightful and disturbing 'factional' account of the trials and tribulations of a neurotic General Practitioner. Williams too was instrumental in setting up the Graphic Medicine website (www.graphicmedicine.org), giving a contemporary face to a story in which the verbal and visual play off each other – closer, then, to the reality of a consultation.

In the tradition of novels, poetry and short stories written by doctors about their work and their patients, which show various levels of autobiog-raphy and confessional content, there is a rash of recent output. Abraham Verghese's (2009) *Cutting for Stone* has autobiographical elements, but his earlier literary works are explicitly confessional, such as *The Tennis Partner*

(1999), a story of moral conflict, and the earlier *My Own Country* (1994), subtitled *A Doctor's Story of a Town and Its People in the Age of AIDS*. Margaret Edson's *W;t* won the 1999 Pulitzer Prize for drama. It was her first play, dealing with a woman academic's diagnosis and subsequent treatment of ovarian cancer. As we have seen, it is a scathing attack on the impersonal side of medical treatment from the perspective of a humanist scholar of John Donne's poetry (Professor Vivian Bearing, the heroine of the play). As Dr Harvey Kelekian, the chief of medical oncology, relays the diagnosis, prognosis and treatment plan to Dr Vivian Bearing, expert in John Donne's poetry, so his objective scientific method and language are meticulously anatomized and dissected by Vivian's scholastic methods drawn from the humanities. 'Words' are, says Vivian, 'my life's work' and she recognizes that words too are the life's work of the doctors who are treating her. But her words, inspired by Donne, are 'Itchy outbreaks of far-fetched wit' (hence the title of the play). 'Wit' is a way of seeing with and through words. Precise words. Yet the doctors too use precise words – 'antineoplastic', 'pernicious' – but, while these refer to the body in the context of medical practice, these words seem to be stripped of body and beauty and employed, in Edson's, account as scalpels rather than poetically or generously.

Mikhail Bulgakov (2012), author of the classic novel *The Master and Margarita*, a satire on Soviet bureaucracy, published a series of stories in Russia in 1925–26 about his work as a young doctor set at the eve of the Russian Revolution. This set the standard for the genre of personal confessional tales of doctors and surgeons, where standouts include the work of Richard Selzer (1996: 7) a surgeon who claims that 'I have always been intoxicated by words' and that 'There is no one way to write'. John Murray (2000) and Vincent Lam (2006) both write about intensive care, where their work as doctors is based. Lam is a talented novelist (e.g. *The Headmaster's Wager*, 2012). The surgeon Atul Gawande (2002, 2008) is a fine journalist and a regular columnist for the *New Yorker,* developing the ground-breaking work of Richard Selzer to engage more with the limitations of surgery. This, too, is the subject of the surgeon Gabriel Weston's (2009) confessional *Direct Red* and her novel *Dirty Work* (2013). Both of these books deal with issues of women in a male-dominated surgical world. Lisa Sanders (2010) is a regular columnist for *The New York Times* and writes factual but literary accounts of medical practice as 'patient's stories' told by her as a doctor, illustrating the potential for holding the twin narratives of layperson and medicine. And Henry Marsh (2014) is a distinguished UK neurosurgeon who has felt the call of the Muse and sets out a fairly journalistic confessional account not only of his work but of his growing dissatisfaction with the bureaucracy of the NHS and the tempering of, by his own admission, a feeling of self-importance that seems to come with the role of surgeon.

In the face of this growing and diverse interest in narrative-based approaches to medicine, a counterargument has developed, one of scepticism and a warning that 'narrative' has become a weasel word, like 'empathy' and 'creativity'. Narrative approaches seem to always imply good things and are rarely talked about as counterproductive or having unintended negative consequences. Is there a world without narrative? Julia Connelly (2002: 138–40) asks how do we carry out medicine and healthcare 'in the absence of narrative' – for example 'when the patient's mind is severely limited'? This would also be true for care of autistic children or people with severe mental illness who are unable to communicate readily or hypercommunicate with florid symptoms. Connelly also reminds us about the elderly, particularly those with Alzheimer's disease or dementia. Her response is not that these persons are incapable of telling or understanding story, but rather that we must become adaptable and elastic in what we understand 'story' to be. For example, something that Connelly does not discuss is that 'story' need not be confined to words but can be constructed through visual images (such as photography), music and sound.

The philosopher Galen Strawson (2004) takes a different tack by refusing narrative rather than widening its conventions. Strawson bemoans the dominance of narrative thinking in the arts, humanities and social sciences, seeing this as potentially exclusive of other views. Strawson also rejects both the descriptive thesis that our lives and identities are storied, or narrative creations; and the normative thesis that narrative is a 'good thing'. He makes a distinction between 'episodic' and 'diachronic' thinking and experience, where the former is out of time or does not consider time to be important (where place or space may be). The latter thinks in terms of unfolding time. 'Episodics' and 'diachronics' are talked about as two distinct temperaments, even personality styles. However, diachronics do not necessarily subscribe to the view that life is a narrative event or that narrativity is essentially a good thing. There are other ways of experiencing besides narrativity.

Strawson's argument is philosophical and has no basis in empirical research knowledge. However, it does provide an interesting counter to uncritical enthusiasm for narrativity. Angela Woods (2011: 73) has taken up Strawson's argument to question unexamined assumptions about the use of narrative approaches within the medical humanities, or the dominance of narrative-based medicine. She highlights 'seven dangers or blind spots in the dominant medical humanities approach to narrative'. Woods complains that there is difficulty in giving precise definitions to narrative and that 'narratives' are merely academics' dressing up of what laypersons call 'stories'.

Well, both of these complaints are unfounded. I give several clear definitions of narrative above, including Paul Ricoeur's more elaborate one and continue this later with observations by Jerome Bruner and others. Further, 'narrative' and 'story' are used interchangeably across the literature and without prejudice – for example Rita Charon (2006) titles her formative text *Narrative Medicine* but subtitles it *Honoring the Stories of Illness*, and co-edits a text called *Stories Matter* with Martha Montello (Charon and Montello 2002) that is subtitled *The Role of Narrative in Medical Ethics*.

Woods's seven objections to the unquestioned use of narrative in medical humanities are:

1 Authenticity and veracity – can we trust that stories are true?
2 Can narratives promote harm?
3 'Narrative' can act as an umbrella term and is then non-discriminatory or over-inflated – for example can acts of 'creative output' such as dance count as 'narrative'?
4 Distinctions are readily collapsed between different forms of narrative such as anecdotes and autobiographies, thus nullifying discrimination between types.
5 A sophisticated account of genre is missing from the literature on narratives.
6 It is easy to overlook the cultural and historical frames for production of narrative, where stories are often presented as trans-historical and trans-cultural.
7 Narrative has been promoted as a form of agentic, autonomous and authentic expression and identity construction, where there are competing models of selfhood.

Woods asks us to 'denaturalize' narrative approaches, certainly to treat them with caution and critical awareness and pursue 'non-narrative' approaches to inquiry in the medical humanities, such as the uses of metaphor and non-narrative embodied interaction. She recommends the use of non-linguistic forms of expression such as those developed by Deborah Padfield (2003) in her work on visualizing pain through photography. With reference to the performance and visual arts work on bodily transformation and modification of Stelarc and Orlan, Woods notes that such work interrupts 'the principle comforts of narrative – continuity, closure and containment – in pursuit of the paradoxical, the ambiguous and undecidable'. But this is a very limited reading of 'narrative' and goes against the grain of Woods's own seven warnings.

Stelarc and Orlan, for example, within the radical nature of their body modifications do actually follow a conventional narrative line – for example, Orlan charts out body modifications through her own chronology that deal first with bottom-line feminist issues of standard representation (what is beauty and who represents this?) and then moves to a future-oriented sense of 'other-world' identity in her later work. Stelarc shows a similar progression, from limited human towards a trans-historical and trans-cultural horizon of prosthetic augmentation or cyborgism. Indeed, both artists can be criticized for the shared normativity of their respective work narratives, where their platform is the healthy human who can be augmented and not the challenged human who can be given an opportunity to live a more fulfilling life through augmentation. In this sense, there is even a streak of Futurism and totalitarianism in their work, despite its outward alignment with the liberal avant-garde.

Narrative cannot be characterized by 'principle comforts' of 'continuity, closure and containment'. This is to ignore a swathe of experimental writing such as the 'prescription culture' authors discussed critically and at length in the following chapter. Angela Woods is right to raise concern about the uncritical and unreflexive use of 'narrative' approaches in the medical humanities, but her seven objections can be readily answered:

1   Authenticity and veracity – can we trust that stories are true? – well, simply read the new wave of anthropologists such as Michael Taussig and Alphonso Lingis who argue for a paradoxical fictional veracity, best illustrated by the novelist William T. Vollman's (2007) *Poor People*. The stories may not be entirely 'true' but their ethical imperative is clear.

2   Can narratives promote harm? Yes, narratives can have unintended and intended 'harmful' consequences. Asking people to recount stories may restimulate repressed, uncomfortable material in a psychoanalytic sense. Further, are stories not meant to stir us up? Does 'harm' cover feeling ill-at-ease or disgusted? While writing this chapter, I have been rereading John Steinbeck's *East of Eden* and I feel, once again, fundamentally shaken and stirred by that story. Does this discomfort stop me from reading it? No – it makes me want to dwell on the issues Steinbeck raises about 'pure' good and evil.

3   'Narrative' can act as an umbrella term and is then non-discriminatory or over-inflated – for example can acts of 'creative output' such as dance count as 'narrative'? Well, structures of narrative can of course be applied to performance. What is at question is surely the quality and impact of the narrative and the art work.

4   Distinctions are readily collapsed between different forms of narrative such as anecdotes and autobiographies, thus nullifying discrimination between types. Yes, fine, but this can be approached from another perspective – that of genre. As explored above, Minimalist art can collapse down to the equivalent of an anecdote in form, but still retain richness of experience.

5   A sophisticated account of genre is missing from the literature on narratives in medicine and healthcare. This may have been rectified by Schleifer and Vannatta's (2013) work on narrative (their Chapters 3 and 8 discuss genres), and see later in this chapter.

6   It is easy to overlook the cultural and historical frames for production of narrative, where stories are often presented as transhistorical and transcultural. This is readily rectified by reading fictional work that is sensitive to such issues, such as Abraham Verghese's *Cutting for Stone*.

7   Narrative has been promoted as a form of agentic, autonomous and authentic expression and identity construction, where there are competing models of selfhood. I would suggest that this is only true for a segment of the literature – for example poststructuralist feminist work

such as that of Hélène Cixous (discussed in Chapter 3) and postmodern writers discussed in Chapter 8, do not fall foul of this self-referential trap.

A further danger, not mentioned by Woods, is the tendency to see 'narrative' as the flipside of 'scientific' thinking. Once scientific medicine and narrative based medicine are divided, then they have to be brought together again, with extreme effort, in a stereoscopic method (Meza and Passerman 2011). Why they were divided in the first place is perhaps a more interesting question, and this is usually laid, unfairly, at the door of C.P. Snow's 'Two Cultures' 1959 Rede Lecture. While Snow diagnosed the emergence of a division between two cultures of science and the humanities, he did not support this division, later writing a book promoting a 'third culture' of integration (Snow 1963).

Two kinds of thinking? Narrative and science

The eminent American psychologist and philosopher William James (cited in Bruner 1986: 1) noted, rhetorically, that 'To say that all human thinking is essentially of two kinds – reasoning on the one hand, and narrative, descriptive, contemplative thinking on the other – is to say only what every reader's experience will corroborate'. Recognizing these two modes of being – on the one hand logic and analysis, now raised to a supreme level as the dominant discourse of scientific method and the search for truth or fact; and on the other descriptive story, by definition anecdotal but raised to the lofty heights of a cultural myth or a great novel, as the search for meaning – is one thing. Placing them into oppositional camps reflects a third discourse – that of structuralism, working through the logic of oppositions and often competition or even hostility. As contemporary feminists have pointed out in particular, such oppositional thinking tends to promote dominance of one pole over another – for example, the gender bias of men over women; the age bias of adults over children; the race bias of white over black; and so forth. Better to promote a post-structuralism in which structures potentially do not work oppositionally but collaboratively, as complex conversations. The art and the science of medicine can be engaged in this more productive way.

The psychologist and educationalist Jerome Bruner (1986: 11) also suggests that narrative and scientific ways of knowing – 'a good story' and 'a well-formed argument' are 'complementary', 'but irreducible to one another'. Notice that Bruner has introduced another factor here – quality – by talking about a 'good' story and a 'well-formed' argument. Narrative and scientific thinking differ primarily with how they represent causality, summarized in the word 'then'. A logical proposition, common to science, says 'if x, then y'. In a narrative, there is not a generalization or universal law, but a particular case: 'the woman died suspiciously, then a man she was having an affair with suddenly leaves town'. We do not know if the two events are causally connected, but in juxtaposing them, there is already a story with intrigue, in the genre of the murder mystery, with characters and with a skeleton plot. A patient does not visit his or her general practitioner and say 'I had an episode of haematuria this morning'. Rather, he or she, probably anxiously, tells an episodic story of noticing blood in his or her pee.

Bruner (1986: 12) calls the scientific way of knowing 'paradigmatic' or 'logico-scientific' – how to know truth rather than 'how to endow experience with meaning' – the latter characteristic of narrative knowing. Paradigmatic thinking, on the other hand, employs typical strategies such as hypothesis forming and testing; strict implication (one thing predictably leads to another); conjunction and disjunction (things logically match or fall apart); hyperonymy and hyponymy (semantic relations between two things, such as a larger class – trees – as hyperonym and a specific example – larch – as hyponym). This kind of thinking relies on typical methods – the verification of truth or fact through replicable, well-designed experiments. The point of scientific thinking is to reduce uncertainty or ambiguity for predictable laws and operations. The point of a narrative is that it generates ambiguity, purposefully, where contradiction reflects the messiness of life itself. Hence, appreciation of narrative requires tolerance of ambiguity.

The subjunctive mood and narrative tension

Here is a radiologist's diagnosis given at a clinical meeting, where objective, tight, formalized case presentations are required. The radiologist is reading an X-ray from a test – a double-contrast barium enema – that shows an 'apple core lesion' (see Figure 6.2, page 141), a readily identifiable pattern indicating colonic cancer: 'There is an area of narrowing in the sigmoid. The undercut edges give an apple core appearance. This is colonic carcinoma.' The language is indicative, or points to certainties. Also, the patient is not mentioned but is reduced to symptom description. For the sake of illustration, let us present this grim diagnosis as a poem:

There is an area
of narrowing
in the sigmoid

The undercut
edges give
an apple core appearance.

In contrast, here is a poem, first published in 1923, by William Carlos Williams, a famous poet at his peak in the mid-1940s, but also a paediatrician and family doctor working in New Jersey. Williams was the originator of 'minimalist' poetry – poems stripped back to bare essences verbally but not stripped of meaning – and would write poems on his prescription pad between house calls:

> so much depends
> upon
>
> a red wheel
> barrow
>
> glazed with rain
> water
>
> beside the white
> chickens.

While the 'imagist' and minimalist description seems plain and uncomplicated, it is completely thrown by that opening line: 'so much depends'. So much depends upon what? Williams tells us what – a red wheel / barrow'. But this just deepens the mystery. Like seeing a 'readymade' sculpture, first presented by Marcel Duchamp in a gallery setting such as the infamous 'Fountain' (a porcelain urinal), we are presented with an idea or concept wound into the object or words of the poem. As the Minimalist sculptor Robert Morris said: 'Simplicity of shape does not necessarily equate with simplicity of experience' (Morris undated). The poem sets an immediate conundrum, a tension and an ambiguity. While the language of the radiologist could be set as a concrete, minimalist and imagist poem, it does not work because it is highly indicative – pointing exactly to what it means and squashing all ambiguity or uncertainty. Williams's poem, however, adopts a subjunctive mood – that of ambiguity: 'possibly', 'maybe', 'perhaps'. Again, 'so much depends'. This opening immediately creates narrative tension, where the radiologist's description offers a refusal of the subjunctive mood and narrative tension. Of course, it is unfair to suggest that the radiologist does anything other than resort to plain speaking where the diagnosis is clear – but in many clinical encounters and especially in patients' stories of their symptoms in the context of their lives, 'so much depends / upon'.

Medicine's self-acknowledged symptom of intolerance of ambiguity (Ludmerer 1999) shows in linguistic and semantic biases such as preference for the indicative over the subjunctive mood. This narrative strategy is read as counterproductive and another way that medical students are inadvertently rendered insensible rather than sensible – an-aesthetized or dulled through medical education, rather than aestheticized or sharpened. The indicative bias also refuses narrative tension and then makes it harder to hear a good story, having implications for listening closely to patients. Close observation (Chapter 6) must be twinned with close listening.

Again, patients' stories are generally full of narrative tension, where, for example, issues of impending or ongoing illness may remain unresolved. Patients are often in the midst of an illness story, where the beginning may be known (and is informed by a diagnosis) but the end of the story may be unknown, where prognosis is unclear. Patients' stories then remain largely open-ended and future-oriented, geared to the subjunctive forms of verbs rather than the indicative, where a patient may say 'I'm not sure what will happen' while the doctor says 'you have ovarian cancer', as illustrated in Margaret Edson's *W;t*. In the first, the chief complaint is buried within a mass of other concerns and the patient represents these through 'subjunctivizing' or using language that is open-ended, mood oriented, ambiguous, and may reference wished-for states rather than actualities. This brings narrative tension and makes a 'good' story in that it is gripping through its open-endedness; but of course this may be a 'bad' story to the person who tells it as patient. When critics of narrative medicine point out that narrative is often used uncritically or seen as 'good thing' they forget that the narratives themselves are usually based in illness and suffering. And in uncertainty – the subjunctive in everyday speech is often replaced by modal verbs or modalities. Modal auxiliaries for the verb such as 'might', 'could', 'maybe', 'possibly' and 'probably' retain ambiguity, tension, future orientation and colour or mood even as they are set in scenarios of illness and suffering.

As Bruner (1986: 26) suggests: 'To be in the subjunctive is, then, to be trafficking in human possibilities rather than in settled certainties'. Medicine's refusal of ambiguity through privileging the indicative over the subjunctive is also a refusal of affect, effectively claiming that medicine could be practiced with flat affect. The classic – or 'indicative' – case study is then told as a story stripped of all narrative tension (and then is degraded to a 'report' rather than a story). There is no mood in a case study, despite the fact that real clinical exchanges in consultations often engage affect or mood.

Drawing on the previous discussions of Jacques Rancière's (2006, 2010, 2013) model of the distribution of sensibility and its relationship to dissensus, we might characterize the dominance of the indicative in medicine as the refusal of subjunctivizing or creating mood and narrative tension (and then a particular depth of *engagement* and *interest*). This refusal, in turn, can be read as a parallel impulse to the production and distribution of insensibility, where mainstream medicine and medical education produce and distribute indicative rather than subjunctive moods through emphasis upon stripped back, objectifying 'cases' as opposed to complex persons in context. The (mal)distribution of the sensible – producing insensibility – is paralleled by the distribution of the indicative – refusing mood, narrative tension and ambiguity, for 'safe' but decontextualized clinical judgements.

Byron Good suggests that:

> If literary works call forth an imaginative response from the reader as plots are broken off suddenly or continued in unexpected directions, as relations among elements are left unspecified, and as doubt is cast on

elements of the reader's interpretive repertoire, so surely does illness, particularly psychotic illness, share these characteristics and call forth an imaginative response.

(Good 2000)

Therefore, suggests Good, 'The narratization of illness draws on subjunctivizing tactics as a means of maintaining openness, sources of potency and hope' (*ibid.*). In other words, the way that stories of illness are structured may offer a source of hope for patients, where uncertainties are evident. This of course can also be a false hope. If we are to makes sense of, or give sense to, illness, then we must understand that illness for each individual patients spins out as a story that has unexpected twists, especially in the field of mental health. Gay Becker's ethnography *Disrupted Lives* gathered narratives from Americans undergoing minor to major disruptions such as unexpected illness. She reports that:

> Sometimes the storyteller presents several possible scenarios from which he or she is attempting to engineer the desired end. This phenomenon is referred to as the subjunctivizing element in narratives, which engage in human possibilities rather than certainties. Stories have subjunctivizing elements when narrators are in the midst of the stories they are telling.

(Becker 1997: 28)

Those telling stories of their own illnesses, especially chronic illness, are often in the middle of that story and not at its end. Therefore stories looked forward and backward simultaneously and remained suspended, incomplete. Such stories subjunctivize reality, or create a mood of ambiguity, through implicit rather than explicit meanings, subjectification or self-referential meanings and description from multiple perspectives. This creates a world of contingencies not certainties.

Genres

Genres are broad categories or types. The classic genres in literature are epic (such as Homer's *Iliad*; see Allums 1992), tragic (such as Shakespeare's *Macbeth*; see Arbery 2003), comic (such as Douglas Adams' *The Hitchhiker's Guide to the Galaxy*; see Cowan 2011) and lyric (such as Virgil's *Georgics* and *Eclogues*; see Cowan and Cowan 2012). Other genres include detective, thriller, science fiction, historical fiction, children's, young adults, romance, erotic, pornographic, comic books, graphic novels, fairy tales and horror. As discussed above, in the case of the medical diagnosis, for example, given in a sombre, dry affectless voice, this can seem to be in the genre of Minimalism. But when William Carlos Williams's poem was compared with the radiologist's diagnosis, we saw that the medical diagnosis merely imitated the genre. Williams, in contrast, introduced the poem with 'so much depends / upon' which made complex what would otherwise seem like a straightforward descriptive account. Minimalism explicitly cultivates flat affect, clean and simple lines, reduction to essences and so forth, but as a cultivated style underneath which complexity boils. The medical version of minimalism is more like flat packing, producing a reduction but without the style – the opposite of elegant reduction in literature such as Raymond Carver's economical stories or Lydia Davies's 'flash fiction'.

On first reading Kathryn Montgomery Hunter's (1991b) account of 'medical sleuthing', medical narrative work makes sense through knowledge of the genre of the detective story. Medical telling and listening is so natural-ized within medical culture that stories are not even noticed as typically within the genres of the epic, tragic or dark comic. Proximity to death is everyday, but this dulls sensitivity to the epic and tragic nature of tales of medicine. Dark comedy is used as a perfectly understandable functional defence against proximity to disease and death, but is not valued for its aesthetic purposes. Further, the heavy reliance on these three genres denies the presence of the lyrical in medicine – the more gentle, song-like aspect of care.

The agenda for democratization of medicine discussed throughout this book is linked with the need to transform medical practice from domina-tion by tough-mindedness within an epic mode to release what is repressed by that mode – lyricism, a more tender-minded, sensitive medicine. Medicine's 'front stage' has historically involved the epic, heroic dragon-slaying doctor; the tragic, which is given with the territory of illness and death; and the dark comic. Black humour develops in hospital subcultures, such as intensive care, as a way of blowing off steam (out of families' earshot). What is missing (and repressed) however is lyricism in medicine. Repressed lyricism returns as cynicism, hostility, arrogance, sarcasm and bullying, felt as disillusion and burnout, dry cinders and bitter ash.

Lyricism can be characterized as tending the garden, vocation, devotion, tenderness, joy, fecundity, abundance, generative, songlike, rhythmic, poetic, rhapsodic, erotic, celebrating the beauty of the mundane (the extraordinary in the ordinary) and providing genuine hospitality (which has the same root as 'hospital'). Doing lyrical work fashions a sensitive self. Lyrical medicine is a no-brainer: elegant, inspiring, beautiful, imaginative, animated, dignified, graceful, sensitive, distinctive, passionate and expres-sive, or 'aesthetic'. Non-lyrical medicine serves as an anaesthetic – blunting, souring and dulling, leading to uninspired, flat, ungracious, insensitive and restrictive practice. Which doctor would you rather have?

The lyricism I am calling for is not 'lite', but intense or full of passion. The poet Saint-John Perse (1961) described such lyricism as 'passionate action' that 'does not raise cultured pearls (but) is intimately related to beauty'. In other words, an 'everyday' beauty, seeing the mundane in a new light. In medicine, the lyrical often meets the tragic. The radiologist's description of an 'apple core' lesion is the revelation of a bitter fruit.

The switch in genre from the epic to the lyric again suggests a switch in metaphor and style: from the lecture to the song, from the individual to collaboration, from martial metaphors (curing) to pastoral metaphors (caring) and from intolerance of ambiguity (dragon slaying) to tolerance of ambiguity (dialogue). Within the lyrical mode, we might find doctors seeing their work as ballads, where the response to the patient is not blunt but tender and sensitive; or as Georgics, traditionally an ode to agriculture and the pastoral life, but in medicine perhaps a celebration and recognition of the fruits of hard labour.

Eclogues (bucolics), championed by Virgil, celebrate the mundane in work – finding the extraordinary in the ordinary. The everyday round of medical work is like this. Not the crash and bang of 'boys' medicine' (accident and emergency or the operating theatre), but the slow pulse of the ward at night, the everyday symptoms brought to the general practitioner: colds and flu, sprains and knocks, a persistent pain, light anxiety and depression. Pindaric odes celebrate the feats of athletes, where attention shifts from heroic individualism and competition to collaboration, team games, echoing the need for doctors to sing the praises of the interprofessional clinical team. Epithalamia are songs in praise of the bride or bridegroom – the junior doctor loses his or her work virginity as s/he gradually gains expertise, undergoing a series of rites of passage. S/he learns 'professional intimacy' – typical of psychotherapy – with a range of patients whom s/he must accommodate, regardless of her personal feelings, managing disgust through counter-resistance or erotic feelings through counter-transference. Finally, epitaphs honour the deceased, where the doctor does not sing the praises of the dead white males of medicine, but rather, through his or her lyrical work, re-members patients who die, in a liturgy of clinical stories.

8 Writing out prescriptions

Hyper-realism and the chemical regulation of mood

Introduction

This chapter offers a case study to show how the more conceptual arguments of previous chapters can be applied: first, to a public health issue and second as a way to do medical education through the medical humanities. This will become clear as the chapter unfolds.

The first wave of the medical humanities whose focus was the academic study of medicine and medical cultures (such as the history of medicine) did not promise much in the way of translation into improving patient care. Rather, it gave a deeper understanding of the contexts in which medicine has developed and can be both appreciated and understood conceptually. A second wave of this approach to the medical humanities promises greater application. This current wave of interdisciplinary medical humanities engages critically with medicine as an ethical practice, ontologies of clinical practice, articulation of the historical conditions of possibility for the emergence of particular medical practices and approaches to health, development of an historical and cross-cultural appreciation of the body and critical evaluation of the medicalization of everyday behaviour. It is this last area of concern that is the focus of this chapter and here, the two streams of the historical–cultural medical humanities and the medical humanities in medical education, discussed in Chapter 2, engage in dialogue.

The focus of the chapter is the development of a 'prescription culture' and its (often unreflexive) representation in contemporary novels and self-help books. By a 'prescription culture' I mean a culture in which taking prescribed drugs for common mental health symptoms such as anxiety and depression becomes an unquestioned or naturalized part of the cultural fabric. In the northern hemisphere certainly, we live in a culture in which prescription drugs are discussed as separated out from the persons who are taking them, to become recognizable artefactual 'actors' in their own right with 'personalities'. This is achieved through three main texts: medical pharmaceutical formularies, online confessional accounts such as YouTube videos and contemporary novels.

Continuing the argument from Chapter 3 on the distribution of the sensible, the development, administration and evaluation of commonly taken anti-depressant and anti-anxiety drugs is part of the political regulation of sensibility. A critical view suggests that, largely driven by the profit motives of the pharmaceutical industry, psychological conditions continue to be medicalized and treated as if they were neurological. As the fabric of the sensible (the aesthetic life) is patterned according to vested interests (the political and economic life) so an aesthetic of everyday life is shaped in which prescription culture has become a normal part of that fabric of the sensible. Indeed, although prescription drugs can be seen to be part of a cultural production of insensibility, they are advertised as producing precisely the opposite effect. They are promoted as relieving debilitating symptoms of depression and anxiety. This treatment of symptom misses the cause – that, for example, living in a manic, sound-bite culture is bound to lower the threshold for what is considered to be a state of depression or one of anxiety.

As discussed in previous chapters, Jacques Rancière (2013: ix–x) suggests, following Walter Benjamin, that 'forms of sensible experience' or 'ways of perceiving and being affected' are subject to historical fluctuations. Those who exert power (authority figures or institutions, such as medicine and the pharmaceutical industry) constitute the historical forces that shape or dictate legitimate forms of sensible experience. The fabric of the sensible, or how we shall perceive, is regulated. The major form of regulation is to produce insensibility in the general population as a form of policing, to dampen down the possibility of dissension or speaking out about ownership of the means of producing sensibility (sensibility capital such as forms of education that are in the hands of the few rather than the many). In other words, sensibility is still open to democratizing. In the purely aesthetic realm, works of art do not simply appear as autonomous products received by a naïve public, but are produced within 'modes of perception and regimes of emotion, categories that identify them, thought patterns that categorize and interpret them' as well as within material modes of production owned by large corporations such as pharmaceutical industries. Just as art/efacts and 'taste' in art are shaped by a material infrastructure such as galleries and their sponsors, so industrially generated advertising, marketing and packaging shapes the fabric of modes of perception in a prescription culture. Modes of education then replicate this structure of inequality.

The topic of the regulation of mood through prescribed medications is of great interest to medical students. However, they tend to be introduced to this topic in a highly mechanical and literal way – through a reductive pharmacology, noting how drugs work instrumentally for generalized populations. The politics and aesthetics – the production and distribution of sensibility and insensibility and forms of resistance to this production – are rarely discussed, but make for excellent content within a medical humanities curriculum. For example, prescribed drugs can be discussed as a key aspect of what Michel Foucault described as 'governmentality' – the production and regulation of 'docile bodies'. The students' text for the study of prescriptions is the national formulary – pharmaceutical reference books produced nationally containing instrumental information and advice on prescribing, and pharmacology related to populations, such as the *British National Formulary* (*BNF*) (a biannual joint publication of the British Medical Association and the Royal Pharmaceutical Society) and *The United States Pharmacopeia and The National Formulary* (*USP–NF*). Formularies do not address individual responses, tastes and tolerances; the contexts in which drugs are prescribed; whether or not they 'work'; how they might be abused; and whether or not they become habitual and naturalized, or part of a cultural fabric. Such contextual insights are provided by academics and now, as we shall see, contemporary novelists.

If medical students are lucky they will discuss issues of 'prescription behaviour' beyond technical knowledge of the drugs that are prescribed with GPs, psychiatrists and pharmacists in particular. But their education in this field normally revolves around a good deal of rote learning based on a drug formulary. Such a compendium of drugs and their effects is written like a car manual. There are no patient case studies – indeed human presence appears to be excluded from the formulary that provides only technical or instrumental descriptions of the drugs, their main effects and side effects. Also, the drugs themselves are described in terms of flat affect, although of course many of them produce strong affective responses in patients. The style of the formulary as a text is then an interesting study in its own right.

Where the formulary resists literary analysis, as it is more like a shopping list, contemporary literature is a powerful entry route into understanding prescription culture. Introducing medical students to the writers and literature discussed in this chapter for example and opening this up for critical discussion in intensive small group settings extends students' education, providing a counterpoint to the literal pharmacology that they learn largely from pharmacists. In conversation with GPs and psychiatrists on placements, students can further develop an understanding of, and insights into, prescribing behaviour or doctors' performances. But it is in conversation with particular patients that students may best develop insight into prescription culture, and the creative writing associated with this culture detailed below fleshes out this understanding and insight.

YouTube has a raft of examples of patients talking about their relationships with prescription drugs that includes discussion of lifestyle, habits, identity, withdrawal, disorder and differing drug 'personalities' or identities. This is a rich source of educational material for the medical humanities.

Prescription culture

In his quasi-autobiographical novel *Lunar Park*, Bret Easton Ellis (2005: 10) goes shopping in his gentrified, surburban neighbourhood. It features 'gourmet food stores, a first-class cheese shop, a row of patisseries, [and] a friendly pharmacist who filled my Klonopin and Xanax prescriptions'. On Main Street anywhere, such drug transactions are happening in broad daylight. Some involve drugs for pre-school age children such as Ritalin, for control of 'attention deficit' and 'hyperactivity'. Most are for adults who do not need psychiatric intervention or hospitalization, but are the 'worried well,' working long hours, possibly unhappy, certainly anxious, and now paranoid about security, in an age where 'the terrorist' is demonized. And many of these drugs, such as Xanax for control of free floating anxiety, are designed to engineer wellbeing – mainly 'stabilizing' moods considered manic or 'enhancing' moods considered depressive.[1]

Later, Ellis (*ibid.*: 159) describes taking his 6-year-old stepdaughter and 11-year-old son to a party. In the car, the girl 'took a small canister and started popping Skittles into her mouth and throwing her head back as if they were prescription pills'. 'Why are you eating your candy that way, honey?' asks Ellis. 'Because this is how Mommy does it when she's in the bathroom' replies the girl. 'Popping' the rainbow-coloured sugar may remove its taste but gives it the status of adult sweets. Once they arrive at the party, Ellis 'started noticing that all the kids were on meds (Zoloft, Luvox, Clexa, Paxil) that caused them to move lethargically and speak in affectless monotones' (*ibid.*: 161). One parent comments that his son is:

> 'taking methylphenidate' – Adam pronounced it effortlessly – 'even though it really hasn't been approved for kids under six,' and then he went on about ... attention-deficit/hyperactivity disorder, which naturally led the conversation to the 7.5 milligrams of Ritalin administered three times a day.
>
> (*Ibid.*: 201)

Note Ellis' use of 'naturally.' There is no particular moral tone in Ellis' report; indeed, his exact observation suggests if anything, coming to terms with the apparently inevitable. Prescription culture has become naturalized and normalized.

In a review of *Lunar Park*, Thomas (2005) notes that pharmaceuticals pervade the book. But the 'pharmaceutical' work goes beyond content to pervade style. Conversation specifies '7.5 milligrams of Ritalin administered three times a day', speaking in the tones of the various drug formularies that inform the prescribing behaviour of doctors, such as the *BNF* and the *USP–NF* mentioned above. While trade names for drugs may differ, the text styles of these 'drug bibles' are identical. Where the formulary becomes the style of conversation adopted by Ellis's characters, it acts as a simulacrum preceding and forming reality. Further, while the text ostensibly describes symptoms to be cured, it comes to model such symptoms, inscribing rather than describing through the same 'affectless monotones' as the medically doped children at the party.

The Guardian for 11 February 2006 carried the following front-page headline: 'Ritalin heart attacks warning urged after 51 deaths in US' (Boseley 2006). The article warns of a statistically small chance that drugs prescribed for attention deficit hyperactivity disorder (ADHD) may increase risk of death from a heart attack. Ritalin and similar drugs are amphetamine-based and raise blood pressure. A handful of children have died this way in the UK since methylphenidate hydrochloride has been used to treat ADHD. The article goes on to say that two million prescriptions for drugs treating ADHD are written every month in the US. Over 30,000 prescriptions a month were written in the UK in 2005. By 2014, ADHD had grown to become the most common behavioural disorder in the UK, affecting 2–5 per cent of school-aged children and young people (NHS Choices undated).

The Guardian article goes on to say that 'In the UK, nobody knows how many people are on the drugs, which are licensed for children as young as six – although there are reports of them being given to children as young as three' (Boseley 2006). By 2014, just over 132,000 children and young people (1.5 per cent) were diagnosed as having 'severe ADHD' in the UK (YoungMinds 2013). The National Institute for Health and Clinical Excellence (NICE) guidelines on ADHD in 2009 (no longer accessible on their website) noted that a 1986 estimate of incidence of ADHD in the UK of 0.05 per cent of children actually receiving medication for ADHD rose to more than 0.3 per cent by the late 1990s – a sixfold increase. In the USA during the same period, the incidence rose from 1.2 per cent to 3.5 per cent – a threefold increase, but from a much higher base. This suggests at least three readings:

- ADHD is a biological condition whose epidemiology was not fully understood but is now unfolding;
- ADHD is a socially constructed condition and then cultural differences in diagnoses would be expected; and/or
- ADHD is a condition wholly or partly shaped by the drug companies who provide Ritalin, Focalin and so forth, amphetamines that 'treat' the condition or contain it.

Whatever the case, mental health epidemics such as the rise in incidence of ADHD must be understood more widely than the somatic to include cultural factors, and then may also be understood and treated through humanities interventions.

The respectable use of prescription medicine is no secret, then. Accounts such as the *Guardian*'s are matched by regular scandals as the side effects of drugs emerge and nobody is surprised to learn that drug companies are making huge profits. Yet any doctor can testify to the public's demand for this grown up 'candy', in a world where so many are stressed, depressed and vulnerable. Again, a scan through the host of YouTube video confessions, primarily by young people, will attest to how complex this issue is.

Many of these confessional videos concern withdrawal symptoms that outweigh the severity of the symptoms that were supposedly treated by the drug prescriptions in the first place.

But Ellis unfolds a subtler diagnosis of prescription culture in *Lunar Park*. As much quasi-anthropological as literary, his deadpan life story shows medicine to be a privileged currency of family life. It binds relationships together, defining obligation, duty, guilt and love. This can be summarized in the moment when Ellis unexpectedly restores a (fictional) relationship with a girlfriend of twelve years previous, along with their son and her daughter by another relationship. 'The summer', he says, was spent 'getting acquainted with the wide array of meds the kids were on (stimulants, mood stabilizers, the antidepressant Lexapro, the Adderall for attention-deficit/hyperactivity disorder and various other anticonvulsants and antipsychotics that had been prescribed)' (Ellis 2005: 42). Even the household dog is on 'meds' after a spell in canine behavioural therapy. The dog therapist had 'prescribed Cloinicalm, which was basically puppy Prozac'. But a side effect of this drug, 'compulsive licking', had kicked in, and the dog was now taking 'a kind of canine Paxil . . . the same medication Sarah [his 6 year old stepdaughter] was on, which we all thought was extremely distressful' (*ibid.*: 47)!

Grotesque though the sight of their dog's compulsion may be, the family is principally worried by the fact that dog and child share the same prescription. Roles must be preserved in this carefully assembled family unit, and getting to know each other's 'meds' is part of their commitment to each other's happiness. Indeed, identities are now intimately linked with those 'meds' and the 'family physician' is enrolled as part of the extended family, a kind of benevolent aunt or uncle promising sweets for all.

Prescriptions, particularly for children, emerge in this literature to offer contemporary rites of passage as normalized as the illegal drug taking of adolescents and the pharmaceutical industry facilitate this convenience. McGough and colleagues (2004) describe 'extended-release capsules' for ADHD favoured by physicians because of 'increased convenience'. The extended-release form of dexmethylphenidate has the trade name of 'Focalin'. In the USA, the most commonly prescribed of this group of drugs is Adderall, which is not licensed in the UK, but the three brands which are licensed conjure images of their promised effects: Ritalin = right/align; Concerta = in concert; Equasym = equal/symmetrical. What is out of kilter must be adjusted.

Doctors and health care professionals are widely consulted to suggest such snappy trade names. They thus contribute to powerful metaphors of what parents wish from their children, what partners expect from each other, perhaps precisely because they are semiotically so facile. 'Focalin' echoes the 'alignment' suggestions of Ritalin. A popular drug for male erectile dysfunction is called 'Muse'; an appetite suppressant treating obesity is Reductil; an anti-depressant aimed specifically at women is Lustral (implying that you regain your shine) and so forth. Of the free gifts offered by drug companies to doctors, pens are the most common. The design of such pens is to catch the eye, so that a potential client remembers the name of the product. A variant of the Lustral (anti-depressant) pen has a large yellow smiley face on the clip. This bargaining between pharmaceutical companies and doctors is quite obvious. It is the complicity between patient and doctor that is the real hallmark of prescription culture, and the parallel between the crass imagery of Lustral and that of the illegal drug ecstasy makes this plain.

We can find a precise analogy to the Lustral plot in Jonathan Franzen's (2001) saga of nuclear family implosion, *The Corrections*. Here a parallel between recreational drugs and the medication of the elderly is the joke. A hopeless literature lecturer loses it all for a weekend of sex with one of his students, who brings along a supply of what she calls 'Mexican A'. Later, we find out his elderly mother Enid is prescribed the same thing by a doctor on her retiree cruise ship, when she finds herself insomniac with worry over her Parkinson's disease-afflicted husband – only here it goes by the name of Aslan, after C.S. Lewis's redemptive lion in Narnia. When Edith asks what 'ASLAN® CruiserTM' does, the doctor replies 'Absolutely nothing, if you are in perfect mental health. However, let's face it, who is?' He explains that 'Aslan provides a state-of-the-art factor regulation. The best medications now approved for American use are like two Marlboros and a rum-and-Coke, by comparison'. Enid asks if it is an antidepressant, to which he replies: 'Crude term. 'Personality optimizer' is the phrase preferred' (Franzen 2001: 369–70). Manufactured by a company named 'Farmacopea', Aslan's plentiful varieties are each optimized for a particular activity or mental state. Besides Aslan 'Basic' there is Aslan 'Ski', Aslan 'Hacker', Aslan 'Performance Ultra', Aslan 'Teen', Aslan 'Club Med', Aslan 'Golden Years' and Aslan 'California'. The company also plans to bring several other blends to market, namely Aslan 'Exam Buster', Aslan 'Courtship', Aslan 'White Nights', Aslan 'Reader's Challenge', Aslan 'Connoisseur Class' and several others. The drug is 'not available' in America. When Enid asks if she can get it in her hometown of St Jude, he advises her to get her Aslan from Mexico.

More chilling than Franzen's spoof, prescription culture is most thoroughly charted in the late David Foster Wallace's (1996) *Infinite Jest*. This darkly comic novel centres on the narrative of a videotape said to be so entertaining that it guarantees compulsive viewing leading to loss of desire for any other activity. Viewers die happily watching the tape in endless repetition. The parallels with prescription drugs discussed here are obvious. Part of the novel is set in a halfway house for recovering addicts and Wallace uses this setting in particular to explore some of the contradictions inherent in the culture of prescribing, including the recreational use of such drugs – in Wallace's phrase, 'abusing prescribed meds'. But where Wallace talks of 'abuse' he is being descriptive not prescriptive. In one scene, a woman has been admitted to the 'psych ward' of a hospital after an overdose and is being interviewed by the psychiatrist. She starts in a matter of fact way: 'I took a hundred-ten Parnate, about thirty Lithonate capsules, some old Zoloft' and then, 'I took everything I had in the world'; that is, the drugs took everything, consumed her whole being. The doctor's reply is flat, technical, missing the point of her admission to total annihilation: 'You really must have wanted to hurt yourself, then, it seems' (Wallace 1996: 70).

She continues with a vivid description of the overdose in which we sense that she has sought rebirth within the suicide attempt:

> They said downstairs the Parnate made me black out. It did a blood pressure thing. My mother heard the noises upstairs and found me she said down on my side chewing the rug in my room. My room's shag-carpeted. She said I was on the floor flushed red and all wet like when I was a new-born; she said she thought at first she hallucinated me as a newborn again. On my side all red and wet.
>
> (*Ibid.*: 70)

The doctor's response to this vivid memory is merely informative (also giving Wallace an opportunity to show off his technical interests): 'A hypertensive crisis will do that. It means your blood pressure was high enough to have killed you. Sertraline in combination with an MAOI will kill you, in enough quantities. And with the toxicity of that much lithium besides, I'd say you were pretty lucky to be here right now'. She tries to re-engage the memory of the near-death: 'My mother sometimes thinks she's hallucinating', but Wallace has the doctor bundling on through with weakly disguised prescription: 'Sertraline, by the way, is the Zoloft you kept instead of discarding as instructed when changing medications' (*ibid.*). She has one more attempt to engage him affectively even adding a rhetorical question: 'She says I chewed a big hole out of the carpet. But who can say?' But the psychiatrist's attention is already elsewhere – focused on his freebie drug company pens in fact: 'The doctor chose his second-finest pen from the array in his white coat's breast pocket and made some sort of note on Kate Gompert's new chart' (*ibid.*: 70–71). These descriptive and then weak prescriptive gestures finally become inscriptions: writing out and reinscribing the patient's identity. Wallace himself struggled with depression throughout his adult life and moved back and forth between drug treatment regimes. He tragically committed suicide in 2008 at the age of 46, at the peak of his writing powers. For Wallace, prescription drugs seemed to help to keep his depression at bay, but eventually the 'black dog' overwhelmed him. We suspect that writing – and Wallace was among the most talented fiction and non-fiction writers of his generation – offered the main therapy in Wallace's life. Certainly, nearly two decades after the publication of *Infinite Jest*, the content remains topical.

Doctors in general write in linear, instrumental and non-literary ways through prescribing, where the act of writing a drug prescription is also the inscription of identity through a 'habitus' (Bourdieu 1977) or typical pattern of practice. Such prescribing then carries over the complications and contradictions inherent to the drug – particularly side effects – to the identity of the patient. Ironically, significant numbers of young women are found to self-harm when taking Seroxat, a drug that promised to reduce psychological harm, thus transforming the cure into symptom. This has been read as an instrumental side effect of the drug. Similarly, drug companies admit the possible occurrence of what they term 'paradoxical effects', in the control of 'hyperactivity'. In the *BNF*, a listed side effect (albeit 'rarely occurring') for Ritalin is 'hyperactivity'! The most commonly reported side effect of extended-release Focalin is its inverse, insomnia. Kids then need another drug to help them sleep: Ellis is informed blankly by his son that his friend Ashton 'took a Zyprexa and then fell asleep'. He responds, 'Well, I suggest you take one too, buddy, because tomorrow's a school day' (Ellis 2005: 69). Zyprexa is an antipsychotic, causing drowsiness.

In prescription culture, the relationship between natural life and prescribed chemical life becomes increasingly blurred. But these writers do not protest. Much like the chemical hall of mirrors with which they jest, they mimic the bad faith of their self-harming characters. Their drawling satires refuse to confess their addictions, rather, laconically describing their own pleasure–pain complicity in the synthetic reality of prescription culture.

Deconstructing drugs

Brett Easton Ellis, David Foster Wallace and Jonathan Franzen are often seen as second-generation postmodernists. Along with others such as Jay McInerney, Rick Moody, Tama Janowitz and J. Robert Lennon, they perpetuate an urban knowing and savvy reflexivity that sees through (in both senses) the institutionalized games of insight that have come to characterize contemporary life. Unlike earlier writers who have explored the social construction of drug culture, they undermine the markers for even an ironic morality on drugs.

Pointing out the continuities between illegal and legal drug taking is not new, any more than accounting for the ordinariness of 'madness'. But these writers do not romanticize mental instability as an alternative to prescribed drugs, as Ronald Laing, David Cooper and the anti-psychiatry movement did in the 1960s. Nor do they romanticize pharmaceuticals, or explicitly condone the abuse of prescribed drugs, as did the Beat generation of the 1950s and early 1960s (Alex Trocchi, Alan Ginsberg, William Burroughs); and the Acid generation of the mid-1960s onwards ('Gonzo' writers inspired by Hunter S. Thompson), who tend to write hysterically. Even compared to the satirical surrealism of the first generation of postmodernists, J.G. Ballard, Thomas Pynchon and Don DeLillo, these information age writers are more detached, mirroring the plain descriptions of the pharmaceutical world itself. Compare Ellis's desultory account of his children's consumption of Zyprexa with the entry for this drug in the *BNF* of the same period (volume 51, 2006):

Zyprexa® (Lilly) PoM
Orodispersible tablet (*Velotab*®), yellow, olanzapine 5 mg, net price 28-tab pack = £56.10; 10 mg, 28-tab pack = £91.37; 15 mg, 28-tab pack = £137.06; 20 mg, 28-tab pack = £182.74. Label: 2, counselling, administration. Excipients include aspartame (section 9.4.1).

The powerful physical substance is abstracted as measurements of quantity, weight and (detailed) cost, while the subsequent 'counselling' on how to administrate Zyprexa is set out as child's play: '*Velotab*® may be placed on the tongue and allowed to dissolve or dispersed in water, orange juice, apple juice, milk, or coffee.'

Note that the technical 'Zyprexa' is now referred to by the user-friendly (and more zippy) company's trade name 'Velotab'. Note too, that the passive tense 'may be placed' avoids any complicating contexts of relationship: we don't need to know whose 'tongue', for example, receives this beneficence. Where Zyprexa is an antipsychotic, causing drowsiness, so the 'dissolving' and 'dispersing' become signifiers for the prescribed state of calm sleep. The tongue upon which we place the dose (or coinage, because all drugs have a cost, meticulously detailed) is metaphorically that of Cerberus, guarding the entry to Hades. Finally, we might note the reference to 'Lilly', appended directly to the drug's name in the entry. This is cross-referenced to the address of the drug manufacturer, Eli Lilly Co Ltd. It was this company that authored Prozac, the most widely used antidepressant in history, though before Lilly found their market, they had tried the same drug as a treatment for high blood pressure, anti-obesity and psychosis (Moore 2007).

It is the medical formulary's sober semiotics, instrumental listing and clipped voice with which the chroniclers of prescription culture play. Coolly witnessing the world, yet simultaneously exaggerating its detail, they implode the moral bounds of earlier postmodern drug reverie. 'N.B. narr tone here mxmly flat/ affectless/ distant/dry', where there is 'no discernible endorsement of cliché', remarks David Foster Wallace (2001: 159) in a short story titled 'Adult World'. But there is a discernible cliché here: that of clinical formulae. The central character in Wallace's short story 'The Depressed Person' (*ibid*.: 31–58) is introduced simply through her anti-depressant drugs' history, as a flat list: 'Paxil, Zoloft, Prozac, Tofranil, Welbutrin, Elavil, Metrazol...Parnate both with and without lithium salts, Nardil both with and without Xanax'. This can be read as a satire on the reductionist style of the case history taught to medical students in every medical school where the patient is boiled dry to a set of symptoms, transmitted with flat affect to produce further objectification. Here is the advice from Weill Cornell Medical College:

> Summarize the case: this is important! The summary should include a few well-crafted sentences, perhaps 3–5 in all. A concise, accurate summary shows that you have grasped the essentials of the case and can distill the clinical data into its essence.
>
> (Weill Cornell Medical College undated)

Here, the patient's 'chief concern' is reduced to the 'chief complaint' (Schleifer and Vannatta 2013) that, as we have seen in previous chapters, may mask or miss the chief concern.

The fiction writers we discuss here bolster this disembodied hyper-realism with pseudo-erudition and the (ab)use of academic trappings, such as Rick Moody's (2002) quotations from historians of American Puritanism – italicized, suggesting sarcastic emphasis. David Foster Wallace literally attaches pages of footnotes on the drugs his characters navigate and in the process personifies the drugs, thus emphasizing their role in identity construction, such as 'Oxycodone hydrochloride w/ acetaminophen, C-II Class, Du Pont Pharmaceuticals' (Wallace 1996: 996); or the post-operative pain killer, 'Ketorolac tromethamine, a non-narcotic analgesic' personified as 'little more than Motrin with ambition' (*ibid.*: 1076). Substituting drug discourse for character, quotation for expression, they avoid even the depth of metaphor, preferring the metonymic technique of offering part for whole, or, we might say, symptom for aetiology. Moody muses that lists themselves are suggestive of an ethical paralysis, but one which he dryly witnesses without being able to stop – a sure sign of addiction: 'The list itself, the catalog, as a journalistic gesture, generates further lists. In fact, the list itself becomes a frequent compositional trope of murderers' (Moody 2002: 223).

Thus, they deconstruct prescription culture simply by citing it. This becomes clear when we pose it against the more common alternative to medical treatment, the 'talking cure' of psychoanalysis. These writers have little but contempt for its acceptance of the 'given', literal body, sceptical of any claim to be able to restore some authentic experience which drugs cannot. Indeed, their own extreme reflexivity appropriates the language of talking cures to subvert and parody such therapies as well. More obviously, they suggest that prescription and therapy cultures are in cahoots in scenes where doctors act as quasi-therapists, therapists prescribe anti-depressants and patients seek both therapy and drugs in turn or simultaneously.

Moody's memoir, titled *The Black Veil*, is perhaps the most pointed in this regard. Moody charts his youthful ambition to self-destruct through drug-taking and drinking, weaving this alongside the story of his forbear Joseph Moody, a seventeenth-century preacher who wore a black face veil through life in shame of having killed a friend as a child. Moody's dry conclusion that 'concealment is necessary to identity' (Moody 2002: 298) thus checks his own confession of shame at addictions and breakdown. It also checks any acknowledgement of his therapists, who are glimpsed as either sharks or fools:

> Beyond stories, my principal interest in these expensive consultations with the mental health professional was not the back and forth of conversation, to which I offered as little as possible, but rather *the drugs*, because, by virtue of the *unexplained panic event*, I had been given a certain prescription, and I carried the vial of it with me wherever I went.
>
> (*Ibid.*: 139)

Later, attending a rehabilitation programme as partner to his equally alcoholic girlfriend, he is pulled aside by a counsellor 'in her late thirties, with a red bob', whose sweaters were *'excessively colourful'* (*ibid.*: 178):

> It was naïve to have failed to see that I was going to look *appetizing* to the employees at the rehabilitation center, especially when my mental health professional back home, in a strangely paranoid outburst, had warned me to be on the alert for this very possibility. *These AA people will try to convert you.*
>
> (*Ibid.*: 179)

Even when he spontaneously checks himself into a psychiatric hospital and stops drinking, Moody maintains his arid performance. Rather, and in this way he also marks out the deconstructive approach to drugs, he suggests that poststructuralist 'Theory' had been his true turning point:

> in junior year, I took a couple of film courses in the department known as *semiotics*. This brought me, at last, to 'Foundation of the Theory of Signs,' or Semiotics 12. *Where the school of deconstruction welcomed its fresh prospects.*
>
> (*Ibid.*: 95)

This period was near Moody's twentieth birthday 'and a number of crises were in the midst of their germination'. He had broken up with a long-term girlfriend and fell in with 'not one but two mercurial, dark, undependable women'. The first introduced him to cocaine. He also started taking large quantities of a 'prescription medicine' that 'a friend...referred to as *Australian quaaludes*. They were probably strong anti-histamines, not much more'. However:

> Taken in large enough doses...or combined with beer, they made my friend's customers, myself among them, thoroughly confused. I experienced my first regular blackouts on these pills, and whole days were

lost. Or I came to at some party having shredded articles of my clothing and talking like a reptile.

(Ibid.: 96)

When his second 'mercurial, dark, undependable' woman ditched him,
Moody 'decided to take *all* the quaaludes, with some Jack Daniel's' that he
refers to as 'my *unconvincing suicide attempt*' (*ibid.*: 96).

He remembers taking maybe 15 pills and then falling asleep, waking 12
or 14 hours later to realize that he was '*missing my discussion section of
semiotics*'. The set reading is Michel Foucault's (1991) *Discipline and
Punish*. Moody arrives at the class but 'I put my head down on my desk and
went to sleep. I didn't wake again until the stirring of the rest of the class at
lunchtime. You'd think a *conversion*, a battering of the heart, couldn't
possibly have firm tread on such lassitude, but sometimes conversion is like
pines that grow on glacial outcroppings' (Moody 2002: 97).

Moody goes on to describe the trajectory of this surprisingly rooted
conversion: 'when I had expelled the quaaludes in me, *Discipline and
Punish* looked entirely new'. He suddenly *saw* Foucault's 'extremely artful
and generous' theory about the displacement of sovereign power by capillary power, where '*The body is directly involved in a political field; power
relations have an immediate hold upon it; they invest it, mark it, train it,
torture it, force it to carry out tasks, to perform ceremonies, to emit signs*'.
The body is both disciplined and resists governance in new ways.
Importantly, 'The theories of Foucault...seemed to have...more in
common with novels than with the dry social theory that I had found in my
philosophy classes. And it was this novelistic dimension that kindled in me
the *zealotry of the newly converted*' (*ibid.*).

For Rick Moody, conversion to the new semiotics comes to displace his
suicidal wishes. The deep semiotics of theory replaces the surface semiotics
of mood design by chemistry. Moody's 'conversion' centrally involves his
insight into the power of Foucault's suggestion that the replacement of
sovereign power by capillary power does not represent the progress ('freedom from') claimed by liberalism but offers a pervading governmentality.
This translates our prescription drugs into pharmaceutical prisons, ongoing
forms of surveillance and control. Where, again, moral injunctions or
imperatives may be disguised as invitations to freedoms ('Enjoy!', 'Have a
nice day!'), supposedly liberating prescription drugs may then become literally prescriptive, a cultural injunction. But this insight does not in fact stop
his drug habit, which is merely deferred. Moody's post-ironic response is to
live that injunction out, to explore its terrible shame, to refuse to confess
what he suggests, in the end, is American culture itself.

From this perspective, we might interpret these writers' refusal to moral-
ize as a protest against prescription culture's own hypocritical plot of
conversion and cure. Their apparent detachment offers commentary without prescribing, thus smuggling in critique at the level of style which they

do not offer at the level of plot. Ironically, then, as they themselves 'write out prescriptions', medical handbooks such as the *BNF* come into relief as exercises in the hyper-real of their own.

The *BNF*, designedly instrumental, is also a descriptive catalogue that strains to bracket out the contexts in which the consumption of its contents actually takes place. From its terse notices of 'contra-indications' and 'side effects', in the people-ness landscape of its passive tense and in appendices where its classifications blur, we sense repressed scenes of parents organizing their kids' medications, or students' swapping drug stories. The following, under the heading of 'Borderline Substances', is appended to the entry on Zyprexa discussed above:

> In certain conditions some foods (and toilet preparations) have characteristics of drugs and the Advisory Committee on Borderline Substances advises as to the circumstances in which such substances may be regarded as drugs. Prescriptions issued in accordance with the Committee's advice and endorsed 'ACBS' will normally not be investigated.
>
> (*BNF* vol. 51, 2006)

The absence of a human(e) voice in the text of the *BNF* reflects the search for perfection through new levels of biotechnological intervention, but in its marginal appendices and footnotes, we glimpse its own borderlines. The BNF acts as superego, Freud's infamous 'absent presence' that frames invitation as imperative ('Enjoy!', 'Have a Nice Day!', etc., leading us to face the world with a Klonopin rictus, a Duchenne smile, empty ecstasy). There is no reflexive voice, simply flat prescription. Its monologue describes a world in which the simulacrum has come to precede the real, or the map displaces the territory.

In the culture of the simulacrum the diagnostic label precedes and comes to form the condition or illness it supposedly only describes. This is also the standard 'anti-psychiatry' critique. An insert in *BNF* 51 (March 2006) offers a warning about Atomoxetine, where prescribed for ADHD: 'In September 2005, the Committee on Safety of Medicines...wrote to health professionals about the risk of suicidal thoughts and behaviour in children taking Atomoxetine for Attention Deficit Hyperactivity Disorder'.

In advising that patients and their carers should look out for and report adverse changes of mood or behaviour as the child takes the drug, the drug itself is policed, but not the diagnostic category 'ADHD', without which such drugs would not be produced.

In summary of this section, the deconstructive novelists we have considered chart their responses to the creeping pharmaceutical culture in the backhanded manner of Jacques Derrida's philosophy, attempting not so much to judge as to both violently differentiate and tenderly defer. In this way, such deconstructive writing does not offer a 'cure' for prescription culture at all, but an exaggeration of its symptoms, the diagnosis of a diagnosis, the double 'writing out' of its paradoxical effects. However, in the final section, we argue that this rather tortuous approach does have benefits.

The value of literary deconstruction in understanding health interventions

We have explored a literary rather than sociological response to the prescription of mood-altering drugs as a 'health' intervention, because we consider that literature plumbs the social unconscious in a different and powerful way. The novels we have discussed deconstruct the objectivity of medical texts and expose the contrary injunction to 'be happy!' which sustains prescription culture, but they do this in the form of imaginative symptoms, rather than explications, of a condition that they themselves share.

No doubt many readers will find these writers overemphasize the determining aspects of 'prescription' as habitus. The synthesizing research by Pound and colleagues (2005: 1) on patients' actual behaviour in relation to prescriptions reveals there is 'widespread caution about taking medicines', that they do not just 'accept their medicines . . . passively', but 'actively, or . . . reject them'. This is as true in relation to mood-altering drugs as it is with others, and, moreover, is also the case in the United States as well as in Britain that not only has an exceptionally high consumption rate but the highest drug prices in the world, towards which most patients are making co-payments. 'The main reason why people do not take their medicines as prescribed is not because of failings in patients, doctors or systems, but because of concerns about the medicines themselves' (*ibid.*).

It would, of course, be foolish to overstate the powers of prescription as a cultural injunction. We only have to contrast national formularies with the very different handbook for women's health and sexuality, *Our Bodies, Ourselves* (Boston Women's Health Book Collective 2005), which has been arguing against the over-medicalization of social problems since 1970, when the Boston Women's Health Book Collective first produced it (the most recent edition was published in 2011). This classic of second wave feminism has been republished nine times in the US and translated into 19 languages, representing an alternative stream of American influence abroad. Along with a website (www.ourbodiesourselves.org), it aims to empower women as their own health experts, emphasizing 'That a pathology/disease approach to normal life events (birthing, menopause, aging, death) is not an effective way in which to consider health or structure a health system'.

If that is its own 'diagnosis of the diagnosis', it also challenges the stark post-industrial vision of authors such as Ellis, Wallace and Moody in stylistic method. Unashamedly modernist in contrast to the latter's postmodernist hyper-realist satire, *Our Bodies, Ourselves* is not merely realist, but autobiographical, weaving 'first-person stories' collected from conversations, letters and email messages through its chatty text (Boston Women's Health Book Collective 2005: xi). These personal narratives express the struggle to take control within complex social landscapes, as an example from 'Women Growing Older' in the British edition suggests:

> A psychiatrist gave me valium when I was in my forties. I took it regularly or fairly frequently for about five to ten years. Now I think that tranquillisers suppressed or sent underground the pains of that period (divorce, death of mother, betrayal by a lover). These pains still surface with agonizing strength. Maybe if I had fully faced them and 'digested' them at the time they happened this would not be the case.
>
> (Phillips and Rakusen 1996: 453)

Like Ellis, Wallace, and Moody, *Our Bodies, Ourselves* does invoke the lists and maps of national 'formularies' and chemical guides, yet announces its humane intention to people that landscape. Its storytelling challenges, individualizes and reanimates the flat affect of the written prescription and its writing family, restoring a narrative shape that is basic to the conception of a life story as a frame of change, argument and development, though not necessarily the conversion of absolute cure. This methodology also acknowledges that good doctors can and often do encourage a patient's sense of agency in this respect, particularly in the oral genres of case-history taking reception and diagnosis, despite the affectless mode of the written prescriptions they may then produce.

Our Bodies, Ourselves suggests that there is something deeply astray in both the ideas and the feelings of the novelists we have discussed, in their strange submission to prescription and, moreover, in the masculine terms in which they perceive their alienation. We propose, nevertheless, that deconstructive literature retains a unique value for anyone interested in the ideological aspects of prescription. This is precisely because of its sophisticated addiction combined with a fear of dependency, its inside-outside relationship. Deconstructive literature rejects the romanticism of earlier literary drug-users, but it also exposes a more covert romanticism in therapeutic alternatives that promote their own ideologies of conversion and cure.

The style of the deconstructive writers we have discussed models the paradox (and double bind) of the *pharmakon* – the drug as both 'poison' and 'cure'. Jacques Derrida (1993), deconstruction's inventor, if it can be said to have one, argued in 'The Rhetoric of Drugs' that we should stop scapegoating drug-taking, noting the artificial line drawn between the *pharmakon* as remedy (*prescription pharmaceuticals* are social, authentic, natural, demanding and productive) and poison (*illicit drugs* are solitary, fantastical, unnatural, effortless and unproductive). Boothroyd (2000) argues that deconstruction presents the possibility of an alternative thinking of the relation to 'drugs'. If we take Boothroyd's case to refer to prescription culture as well as recreational drug culture, and then to include anti-depressant, anti-anxiety and ADHD medications, it raises very important questions about prescribing as a 'health' intervention:

> drugs may be taken *otherwise* – in a sense for which there is as yet no concept, on the basis of a non-authoritarian, deregulated understanding of their *multiple* effects, in *several* senses. In other words, the force of the dominant drug rhetorics may be countered by the deratiocinatory force of a reinscribed notion of drugs. Could there be a *measure* for drugs, unfettered, for example, by such rhetorics as those of authenticity and inauthenticity, of health and illness, of use and abuse, etc.?
>
> (Boothroyd 2000: 58)

This characteristically displacing quote suggests in fact that deconstruction can be *equated* with drug taking, for both of them undo notions of truth and order which are naturalized in prescription culture. Much the same could be said of Sadie Plant's (2001) *Writing on Drugs*, which invokes Foucault to map out how the conventional prohibitions against illegal drug taking only incite its practice – with ironically creative effects.

Deconstructing arbitrary distinctions between medicine and drugs, then, has little to say about the free will lost in addiction, and nothing about the evidence of patients' control over, or even rejection of, prescription drugs in the pragmatic politics of texts such as *Our Bodies, Ourselves*. But this is not its point, nor its usefulness to those working in the everyday of healthcare. Rather, it is precisely its doubt about individual agency that so powerfully dramatizes prescription culture's micro-disciplining effects and the wider dissolution of a belief in free will that permits it. A warning and a seduction in one, it exemplifies the same psychology that, without self-consciousness, offers doctors, who offer patients, the *BNF*.

Coda: development of a humanities-based formulary

It is not enough to simply point out that there are striking similarities between the flat affect of the *BNF* (or any other, similar pharmaceutical formulary) and the stylized hyperrealism of the postmodern novelists whose work we discuss above. What should be done about this that may improve medical education with a view to a knock-on effect on patient care and safety? Our argument above is that such postmodern writers, who have a cultivated and developed technique of presenting the world as marketplace shaped partly by 'Big Pharma' interests (Law 2006), do so in a highly detached and very articulate manner that is gendered male. In striking contrast, many of the confessional YouTube videos show young people who are struggling to articulate their symptoms and the side effects of drugs often in claustrophobic confessions.

The smart postmodern writers we catalogue in this chapter model an ironic style that is in part a deliberate attempt to recreate through literature a consciousness that is in part shaped by regular use of antidepressants, anti-anxiety and mood controlling drugs such as the amphetamine-based medications for ADHD. However, we also pointed out that such literature appears to have misplaced its heart, interested more in the cold mechanics of deconstructing society than in the warm art of constructing humane relations and activities. Feelings are not missing from such literature; it is just that these feelings tend to be ones of colder detachment and observation rather than warm attachment, empathy and concern.

Of course, the argument throughout this book has been for a reconstruction of medical practice that, historically, has suffered from over-detachment and objectification of patients. We noted that humanistic approaches such as the long-running *Our Bodies, Ourselves* provide an antidote to the colder detachment of the deconstructive postmodern novel, as a reconstructive engagement. This is also gendered female. However, such an approach bears its own intrinsic faultlines such as a potentially cloying sentimentalism. There is a middle way between medicine's traditional masculine gaze and what many doctors dismiss as 'warm and fuzzy' relationship-centred medicine – a 'warm objectivity' based on authentic patient-centredness (Bleakley 2014).

How then, might we respond in medical education to the issues raised by this chapter? We have already said in the introductory paragraphs that in our experience medical students appreciate the opportunity to discuss 'prescription culture' beyond their technical knowledge of pharmacology and prescribing behaviour. The postmodern novels we discuss above offer a unique way into prescription culture and an aspect of population medicine that invites students to read beyond the *BNF*, but, paradoxically, to draw textual parallels between the *BNF* and postmodern, deconstructive novels. But there is another step that we have experimented with tentatively in undergraduate medical education but have not fully developed – to invite students to begin to construct an 'alternative' or 'critical' *BNF*.

Here is a challenge for medical educators interested in the humanities – how might we develop a limited electronic *BNF* (based, say on a few mood altering drugs used regularly by GPs and psychiatrists) in which we do two things? First, we develop profiles of patients (case studies) that accompany the technical descriptions of drugs, their effects and side effects. At the heart of this part of the alternative formulary are patients' stories concerning their relationship to prescribed drugs. Indeed, as already noted, a bank of such visually enhanced stories is already available on YouTube. Here, mainly young people talk about their individual experiences with anti-depressants, anti-anxiety and other mood regulating and mood enhancing drugs. Many of these stories stress 'regulation' over 'enhancement'.

Second, we develop 'character profiles' of the drugs themselves, treating them as active agents. Actor–network theory is slowly becoming an influential model in medical education research and pedagogy, both as a conceptual framework and a research approach using ethnography

(Bleakley 2014). Actor–network theory proposes a radical symmetry between persons, ideas and material artefacts where the latter are given agency. This is not too hard to comprehend if we think of computers as extending our cognition and a variety of pharmaceuticals as extending our senses, affects and cognitions or regulating potential disruptions. Developing a character profile of a drug in concert with a character profile of a patient gives a way for medical students to better imagine the potential interactions between persons and drugs, where the latter can act as allies or foes. The alternative formulary can then be developed as a mobile device application. The elements in the learning network for understanding more about prescription culture are then: novels such as those described in this chapter, counter-literature on psychological health such as the Boston Women's Health Book Collective's series of books, patients with mental health issues related to prescribed anti-anxiety and anti-depressant drugs and/or YouTube confessional videos, a 'living' mini *critical formulary* in which the drugs are not only described in functional terms, but case studies are provided to give a human face to the mechanics of the pharmacopoeia. This would be the medical humanities in action in medical education.

Note

1   This section of the chapter ('Prescription Culture') was written in collaboration with Dr Margaretta Jolly, University of Sussex.

9 Evaluating the impact of medical humanities provision

Introduction

There is still considerable resistance to accepting that the medical humanities could play an important role as core and integrated provision in an undergraduate medicine curriculum as argued throughout this book. Sceptics towards this curriculum innovation are usually strong proponents of evidence-based medicine, where what counts as 'evidence' is constrained by the scientific paradigm. Arts practitioners and humanities scholars are not used to working within such a paradigm that appears constrictive. Second, theoretical rationales for including the medical humanities in medical education are generally flimsy. This book has set out to challenge this in developing a robust and well-informed theoretical framework for including a strong medical humanities curriculum component. Third, curriculum planners seem unable to get over a hurdle of how to incorporate the medical humanities. Instead of, for example, conceiving the curriculum as a text, and then asking to what extent is the curriculum an aesthetic text teaching an art and craft of medicine – a process approach – curriculum planners get bogged down in content, in planning a syllabus rather than an educational experience.

It is shameful that medical educators have not fully taken on board the most important contemporary revolution in curriculum thinking – the curriculum reconceptualization movement (Pinar 2012). This models how a curriculum can be planned and implemented in an integrated fashion – for example where science teachers 'think aesthetics', just as medical humanities faculty might, without the burden of planning 'content' but rather with the challenge of related staff development. It is not such a big leap to imagine how, for example, living and surface anatomy can be learned much more deeply through collaborations between artists, computer games and software designers, medical illustrators and anatomists. Basic clinical skills such as the physical examination can be greatly enhanced through arts-based observation (Chapter 6), while taking a history can be enhanced through learning narrative capabilities. These approaches require thinking medicine with the arts and humanities.

Supporters of the medical humanities point out that it is in the arena of patient-centred, narrative based medicine, rather than population-centred, evidence based medicine, that the medical humanities play a significant role. Yet sceptics, who see the medical humanities as 'fluffy', continue to demand evidence of the effect of medical humanities as medical education interventions. Such sceptics also point to the controversies within the medical humanities, discussed particularly in Chapter 1, as evidence that proponents of the medical humanities do not have their house in order – forgetting that similar controversies, contradictions, rifts and tensions exist in the worlds of biomedical science and clinical practice as these apply to medical education.

However, the question of impact of medical humanities interventions in medical education should be addressed and in this chapter I look – if at times, with a sideways glance – at evaluation or proof of impact. I do not wish to simply repeat what a literature review of evidence of impact of medical humanities interventions has found (Ousager and Johannessen 2010). Rather, I wish to problematize the whole issue of 'measuring impact' to suggest that 'evaluation' of the impact of medical humanities provision through current dominant models itself needs to be critically evaluated and problematized.

Measuring the immeasurable?

In order for the medical humanities to establish greater traction in the undergraduate medicine curriculum, sceptics press advocates to work harder on demonstration of impact on learning. Polianski and Fangerou (2012) describe a 'vehement debate' about the purposes of medical humanities in medical schools, with sceptics placing the burden of proof of effectiveness on the shoulders of advocates. In contrast, advocates – even where sympathetic to outcomes-based learning – suggest that measurement of impact is confounded by complexity of input, culminating in attempting to measure the immeasurable. This is not a new debate – a quarter of a century ago McManus (1995: 1144) suggested that 'Any serious evaluation of the humanities in medicine . . . must bite the bullet of definition and measurement, even if it seems to be "defining the indefinable".'

Ousager and Johannessen (2010) conducted a literature review of impact studies within the field of the medical humanities, consulting 245 articles and finding only nine that measured longer-term impacts of interventions, such as longitudinal scores on attitude scales and surveys. The authors tersely conclude: 'Evidence on the positive long-term impacts of integrating humanities into undergraduate medical education is sparse'. An earlier, less comprehensive, review (Wershof Schwartz *et al.* 2009) raises a wider set of conceptual issues, but is no less pessimistic in its conclusions. Across studies reviewed, effects of interventions were claimed in three areas: medical humanities input promotes empathy, professionalism, and self-care in medical students. However, lack of control over interplay of variables, biased populations, and poor conceptualization were seen to confound such studies and to reduce the power of their claims. The review offers a pessimistic conclusion: 'few data are available to support the hypothesis that humanities affects professional behaviour'. More worryingly, the problematic and contested terms 'empathy', 'professionalism' and 'self-care' remain untouched.

In a systematic, key-informant review of medical humanities provision at 14 of Canada's 17 medical schools, Kidd and Connor (2008) note a gap between the convergent evidence-based approach towards teaching the clinical sciences and an 'anarchic' approach of medical humanities teaching. The authors suggest that the continuing presence of such a gap explains why the medical humanities are commonly marginalized and urge providers to consider how they might close this gap, while noting that this presents a challenge, where the medical humanities 'defy easy metrical appraisal'. Given the attention that I have given to the use of language in medical encounters throughout this book, such as the resistance within medicine to the subjunctivizing mood (Chapter 7), 'defy easy metrical appraisal' simply plays straight into the hands of sceptics towards the medical humanities. Do those whose hearts and passions are in providing a genuinely deep experience for students in linking clinical practice to humane care really think about the 'easy metrical appraisal' of what they do?

How trustworthy, however, are these meta-reviews in their own right? Are 'easy metrical appraisal' instruments themselves inherently flawed? The review of Ousager and Johannessen (2010) was sharply critiqued by both Belling (2010) and Charon (2010). Belling (2010: 940) suggests that empirical studies of the impact of medical humanities provision offer reductionist approaches, where the instrumental tools used for evaluation are currently so blunt that 'the medical education establishment should be challenged to continue investing in immeasurable outcomes'. Can we then sharpen our evaluation tools? Charon (2010: 936) suggests a rethink of the nature of outcome studies in the medical humanities by moving away from proxy measures, such as medical students' empathy, to outcomes such as 'the success of their patients to achieve the health goals…they set for themselves'. However, Charon continues to note a conceptual paradox, where she questions the value of applying reductive positivistic methodologies to a field that is so inherently complex: 'One can and ought to wonder whether it is beside the point to try to measure, through reductive processes of evaluation, that aspect of learning which is meant as an antidote to the reductiveness of the curriculum itself' (*ibid.*).

Are there other, more pressing, issues than measurement of impact?

The current debate about measurement of outcomes following from humanities interventions in medical education may be distracting from a bigger issue that has long been debated – just what is the purpose of medical/health humanities provision, addressed particularly in Chapters 1–3? In any case, as noted above, the outcome measurement debate has been generated by sceptics and not advocates – again, the former placing the burden of proof of effectiveness on the shoulders of the latter. To some in the medical humanities movement, energy is better spent forming a strong rationale for why the humanities should be included as core and integrated provision in undergraduate medical education, such as:

- Serving as a critical counterweight to a reductive biomedical science that dominates the curriculum. Science taught in medical schools often fails to be integrated across specialties and is largely shaped by 'top down' approaches (dictated by specialists) rather than 'bottom up' approaches (drawing on a variety of key stakeholders, including students, junior doctors and nurses; Bull and Mattick 2010). Non-reductive, holistic science, that explores complexity, chaos theory and dissipative structures, is yet to make an impact in the undergraduate medicine curriculum. Science has crowded out learning the artistry of medicine, where doctors are not pure scientists but 'science using' practitioners (Hunter 1991b). The art of medicine has also been reduced to a technical process involving 'communication skills' and 'professionalism' whose worth is judged through evidence gleamed from quasi-scientific studies.
- To educate for empathy. This offers a counterweight to the tendency for medicine to objectify patients and provide inhumane care. Education for empathy includes education for humane, socially aware and responsible practice. Here, the medical humanities are twinned with ethics provision. Where sceptics say 'I'd rather be treated by a competent but brusque technician than a considerate but technically poor doctor', this misses the point. A good doctor is both technically proficient and humane. Lack of non-technical competence is a major cause of medical error (Bleakley and Marshall 2013).
- To provide a realist philosophical alternative to the idealist position of utilitarianism informing medicine's notions of 'healing', 'health' and 'wellbeing'. Sceptical philosophical positions accept the reality that illness is a part of life, but also that illness may have meaning and be productive. Further, one person's 'wellbeing' (for example sadism, cross-dressing, binge drinking, or base jumping) is another's 'illness'. Medicine's unquestioned assumption of the value of an utilitarian position is undermined by persistent and high levels of iatrogenesis – illness and death produced by medical interventions – and by the public's determination to undermine health through risky lifestyle choices such as poor diets, lack of exercise and drug and alcohol abuse; risky sports pursuits; and violence grounded in political and ethnic differences.
- To educate for tolerance of ambiguity and then for democratic practices. The gap between tolerance of ambiguity and engaging with democratic habits may seem large, but the connection is readily justified.

Progressive streams of thinking have developed differing 'critical medical humanities' as described in Chapters 1 and 2 (Bleakley 2013b). These streams critique conventional medical humanities as not only subscribing to the same value system as orthodox medicine, but also to present a 'tame' (Macneill 2011: 86) approach offering students 'soft' relaxation, celebratory supplement, or diversion from the 'hard' stuff of biomedical science and evidence-based clinical practice. Rees (2010) further notes that the medical humanities can be employed non-critically, serving medical dominance rather than used in a more radical politically, aesthetically and ethically interventionist manner. Where the functional limit of the arts and humanities has been to nuance medical practice, rather than fundamentally critiquing such practice, the form of the arts and humanities drawn upon has avoided the critical and political liberal avant-garde, as noted in Chapter 6.

Wear and Aultman (2005) show that while medical students readily tolerate benign plots and characters in literature, transgressive and challenging plots and characters at first produce resistance rather than empathy. Exposing medical students to challenging narratives can produce discomfort, defensiveness and resistance to confronting political issues such as inequality and oppression. This offers a reminder of what is, arguably, the central purpose of art, certainly of the avant-garde – consciousness-raising through creating discomfort, challenge or ambiguity. Such consciousness-raising is a three-step process: first, producing disruption through challenging habit; second, allowing typical patterns of resistance to emerge; and third, analysing such resistance to develop new awareness. In a commentary, Belling (2010: 939) notes:

> Wear and Aultman articulate the limitations of treating (medical) humanities merely as a palatable reprieve from 'hard' work. They argue instead that we must attend to resistance, *even provoke it*, if (medical) humanities teaching is to promote critical inquiry as well as neutral reflection' (my emphasis), where 'rigorous humanities teaching can develop an orientation toward uncertainty, knowledge, and action that characterizes the best physicians.

It is this 'orientation toward uncertainty' – and the dual claim that it both characterizes the 'best' doctors and that it can be developed through 'rigorous humanities teaching' – that provides the focus for this closing chapter. A central interest of the chapter is how 'homeostasis' is viewed in medicine and the arts, where it is a primary aim for medicine but problematic for the arts and humanities. Where medicine aims to maintain bodily homeostasis or internal regulation and balance, working against illness and towards health and wellbeing, the progressive arts can be seen to upset cultural homeostasis to induce a permanent state of questioning of what constitutes cultural 'health' and 'wellbeing'. In short, medicine aims to reduce ambiguity where the arts aim to produce ambiguity, offering different 'orientations to uncertainty' in Belling's phrase above. Such orientations to uncertainty or ambiguity should not be read as an opposition between science and art, but as a productive tension. Where medicine and the arts both share high levels of ambiguity and uncertainty, they have developed differing tactics as a response (Luther and Crandall 2011). Medicine has, historically, refused to accept uncertainty, where the arts and humanities have celebrated ambiguity. What, however, is the value of ambiguity for both the arts and medicine?

William Empson's seven types of ambiguity

Ambiguity as a resource in poetry and medicine

While William Empson was still an undergraduate student at Cambridge University in the UK, at first reading Mathematics and later switching to English, he wrote one of the most influential books in modern literary criticism. Composed when he was not yet 22 and published in 1930 when he was 24, *Seven Types of Ambiguity* founded a school of literary criticism – the 'New Criticism' – characterized by 'close reading' of texts. Empson's (1991) close reading of English poetry revealed seven different kinds of ambiguity as poetic devices – ways in which linguistic ambiguity could be used to bring vibrancy, meaning and impact to a poem, celebrating ambiguity as a resource rather than a hindrance.

When Empson wrote this book, western medicine was characterized by strong paternalism. Men dominated the profession and patients were placed in a passive role of assumed ignorance. Although medical and surgical practices were riddled with uncertainty, the profession, especially surgery, refused to acknowledge such uncertainty. Indeed, the medical historian Kenneth Ludmerer (1999: 325), as noted earlier, describes a 'century-long defect in medical education: the failure of medical education to prepare learners to deal with uncertainty'. One of the major turns in contemporary medicine and medical education is the growing recognition by the profession to admit to high levels of ambiguity and uncertainty and to share this openly with patients and colleagues (Truog *et al.* 2011).

The medical humanities can play a vital role in giving meaning to such ambiguity in medicine. First, admitting to ambiguity is also facing reality. Medicine is complex, inherently ambiguous and uncertain. Medical education must teach students and junior doctors to 'think complexity' (Bleakley 2010; Bleakley and Cleland forthcoming) and to tolerate high levels of ambiguity, especially early in their practice (Bleakley and Brennan 2011; Luther and Crandall 2011). Complexity models challenge naïve versions of homeostasis, where systems are stable only in the sense that they maintain maximum complexity without falling into chaos. Thinking complexity and tolerating ambiguity do not hinder medical practice from providing good diagnoses and appropriate treatments. Such thinking may, however, reduce the load of unnecessary testing currently plaguing medicine, where such over-testing is justified as reducing uncertainty.

Second, admitting to ambiguity marks the profession as non-authoritarian. As noted elsewhere, intolerance of ambiguity is a key trait of the authoritarian personality (Adorno *et al.* 1950). There is a good psychological reason for this – refusing uncertainty allows one to remain in control. However, contemporary health care is intolerant of authoritarian behaviour and the strict hierarchies that result from it, where inter-professional, team-based care is the ideal. In this shift to collaborative healthcare, the model of the heroic, autonomous (and often authoritarian rather than authoritative) doctor is fast disappearing. Third, patients want to collaborate and, while understandably keen to have a clear diagnosis and prognosis, are able to tolerate high levels of ambiguity (Roter and Hall 2006). Fourth, and finally, accepting ambiguity is integral to healthcare practitioners' duty of candour, complementing a duty of care (Truog *et al.* 2011). Medicine is only now admitting to an unacceptably high rate of medical error, with the knowledge that improving communication with colleagues in teams and with patients can potentially halve such error (Xyrichis and Ream 2008). As some level of error is inevitable even where patient safety is at a high level, it is important that the fundamental uncertainty inherent to medical practice is recognized and talked about openly with patients and their families.

It is only in recent years that medical education has recognized the need to explicitly educate medical students for tolerance of ambiguity, for example through patient safety awareness and practices. Typically, intolerance of ambiguity bleeds in to professional communication as a way of defending against the discomfort or anxiety of uncertainty. Hence, despite over 30 years' worth of emphasis upon communication skills training in undergraduate medical education, doctors still interrupt patients in consultations on average after 18 seconds of meeting them and resort to monologue (telling, informing) rather than dialogue (question and answer, debate; Roter and Hall 2006), presumably in order to exercise control. The effects of the anxiety produced by the inability to manage uncertainty may show in the relatively high rates of distress, burnout, suicide ideation and suicide among doctors (British Medical Association 2012) and medical students (Dyrbye *et al.* 2008).

Empson's seven types of ambiguity transposed to medical education

Returning to Empson's (1991) book, his seven types of ambiguity as poetic devices can be transposed to medical education as guides to preparing doctors of the future. This exercise of transposition can get us into the habit of thinking ambiguity (or tolerating uncertainty). Thinking this way produces a healthy scepticism towards the use of naïve measurement of the impact of the medical humanities, reducing the nonlinear complex to the linear (albeit complicated) and translating qualities into quantities as metrics.

1   The first type of ambiguity described by Empson is the general use of metaphor

Chapter 6 describes the place of resemblances, analogies, similes and maxims or aphorisms in medicine. These are linguistic tropes allied to metaphor (Donoghue 2014) describing a likeness that is not literally true, bringing two disparate things together, such as 'right as rain' – a metaphor for wellbeing, or 'greased lightning' – a metaphor for swiftness. An extended metaphor is an aphorism – a pithy saying such as 'power corrupts and absolute power corrupts absolutely'. Resemblances, discussed in Chapter 6 (an 'apple core lesion', a 'bamboo spine'), and aphorisms or 'clinical pearls' ('when you hear hoofbeats, don't think zebras' – or, stick to the obvious when making a differential diagnosis) are, as we have seen, commonly employed in medicine, for example in helping with pattern recognition diagnosis (Bleakley *et al.* 2003a, 2003b; Levine and Bleakley 2012). This occurs across the senses. For example, a coarse crackle in the lungs heard through auscultation, indicating an airway disease, is likened to the slow opening of a Velcro fastener.

2   A second type of ambiguity is where two or more meanings are resolved into one

The original meanings, however, still linger or show through the apparent resolution. For example, two different metaphors may be used at once, such as: 'he is as good as dead' and 'the writing is on the wall'. In medicine, this is a common kind of ambiguity employed in psychiatry, where multiple symptoms are present but the person is characterized by a main descriptor affording meaning, such as 'autism' – while, for example, attention deficit hyperactivity disorder (ADHD) may also be present as part of that syndrome.

3   A third type of ambiguity is where two ideas that are connected through context can be given in one word simultaneously

Thus, lightning may 'crackle' and one's hair may simultaneously appear to 'crackle' in a thunderstorm. The context brings the two together with impact. Indeed, a series of imaginative ideas may 'crackle' in the process, leading to a serendipitous insight, or a plan for action. In the illustrative example above (1), an airway disease may be diagnosed through auscultation, heard as a coarse crackle like slowly opening a Velcro fastener. In the same context (auscultation of the lungs using a stethoscope), a late inspiratory fine crackle may indicate pulmonary fibrosis or congestive heart failure.

4   *A fourth type of ambiguity is where two or more meanings that do not normally align combine, bringing into focus a complex state of mind in the author*

This is the holding of an apparent contradiction, such as 'radical tradition-alism'. For example, in medical education, there is a current call to return to traditions of bedside teaching, first inaugurated in the late eighteenth century (Foucault 1989). However, such teaching is radicalized through contemporary pedagogy, so that, for example, patients, students and other healthcare professionals become collaborators with consultants/attending physicians in a democratic teaching episode.

5   *A fifth type of ambiguity is when an author 'discovers' an idea through the act of writing*

For example, two separate ideas may be written out, at first disconnected, but then coming into focus to reveal a new idea arising from their collision. This is wholly familiar in writing reports or referral letters in medicine. In tracing an ambiguity in a patient case, a general/family practitioner writing a referral letter may suddenly see a connection. For example, a patient referred to an urologist after an episode of haematuria is considered to possibly be bleeding from a bladder lesion. However, the GP recognizes from the patient's history as he is writing the referral letter that the bleeding may be from an enlarged prostate.

6   *A sixth type of ambiguity is when the writer appears to say nothing and 'close' readers have to invent a meaning of their own that may be in conflict with the poorly expressed or underdeveloped meaning of the author*

Here, author and reader collaborate in producing the text. This is a good definition of patient-centred medicine, where patients, especially as experts in their own illnesses, often fill in the gaps left by doctors. Where the patient is often ignorant of the causes of symptoms, doctors act as close readers of the patient's text (Bleakley *et al.* 2011).

7   *A seventh type of ambiguity is when two words or ideas appear that, within the context of the text, are opposites and expose a fundamental and unresolved division in the author's mind*

In medicine, this can be illustrated by the classic slippage from descriptors of certainty such as 'we know this is the case', or 'it is definitely...', to those of varying levels of ambiguity and uncertainty such as 'probably' and 'maybe'. These can be held together in the same sentence: 'I am pretty sure that this is possibly a case of...'. I have also framed this as movement between the indicative and the subjunctive mood in Chapter 7.

As Empson's seven types of ambiguity (as poetic devices) illustrate, in the arts and humanities the production of ambiguity can be used as a device to breathe new life in to tired or outdated conventions. This again conflicts with medicine's desire to reduce uncertainty. However, as the examples above show, medicine in fact regularly deals with the presence of uncertainty and this can be seen as a vitalizing force, just as kinds of ambiguity are used for literary effect, as Empson's classic study again illustrates. Ambiguity is then seen as a resource rather than a hindrance. The primary function of the medical humanities in the undergraduate medicine curriculum may be to educate for tolerance of ambiguity, or to prepare medical students for a professional life riddled with uncertainty (Bleakley and Marshall 2013). Hence, perhaps a sharper instrument for measuring the impact of the medical humanities is to consider the presence of tolerance of ambiguity. Indeed, tolerance of ambiguity has been measured through scales, including a recent new, sharper version (Hancock *et al.* in press).

Issues of 'impact': seven types of resistance to ambiguity

While a 'vehement debate' may be raging about both the need to evaluate the impact of the medical humanities in medical education and the means by which this may be done, there are several existing vehicles for such evaluation, including metrics. These are considered below. However, these seven ways of evaluating impact share a common flaw – they fail to address the overall issue of maintaining ambiguity as a complex resource (to be appreciated through a mindset of complexity), rather than a hindrance to be repressed, displaced, or disguised through reductive measures. Indeed, they set out to reduce ambiguity under a common philosophical stance of utilitarianism. For this reason, they can be considered to be necessary, but not sufficient, for evaluating the impact of the medical humanities in medical education.

1   *Measuring tolerance of ambiguity*

As outlined in earlier chapters, Martha Nussbaum (2010) argues that a primary function of the humanities in culture is to educate for democracy through empathy for others, or tolerance of difference. We can then predict that medical humanities in medical education would also lead to tolerance of difference, or generally increase tolerance of, or for, ambiguity (or lowering of intolerance of ambiguity).

Evaluation of a curriculum innovation at a new medical school – Peninsula Medical School, UK – was conducted through a longitudinal retrospective Likert scale survey questionnaire. The questionnaire was given at entry to the junior doctor programme and nine months later, asking how well the undergraduate programme had prepared the participants in the study on a number of clinical responsibilities and professional behaviours, where one of the questions concerned 'coping with uncertainty'. The Peninsula cohort was compared with a mixed, similar sized, cohort of graduates from other medical schools working in the same Deanery. The largest significant difference in favour of Peninsula graduates across all questions was found on 'coping with uncertainty' (Bleakley and Brennan 2011). Scores on a validated scale of tolerance of ambiguity also showed a difference between the cohorts, with the Peninsula cohort scoring higher, but this difference was not statistically significant.

The importance of this study rests in the fact that Peninsula – only established in 2002 – pioneered the most radical medical humanities programme across UK medical schools and possibly internationally, by introducing the medical humanities as core and integrated in the curriculum. Such limited data do not of course specifically indicate that it is a core, integrated medical humanities curriculum that produces relatively higher levels of preparation for coping with uncertainty. This is just one factor in a curriculum 'brand' and 'climate' (Genn 2001) that has other innovations besides the medical humanities input, but Peninsula had set out to create a climate of innovative learning in which clinical sciences, arts and humanities engaged in productive conversation.

Measuring tolerance of ambiguity as an effect of a medical humanities intervention could be carried out with a controlled intervention within a single cohort of students, but this would need to be a longitudinal measure to gauge lasting effect. Further, such an effect might be predicted from a curriculum where the medical humanities are core and integrated (and then a controlled study within a cohort is not possible), but not necessarily from specific interventions such as a single optional study unit. Also, the measurement of tolerance of ambiguity/intolerance of ambiguity on a generalized scale may not have ecological validity, where ambiguity and uncertainty are experienced in particular, often paradoxical, ways across clinical contexts. Medicine presents many layers of ambiguity presented simultaneously – for example, pressure for clear diagnoses vies with not putting patients through unnecessary examinations and tests.

2   Can we draw on the evidence of impact drawn from the arts and health movement?

In looking for evidence of impact of the medical humanities in medical education, should we turn to the large body of studies within arts therapies that demonstrate impact? In a review conducted for Arts Council England, Staricoff (2004, 2006) cites nearly 400 papers showing a positive impact of arts interventions on health outcomes. In the same year, Ulrich and colleagues (2004) cited nearly 700 peer-reviewed research studies showing beneficial impact of arts interventions on health outcomes. Typical of such studies quoted are beneficial effects on perception of pain for rheumatoid arthritis sufferers through listening to music; and reduction in length of hospital stay and need for pain relief for orthopaedic and trauma patients exposed to an arts-rich environment. Stuckey and Nobel (2010) conducted a review of the arts therapy literature between 1995 and 2007 to assess links between arts interventions and healing and found an impressive array of positive results both in terms of health outcomes and psychological meaningfulness.

Despite these apparently impressive research outcomes, there are three main objections to drawing on the arts for health movement as evidence of the impact of medical humanities in medical education. First, there is a pervasive confounding factor in the studies themselves – it is difficult to separate the effect of the art practice from the effects of other factors such as communication, emotional support and interest provided by the artists or arts therapists. Second, the 'arts for health' approach is not concerned with how we educate doctors and healthcare practitioners. Third, arts for health can be seen to have fundamentally different aims than the medical humanities, drawing on a different philosophical tradition.

An important distinction can be drawn between arts for health/arts therapies approaches and art and the humanities in culture, where arts for health/arts therapies are usually about a patient's therapeutic engagement with a medium (paint, clay, words, music) rather than exposure to an expert artist's production. The patient does not act as expert 'artist' even when active rather than passive with the medium. The medical humanities and arts for health/arts therapies are not clearly aligned. For example, where arts for health practitioners and arts therapists use a medium, such as paint or film, to help restore confidence in a depressed person or to relax a person suffering from Parkinson's disease, artists often use the medium to do therapy on art itself, asking fundamental questions about the nature and purposes of the medium.

Although arts for health/arts therapies approaches may be included as special study units within the undergraduate curriculum, such approaches are not generally about medical education. Medical students do not learn to become arts therapy practitioners with patients. Rather, within medical education the concern is whether or not the arts and humanities change the ways that these students will practice as doctors, so that patients 'receive' the arts and humanities interventions through the medium of the doctor, not the medium of paint or sound. Of course, the distinction is not as tightly drawn as this. The medium of language is shared between doctor and patient and narrative approaches to medicine look at the collaborative production of meaning through shared language.

Finally, there is an important philosophical issue at stake. Despite the distinctions drawn above between the medical humanities and the arts for health approach, historically, the medical humanities have been intimately tied up with the Arts for Health movement as outlined in Chapter 1. For example, as discussed in Chapter 1, in the UK, 'Arts, health and well-being' was the title of the Nuffield Trust-supported report (Phillip 2002) from two conferences held at Windsor in 1998 and 1999 that can be seen to have inaugurated the medical humanities movement in the UK, as noted in Chapter 1. Note the rhetoric of the title of that report – the arts and humanities are linked with 'health and well-being' or the pursuit of homeostasis.

Again, what is not debated in this report is that such an aim is also grounded in a particular and dominant philosophy – utilitarianism. As discussed previously, here, life's purpose is the pursuit of happiness and the greatest good for the greatest number of people. 'Life, liberty and the pursuit of happiness' are ideals embedded in the American Constitution and Declaration of Independence. That happiness is preferable to misery is held to be 'self-evident'. In 1693 the empiricist John Locke wrote: 'the highest perfection of intellectual nature lies in a careful and constant pursuit of true and solid happiness' (Locke 1975: 2.21.51). Modern medicine, with its central notion of homeostasis, follows this philosophical position, but the arts and humanities in general tend to diverge, often wildly, from such a philosophy.

To repeat what has been argued earlier, that the pursuit of happiness is always preferred to misery must be qualified as relative. Utilitarians describe the best possible state of happiness for the greatest number of people, but again, whose 'happiness' are we describing? One person's happiness is another's pain or disgust. Recall the account of Bob Flanagan's performance art from Chapter 2 grounded in sado-masochism. Paradoxically, the greatest pleasures to some may induce high levels of risk. Love may be the most beautiful pleasure but is always close to the pain of loss. Importantly, illness can offer a way into rich experiences that health denies, although for many, illness is an intolerable burden and such a view may seem condescending. Further, notions of pain and pleasure change historically (Elias 2000) and culturally, and are intimately bound with what mass media dictate.

The psychologist James Hillman (1992), while again not valorizing pain and suffering, points to its inevitability and a duty to give suffering meaning rather than denying or repressing it. Hillman follows Freud's view that the repressed returns in a distorted form. Suffering – or as Hillman calls it, an inherent 'pathologizing' of the soul (the tendency to produce symptom against the grain of idealism) – must first be appreciated before it is explained or given meaning. Further, repressed symptom will return in a worse form. This perspective of giving suffering meaning, was not simply voiced by Hillman but enacted. Dying of cancer, he refused large doses of pain relief, living his dying rather than dulling it.

Hillman notes four styles of refusal of pathologizing. First, *nominalism* defends against the impact of pathology by naming and classification, separating the 'pathological' neuroses and psychoses from the 'normal'. Second, *nihilism* cultivates pathology as a lifestyle, which for Hillman is as bad as refusing such pathology (this suggests that artists such as Bob Flanagan are nihilists, not engaging with pathologizing, but cultivating a pathological lifestyle). Third, *transcendence* attempts to get above and beyond pathology, aligning with ideals of health, happiness, wellbeing, wholeness, and so forth – referred to above as constituting utilitarian values. Fourth, *medicalizing*, rather than psychological insight, attempts to rid us of pathology without examining its meaning, purposes or value. Hillman does not want us to cultivate pathology or glorify suffering, rather, he asks us to suspend the four common ways of refusing a voice for pathologizing listed above, to accommodate pathology as an inevitability that can be given meaning. Of the four great genres of literature, the epic, comic, lyrical and tragic, it is tragedy of course that attempts to frame and give meaning to the ambiguity of pathology (Arbery 2003).

3   Evidence through the science of communication

A third possible source of evidence for the impact of the medical humanities is to draw on evidence from rigorous studies of communication in medicine. As discussed previously, patient safety studies show that current approaches to how we educate doctors in communication are not working. Poor communication with patients and with colleagues in healthcare teams leads to high levels of avoidable medical error (Kohn *et al.* 1999). 'Empathy decline' continues among later year medical students and early years junior doctors (Neumann *et al.* 2011). Empathy decline can be stemmed and communication improved through curriculum design in medical education (Wershof Schwartz *et al.* 2009; Rosenthal *et al.* 2011). Pilpel, Schor and Benbassat (1998) suggest that medical error may be reduced not specifically by focusing upon teaching communication skills, but through teaching medical students about the cultural and institutional barriers to acceptance of medical error, primarily 'institutional norms that encourage authoritarianism, intolerance of uncertainty and denial of error'. It is a short step from this insight into symptoms to suggestion of a cure, as this book outlines. The medical humanities in medical education may just offer that cure.

Bleakley and Marshall (2013) describe a model for understanding how the medical humanities can act as the key intervention in a curriculum for improving quality of communication and then patient safety. This draws again on Martha Nussbaum's (2010) idea that the humanities are the main force for democratizing culture, transposing this to medicine. Bleakley and Marshall argue that medical culture is characterized by its undemocratic structures and that the medical humanities can act as the primary force for democratizing medical culture through medical education. Again, drawing on Donald Winnicott's (1971) ideas, Nussbaum suggests that where children learn empathy through the imaginative nature of play, adults must also have a 'potential space' of adult play or creative opportunity to deepen empathy and respect for the 'other', or to learn tolerance of difference and ambiguity. Such adult developmental space can be provided in the medicine curriculum through core, integrated provision of the medical humanities.

However, for many, communication in medicine (along with ethics and professionalism) is not pure medical humanities, or would not be thought of as a medical humanities curriculum innovation or intervention. While there are dangers in lumping together the 'non-technical' sides of medicine (communication, team work, ethics, professionalism, humanism) the overlaps are strong. Further, if the medical humanities are informed by both the arts and humanities, surely communication is just as central to the humanities as it is to the social sciences?

4   Medical humanities outcomes can be measured through cumulative tightly controlled experiments

While one small-scale study may not provide robust evidence of an effect of a medical humanities intervention, if this study is iteratively refined, or if the results of similar studies are combined, the cumulative effect can be significant. For example, a series of differently designed studies with a common aim has demonstrated a significant effect of educating medical students and doctors for visual acumen through educating close observation, collectively termed 'arts-based observation' (for example, Shapiro *et al.* 2006; Kirklin *et al.* 2007; Naghshineh *et al.* 2008; Perry *et al.* 2011), discussed at length in Chapter 6.

5   Humanities and social science graduates perform as well, or better than, science graduates in undergraduate medicine

In a matched cohorts, longitudinal evaluation study over six years at Mount Sinai in New York, the performance of non-traditional 'humanities' students (who enter medicine without traditional premedical requirements through special, intensive science course routes) has been compared with traditional 'science' students (Wershof Schwartz *et al.* 2009; Muller and Kase 2010). Residents from the humanities programme perform just as well as those with a conventional science background on measures of achievement such as National Board of Medical Examiners scores. 'Humanities' students perform as well as 'science' students by year 3 and outperform those students in areas such as communication.

Wershof Schwartz and colleagues (2009) have carried out a critical literature review of studies showing the same effect, although they point out that some studies have been biased by poor design such as inclusion of self-selected students. The finding that 'humanities' medical students are not handicapped by, but may benefit from, their academic history is particularly important because 15 per cent of medical students in the USA are humanities or social science majors.

6   *Basking in the light of an overall 'product', 'brand', or 'identity' success, where the medical humanities offer a key component*

In looking at the evolution of an overall curriculum with a core, integrated medical humanities component, we can share the limelight of any success with other components. We might track the development of a 'product', 'brand' or 'identity' of a particular curriculum and draw, ironically, on metrics such as league tables of medical schools' performances, and popularity through student satisfaction surveys.

7   *The culture of medicine is changing through feminizing*

A number of studies show that women doctors are more empathic than their male counterparts, give more time to patients and offer more sophisticated levels of communication (such as closer listening and better paraphrasing) than their male colleagues (Roter and Hall 2006). As medicine feminizes (Bleakley 2013a), will this major cultural change produce an impact equivalent to or stronger than those claimed by the medical humanities lobby?

So much for the *via positiva* – ways that we might garner evidence for the impact of the medical humanities in medical education without undue scepticism. Each of the seven approaches above has limitations, as noted. However, they may collectively offer a way forward for gathering evidence, some of it from measurement. These seven ways, as noted earlier, may be necessary but lack sufficiency. For example, more work is needed connecting curriculum interventions to patient outcomes.

Now for the *via negativa*. The remainder of this chapter will develop a model of the purpose of the medical humanities not as palliative and aiming for homeostasis, but as provocative, indeed deeply disturbing, but in an educationally positive way. As already noted from the critiques of Belling and Charon, traditional measures of impact of the medical humanities can miss the primary power of medical humanities input, which may be to subvert rather than support homeostasis. Drawing on Empson's model of ambiguity, seven kinds of subversion of homeostasis will be considered as a model for questioning the value of current medical humanities impact studies.

Seven types of ambiguity that question the value of current medical humanities impact studies

A via negativa *and reflective pause*

The *via negativa* approach below does not constitute throwing the baby out with the bathwater, abandoning the seeking of evidence for impact, but rather problematizes the issue by considering the conditions of *impossibility* for gaining such evidence, rather than conditions of possibility. For this reason, this closing section offers punctuation, a point of pause and reflection, in the headlong rush to satisfy the dominant discourse of 'metrics'. This may help us to return to, and to ponder more closely, the critiques of practitioner theorists such as Charon, Belling, Wearing and Aultman, who are first and foremost natives of the medical humanities territory or region, and will not succumb to the imperialistic tendencies of reductive science as the only route to valid 'evidence'.

1   The first type of ambiguity concerns proof of concept

If measurement of a variable is not a concern, then there is no need for a tight definition and variety of definitions might be welcomed in the spirit of pluralism, tolerance of difference and democracy. However, where measurement of impact remains a concern for instrumental outcomes-based approaches to education, what exactly are we measuring when we measure the impact of a 'medical humanities' provision? Before the concept can be operationalized and measured, we must have proof of concept.

As discussed in Chapters 1 and 2, definitions of the medical humanities differ (Kidd and Connor 2008; Shapiro *et al.* 2009; Wershof Schwartz *et al.* 2009), but the descriptor persists 'for lack of a better term' (Campo 2005). Belling (2010) notes that the systematic review of evidence for impact by Ousager and Johannessen (2010) includes studies on both ethics and communication skills training, neither of which are considered to be 'pure' medical humanities. Introduction of the term 'health humanities' is gaining popularity, as a counter to 'health sciences', but may serve to compound the problem of definition as noted earlier.

In earlier chapters I have shown that at least five distinct models of the medical humanities can be drawn from the literature – (i) as arts for health, (ii) as arts therapies, (iii) as humanities disciplines studying the discipline of medicine (such as the history of medicine), (iv) as arts and humanities elements in medical education and (v) as public engagement arts projects taking medicine as a topic (Bleakley *et al.* 2006; Bleakley 2013b). Further, we have seen how the latter three models have passed into a second wave of 'critical' interest.

Self (1993) identified three differing educational philosophies underpinning medical humanities programmes in the USA: the Cultural Transmission Approach, where the humanities in particular ground medicine in a wider cultural perspective; the Affective Developmental Approach, where medical humanities are concerned with education of empathy and tolerance; and the Cognitive Developmental Approach, where the medical humanities educate for ways of thinking or reconceptualizing.

2   *The second type of ambiguity concerns the assumption that*
    medical humanities interventions are necessarily 'good' or
    'liberating'

The medical humanities may show iatrogenic effects such as zealotry and arts snobbery. As for 'liberation', Petersen and colleagues (2008) argue that the medical humanities can function within the curriculum as a form of surveillance – governance and control. In short, this works on the basis of a paradoxical imperative, disguised as an invitation: 'You will be humane!' (as in 'Have a nice day!' and 'Enjoy!').

3   *The third type of ambiguity concerns a central contradiction:*
    the search for impact and effectiveness of interventions
    through reductive measurement of outcomes can be read itself
    as a primary defence against tolerating ambiguity

This turns the aim of evaluation on its head, where evaluation is now a tactic used to avoid facing the harder and deeper realities of the purpose of the arts and humanities to produce, explore and cultivate ambiguity, rather than to defend against it or explain it away. Rather than facing uncertainty and finding ways to educate for tolerance of ambiguity, the scientific mind-set drives us to reduce uncertainty through experiment. The drive to measure impact of the medical humanities can be read as a symptom of the inability to tolerate ambiguity, underpinned by the broader philosophical approach, discussed earlier, of utilitarianism and empiricism. The arts for health movement can be seen to have fallen under the sway of this philosophy and as a result can be seen to have lost touch with the revolutionary value of art to disturb, or challenge social homeostasis (Bleakley 2013b).

A paradox then emerges at the heart of the arts for health movement – while creating 'health' benefits for patients, the body of 'art' itself can be seen to generally suffer, or is slowly killed. Where the art medium is the sole message, reduced to a vehicle for the expression of the patient's symptoms or a cathartic release, the art becomes safe, conservative, dull, stripped of its revolutionary potential, critical force and subversive interests. The art is then stripped of its powers to act on the 'health' of the culture through triggering resistance and reformulation. As the patient improves through the art therapy, it can then be at the expense of both the art and the culture it monitors.

4   *The fourth type of ambiguity concerns a contradiction: where*
    the medical humanities are increasingly developed as
    integrated and core provision, how will they be isolated from
    other elements of the curriculum for purposes of instrumental
    evaluation of impact?

For the medical humanities to achieve legitimacy, two curriculum events must happen – first, the medical humanities must move away from the status of peripheral provision (for example, as optional study), to central participation in the community of practice of medical education. This will promote the medical humanities to core and possibly integrated provision. Second, the medical humanities must provide evidence of impact. However, these two events are not logically compatible. 'Integrated' implies complex, inter-related provision. The more the medical humanities are integrated at core the less easy it is to isolate interventions as discrete variables open to experimental manipulation and measurement. The danger with integration is that the medical humanities can become absorbed into the dominant discourse of biomedical science, failing in its aim to provide a critical counterweight to core science studies (Chiavaroli and Ellwood 2012). This draws out the healing poison or *pharmakon* from the fangs of the medical humanities and mollifies the intervention in a further potential act of production of insensibility.

5   *The fifth type of ambiguity concerns the danger that artists working within the medical humanities in medical education are potentially compromised – they have to suspend the innovation and radical nature of their practices in the service of becoming 'educationalists'*

Contemporary arts practices are often radical, innovative and experimental both aesthetically and politically. Thanks to a combination of instrumental factors such as health and safety, and social factors such as complying with the norms of a practice, artists may find themselves constrained as educators. This produces a dilution of the potential of medical humanities – for example in the area of promoting social justice – that can be seen to compromise 'impact'. If the function of the liberal avant-garde in the arts and humanities is not to simply shock, but to shock for a purpose in challenging the status quo, then this can be compromised by a focus on outcomes based education that effectively cancels risk, surprise and invention. Frustrated artists may become cynical as a conservative medical education comes to colonize their worlds, muting the potential of their paradoxical remedy or *pharmakon*.

6   *The sixth type of ambiguity concerns the many different ways way in which medical humanities are represented in the curriculum, which either afford, or fail to afford, character and status to that medical humanities provision*

Just as there is disagreement about what the 'medical humanities' are, so there is wide divergence about how they appear in the curriculum, which must make a difference to how impact is felt and how it may be evaluated or measured. This may be seen to constitute a strength, offering variety, but it more likely affords an ambiguity. For example, the character and status of the medical humanities differ between compensatory, complementary and fully integrated modes. The medical humanities may be set as opposing, rather than as a complement to or intrinsic to, science delivery. Importantly, in radical models of the medical humanities, *science itself is explored as intrinsically imaginative and artistic* (Bleakley *et al.* 2006).

Also, in more radical models of the curriculum, explicit attention is given to the curriculum as varieties of 'text' (Pinar and Reynolds 1992), such as gendered, ethical, historical, political, economic, phenomenological and aesthetic. An explicitly aestheticized curriculum means that curriculum designers have thought about form as well as function. The aesthetic curriculum encourages 'connoisseurship' of content and process in learning (Eisner 1976, 1979, 1998) and is concerned with issues such as how education of the senses for clinical judgement is best achieved (Bleakley *et al.* 2003a, 2003b), where 'aesthetic' literally means 'sense impression'. Here, the medical humanities act as texts that inform curriculum design and implementation. If we are to be consistent, then curriculum as an aesthetic text should also be evaluated 'aesthetically', that is in an appreciative way, such as a 'holistic grasp', rather than in an instrumental way, such as through metrics. If the medical humanities are performing their function of reconceptualizing medicine through medical education, then 'measurement' of impact would be through effects of principles such as subversion, inversion, irony and so forth.

Where Charon (2010) suggests that a 'health outcome' measure for the success of a medical humanities intervention might be a patient's ability to achieve health goals that they have set for themselves, we might extend this to include education for tolerance of ambiguity in patients, such as acceptance of the uncertainties of illness, as well as valuing certain forms of illness.

7   *The seventh type of ambiguity is the paradox that the arts and humanities cause kinds of illnesses by opposing homeostasis*

The notion that the arts and humanities may produce 'illness' as an antidote to 'wellbeing' and 'human flourishing' is antithetical to models of homeostasis. Such 'illness' may be an 'ill-at-ease-ness' with culture that is realized in critique, reflection, and reformulation or revolution.

A dominant rhetoric shaping the medical humanities has been concerned with the humanities input supporting health, wellbeing and human flourishing. However, once again, is this primarily the function of the arts and humanities? I have forcibly made the argument that such a view is both ideological and rhetorical, guided by an utilitarian philosophy that often remains dormant when such studies are discussed and itself offered forcefully as 'self-evident'. Again, an alternative view, particularly from the liberal avant-garde, is that the role of the arts and humanities is to upset equilibrium, homeostasis and wellbeing and to induce varieties of imbalance or disequilibrium. Again, Felix Guattari (1995: 106) describes this as 'the incessant clash of the movement of art against established boundaries'.

Artists, in the role of Nietzschean diagnosticians of culture (Smith 2005), may see a cultural malaise in middle-of-the-road, sanitized art of conservative popular culture, or in the ideological art preferred by both fascist and communist regimes. I have previously noted that Adolf Hitler was a painter, but his bland art is precisely the kind of facile and decorative work that fails to interest, excite or disturb, except by association with his name and politics. Hitler banned improvisational music such as jazz as depraved, where jazz of course reinvents and extends music through fresh improvisation. The Nazis preferred militaristic marching music played strictly on the beat, which maintained the status quo. Jazz was also associated with Jewish, gypsy and black music and was then banned as culturally depraved.

In May 2012, the Norwegian artist's Edvard Munch's pastel version of 'The Scream' (1895) was sold for a world record of £74 million ($120 million) at auction in Sotheby's, New York. Here is what Munch himself said about the genesis of 'The Scream':

> One evening I was walking along a path, the city was on one side and the fjord below. I felt tired and ill. I stopped and looked out over the fjord – the sun was setting, and the clouds turning blood red. I sensed a scream passing through nature; it seemed to me that I heard the scream. I painted this picture, painted the clouds as actual blood. The colour shrieked. This became The Scream.
>
> (Munch, diary for 22 January 1892, quoted by
> Dangerous Minds undated)

Later, Munch rendered this memory as a prose poem, hand-painted onto the frame of the very 1895 pastel version of the work auctioned at Sothebys:

> I was walking along a path with two friends – the sun was setting – suddenly the sky turned blood red – I paused, feeling exhausted, and leaned on the fence – there was blood and tongues of fire above the blue-black fjord and the city – my friends walked on, and I stood there trembling with anxiety – and I sensed an infinite scream passing through nature.
>
> (Munch, 1895, quoted by Prideaux 2005: 150–51)

Simeon and Abugel (2006) analysed the genesis and imagery of 'The Scream' as comparable with an experience of morbid depersonalization, a psychiatric disorder.

Great works of art – Bosch's landscapes of Hell, Mantegna's distorted perspectival view in 'Dead Christ', Goya's etchings of war atrocities, Schoenberg's atonality, Joyce's sexually explicit stream of consciousness, William Faulkner's multi-levelled texts on big moral themes, Francis

Bacon's paintings of hysterical Popes, the animal savagery in Ted Hughes's poetry, Anselm Kiefer's apocalyptic landscapes, David Foster Wallace's dystopias of prescription culture America – disturb and provoke rather than placate. This does not mean that great art cannot also please in more conventional ways – for example the embracing atmospheres produced by Mark Rothko's abstracts, the perceptually engaging effect of Bridget Riley's op art or Philip Glass's minimalist music, or the purposefully vacuous and imitative nature of pop art such as the work of Jeff Koons offers 'framed irony'. We cannot ignore, however, that important contemporary art explicitly sets out to invoke the sublime and abject and to promote critique and debate about the human condition and social habits. The purpose of such challenging art is not necessarily to be pessimistic, but rather to encourage scepticism. Indeed, deeply challenging art should make us feel uncomfortable, as it reveals optional ways of thinking and experiencing, returning us to the argument of Wear and Aultman discussed earlier, that the medical humanities do not simply offer a 'palatable' diversion from the 'hard work' of medical science.

Bibliography

Acuña, L.E. (2000) 'Don't Cry for Us Argentinians: Two Decades of Teaching Medical Humanities'. *Medical Humanities*, 26: 66–70.

Acuña, L.E. (2003) 'Teaching Humanities at the National University of la Plata, Argentina'. *Academic Medicine*, 78: 1024–7.

Adler, A. (2009) *Understanding Life: An Introduction to the Psychology of Alfred Adler*. Oxford: One World.

Adorno, T.W., Frenkel-Brunswik, E., Levinson, D.J. and Sanford, R.N. (1950) *The Authoritarian Personality*. New York: Harper & Row.

Aleinikov, A.G. (1989) 'On Creative Pedagogy'. *Higher Education Bulletin*, 12: 29–34.

Alexander, B. (2011) *The New Digital Storytelling: Creating Narratives with New Media*. Santa Barbara, CA: ABC-CLIO.

Allums, L. (ed.) (1992) *The Epic Cosmos*. Dallas, TX: The Dallas Institute.

American College of Physicians (undated) 'Writing a Clinical Vignette (Case Report) Abstract'. www.acponline.org/education_recertification/education/program_ directors/abstracts/prepare/clinvin_abs.htm (accessed 25 October 2014).

Anderson, R.C., Fagan, M.J. and Sebastian, J. (2001) 'Teaching Students the Art and Science of Physical Diagnosis'. *American Journal of Medicine*, 110: 419–23.

Arbery, G.C. (2003) *The Tragic Abyss*. Dallas, TX: Dallas Institute.

Aristotle (1990) *Metaphysica*, trans. W.D. Ross. In *The Works of Aristotle, Volume I*. Chicago, IL: Encylopaedia Brittanica.

Arnheim, R. (1969) *Visual Thinking*. Berkeley, CA: University of California Press.

Arnold, L. and Stern, D.T. (2006) 'What is Medical Professionalism?'. In D.T. Stern (ed.), *Measuring Medical Professionalism*, 15–37. Oxford: Oxford University Press.

Arnold P. Gold Foundation (undated) 'About Us'. http://humanism-in-medicine.org/about-us (accessed 23 October 2014).

Austin, J.L. (1962) *How to Do Things with Words*. Cambridge, MA: Harvard University Press.

Azer, S. (2011) 'Learning Surface Anatomy: Which Learning Approach is Effective in an Integrated PBL Curriculum?'. *Medical Teacher*, 33: 78–80.

Bachelard, G. (1964) *The Psychoanalysis of Fire*. Boston, MA: Beacon Press.

Bachelard, G. (1983) *Water and Dreams*. Dallas, TX: The Dallas Institute.

Bachelard, G. (1986) *The Poetics of Space*. Boston, MA: Beacon Press.

Banaszek, A. (2011) 'Medical Humanities Courses Becoming Prerequisites in Many Medical Schools'. *Canadian Medical Association Journal*, 183: E441–2.

Banks, S.A. and Vastyan, E.A. (1973) 'Humanistic Studies in Medical Education'. *Journal of Medical Education*, 48: 248–57.

Bardes, C.L., Gillers, D. and Herman, A.E. (2001) 'Learning to Look: Developing Clinical Observational Skills at an Art Museum'. *Medical Education*, 35: 1157–61.

Barker-Benfield, G.J. (1992) *The Culture of Sensibility: Sex and Society in Eighteenth-Century Britain*. Chicago, IL: University of Chicago Press.

Barr, D.A. (2011) 'Putting the Flexner Report in Context'. *Medical Education*, 45: 17–22.

Barron, F. (1988) 'Putting Creativity to Work'. In R.J. Sternberg (ed.), *The Nature of Creativity: Contemporary Psychological Perspectives*, 76–98. Cambridge: Cambridge University Press.

Bates, V. and Goodman, S. (2014) 'Critical Conversations: Establishing Dialogue in the Medical Humanities'. In V. Bates, A. Bleakley and S. Goodman (eds), *Medicine, Health and the Arts: Approaches to the Medical Humanities*, 3–14. Routledge: London.

Bates, V., Bleakley, A. and Goodman, S. (2014) *Medicine, Health and the Arts: Approaches to the Medical Humanities*. Routledge: London.

Batistatou, A., Doulis, E.A., Tiniakos, D., Anogiannaki, A. and Charalabopoulos, K. (2010) 'The Introduction of Medical Humanities in the Undergraduate Curriculum of Greek Medical Schools: Challenge and Necessity'. *Hippokratia*, 14: 241–3.

Becker, G. (1997) *Disrupted Lives: How People Create Meaning in a Chaotic World*. Berkeley, CA: University of California Press.

Becker, H.S., Geer, B., Hughes, E.C. and Strauss, A.L. (1961) *Boys in White: Student Culture in Medical School*. Chicago, IL: University of Chicago Press.

Belling, C. (2010) 'Sharper Instruments: On Defending the Humanities in Undergraduate Medical Education'. *Academic Medicine*, 85: 938–40.

Belling, C. (2011) 'Finding Resonance: The Value of Indirection in a Reflective Exercise'. *Journal of Graduate Medical Education*, 3: 580–81.

Benjamin, W. (1968) *The Work of Art in the Age of Mechanical Reproduction, Illuminations*. London: Fontana.

Benner, P., Tanner, C., Chesla, C. and Benner, P. (2009) *Expertise in Nursing Practice: Caring, Clinical Judgment, and Ethics*, 2nd edn. Dordrecht: Springer.

Berlin, I. (1953) *The Hedgehog and the Fox*. London: Weidenfeld & Nicolson

Bernauer, J. and Rasmussen, D. (eds) (1994) *The Final Foucault*. Cambridge, MA: MIT Press.

Bhabha, H. (2004) *The Location of Culture*. London: Routledge.

Bishop, J.P. (2008) 'Rejecting Medical Humanism: Medical Humanities and the Metaphysics of Medicine'. *The Journal of Medical Humanities*, 29: 15–25.

Bishop, J.P. (2011) *The Anticipatory Corpse: Medicine, Power and the Care of the Dying*. Notre Dame, IN: University of Notre Dame Press.

Bleakley, A. (1999a) 'From Reflective Practice to Holistic Reflexivity'. *Studies in Higher Education*, 24: 315–30.

Bleakley, A. (1999b) *The Animalizing Imagination: Totemism, Textuality and Ecocriticism*. Basingstoke: Macmillan.

Bleakley, A. (2003) 'Essay Review of *Social Construction in Context* by K. Gergen, with a reply by Gergen'. *Journal of Community and Applied Social Psychology*, 13: 409–12.

Bleakley, A. (2004) 'Doctors as Connoisseurs of Informational Images: Aesthetic and Ethical Self-Forming through Medical Practice'. In J. Satterthwaite, E. Atkinson and W. Martin (eds), *Educational Counter-Cultures: Confrontations, Images, Vision*, 149–64. London: Trentham.

Bleakley, A. (2005) 'Stories as Data, Data as Stories: Making Sense of Narrative Inquiry in Clinical Education'. *Medical Education*, 39: 534–40.

Bleakley, A. (2006a) 'Broadening Conceptions of Learning in Medical Education: The Message from Teamworking'. *Medical Education*, 40: 150–57.

Bleakley, A. (2006b) 'Towards an Aesthetics of Healthcare Practice: Learning the Art of Clinical Judgement'. In K. Beedholm, N. Buus, S. Malchau, I. Moos and U. Zeitler (eds), *Theory and Practice in Nursing Education*, 25–39. Aarhus: Centre for Innovation in Nursing Education, Aarhus University.

Bleakley, A. (2010) 'Blunting Occam's Razor: Aligning Medical Education with Studies of Complexity'. *Journal of Evaluation in Clinical Practice*, 16: 849–55.

Bleakley, A. (2013a) 'Gender Matters in Medical Education'. *Medical Education*, 47: 59–70.

Bleakley, A. (2013b) 'Towards a "Critical Medical Humanities"'. In V. Bates, S. Goodman and A. Bleakley. (eds), *Medicine, Health, and the Arts: Approaches to Medical Humanities*, 17–26. London: Routledge.

Bleakley, A. (2014) *The Heart of the Matter: Patient-Centred Medicine in Transition*. Springer: Dordrecht.

Bleakley, A. (forthcoming) 'Introduction' to A. Peterkin, P. Brett-Maclean, *Keeping Reflection Fresh*. Kent, OH: Kent State University Press.

Bleakley, A. and Brennan, N. (2011) 'Does Undergraduate Curriculum Design Make a Difference to Readiness to Practice as a Junior Doctor?'. *Medical Teacher*, 33: 459–67.

Bleakley, A. and Cleland, J. (forthcoming) 'Sticking with Messy Realities: How "Thinking with Complexity" Can Inform Clinical Education Research'. In J. Cleland and S. Durning (eds), *Researching Medical Education*. Oxford: Wiley.

Bleakley, A. and Marshall, R.J. (2012) 'The Embodiment of Lyricism in Medicine and Homer'. *Medical Humanities*, 38: 50–54.

Bleakley, A. and Marshall, R.J. (2013) 'Can the Science of Communication Inform the Art of the Medical Humanities?'. *Medical Education*, 47: 126–33.

Bleakley, A., Farrow, R., Gould, D. and Marshall, R. (2003a) 'Learning How to See: Doctors Making Judgements in the Visual Domain'. *Journal of Workplace Learning*, 15: 301–6.

Bleakley, A., Farrow, R., Gould, D. and Marshall, R. (2003b) 'Making Sense of Clinical Reasoning: Judgement and the Evidence of the Senses'. *Medical Education*, 37: 544–52.

Bleakley, A., Marshall, R. and Broemer, R. (2006) 'Toward an Aesthetic Medicine: Developing a Core Medical Humanities Undergraduate Curriculum'. *Journal of Medical Humanities*, 27: 197–213.

Bleakley, A., Bligh, J. and Browne, J. (2011) *Medical Education for the Future: Identity, Power and Location*. Dordrecht: Springer.

Bleakley, A., Marshall, R. and Levine, D. (2014) 'He Drove Forward with a Yell: Anger in Medicine and Homer'. *Medical Humanities*, 40: 22–30.

Bligh, J. and Bleakley, A. (2006) 'Distributing Menus to Hungry Learners: Can Learning by Simulation Become Simulation of Learning?, *Medical Teacher*, 28: 606–13.

Bliss, W. (1999) *William Osler: A Life in Medicine*. Toronto: University of Toronto Press.

Bohm, D. (1998) *On Creativity*. London: Routledge.

Bohm, D. (2002) *Wholeness and the Implicate Order*. London: Routledge.

Boothroyd D. (2000) 'Deconstruction and Drugs: A Philosophical/Literary Cocktail'. In N. Royle (ed.), *Deconstructions: A User's Guide*, 44–63. Basingstoke: Palgrave.

Borland, C. (2006) *Preserves*. Edinburgh: Fruitmarket Gallery.

Boseley, S. (2006) 'Ritalin Heart Attacks Warning Urged after 51 Deaths in US'. *The Guardian*, 11 February, www.guardian.co.uk/frontpage/story/0,,1707535,00.html (accessed 23 August 2014).

Boshuizen, H.P.A. and Schmidt, H.G. (1995) 'The Development of Clinical Reasoning Expertise'. In J. Higgs and M. Jones (eds), *Clinical Reasoning in the Health Professions*, 24–32. Oxford: Butterworth Heinemann.

Boston Women's Health Book Collective (2005) *Our Bodies, Ourselves: A New Edition for a New Era*, 35th anniversary edn. New York: Simon & Schuster.

Boudreau, J.D., Cassell, E.J. and Fuks, A. (2008) 'Preparing Medical Students to Become Skilled at Clinical Observation'. *Medical Teacher*, 30: 857–62.

Bourdieu, P. (1977) *Outline of a Theory of Practice*. Cambridge: Cambridge University Press.

Bowman, P. and Stamp, R. (eds) (2011) *Reading Rancière*. London: Continuum.

Boyle, D., Dwinnell, B. and Platt, F. (2005) 'Invite, Listen, and Summarize: A Patient-Centered Communication Technique'. *Academic Medicine*, 80: 29–32.

Braude, D.H. (2012) *Intuition in Medicine: A Philosophical Defence of Clinical Reasoning*. Chicago, IL: University of Chicago Press.

Brett-Maclean, P. (2012) 'Use of the Arts in Medical and Health Professional Education'. *University of Alberta Health Sciences Journal*, 4: 26–9.

British Medical Association (2012) 'Fatal Results of Doctors' Burnout Revealed'. http://bma.org.uk/news-views-analysis/news/2012/october/fatal-results-of-doctors-burnout-revealednewsitem (accessed 21 August 2014).

Broadhead, R.S. (1983) *The Private Lives and Professional Identity of Medical Students*. New Brunswick, NJ: Transaction Books.

Brochet, F. and Dubourdieu, D. (2001) 'Wine Descriptive Language Supports Cognitive Specificity of Chemical Senses'. *Brain and Language*, 77: 187–96.

Broom, B. (1997) *Somatic Illness and the Patient's Other Story: A Practical Integrative Mind/Body Approach to Disease for Doctors and Psychotherapists*. London: Free Association Books.

Bruner, J. (1986) *Actual Minds, Possible Worlds*. Cambridge, MA: Harvard University Press.

Bryan, C.S. (1997) *Osler: Inspirations from a Great Physician*. Oxford: Oxford University Press.

Bulgakov, M. (2012) *A Young Doctor's Notebook*. Richmond: Alma Classics.

Bull, S. and Mattick, K. (2010) 'What Biomedical Science Should be Included in Undergraduate Medical Courses and How is This Decided?'. *Medical Teacher*, 32: 360–67.

Campo, R. (2005) 'A Piece of My Mind: "The Medical Humanities," for Lack of a Better Term'. *Journal of the American Medical Association*, 294: 1009–11.

Capra, F. and Luisi, P.L. (2014) *The Systems View of Life: A Unifying Vision*. Cambridge: Cambridge University Press.

Carper, B.A. (1978) 'Fundamental Patterns of Knowing'. *Advances in Nursing Science* 1: 13–23.

Cassell, E.J. (1984) *The Place of the Humanities in Medicine*. New York: Hastings Center Publications.

Chambers, T. (1999) *The Fiction of Bioethics: Cases as Literary Texts*. New York: Routledge.

Charon, R. (2006) *Narrative Medicine: Honoring the Stories of Illness*. Oxford: Oxford University Press.

Charon, R. (2010) 'Commentary: Calculating the Contributions of Humanities to Medical Practice – Motives, Methods, and Metrics'. *Academic Medicine*, 85: 935–7.

Charon, R. and Montello, M. (2002) *Stories Matter: The Role of Narrative in Medical Ethics*. New York: Routledge.

Chen, P. (2009) 'Lessons From the Bedside Exam'. *New York Times*, 12 February, www.nytimes.com/2009/02/13/health/12chen.html?_r=2&   (accessed   4 September 2014).

Chiavaroli, N. and Ellwood, C. (2012) 'The Medical Humanities and the Perils of Curricular Integration'. *Journal of Medical Humanities*, 33: 245–54.

Cioffi, J. (2000a) 'Recognition of Patients Who Require Emergency Assistance: A Descriptive Study'. *Heart and Lung*, July/August: 262–8.

Cioffi, J. (2000b) 'Nurses' Experience of Making Decisions to Call Emergency Assistance to Their Patients'. *Journal of Advanced Nursing*, 32: 108–14.

Cioffi, J. (2002) 'What Are Clinical Judgements?'. In C. Thompson and D. Dowding (eds), *Clinical Decision Making and Judgement in Nursing*, 47–66. Edinburgh: Churchill Livingstone.

Cixous, H. (1981) 'The Laugh of the Medusa'. In E. Marks and I. de Courtivron (eds), *New French Feminisms*, 253. New York: Schocken.

Cixous, H. (1991) *Coming to Writing and Other Essays*. Cambridge, MA: University of Harvard Press.

Cixous, H. (ed.) (2004) *The Hélène Cixous reader*. London: Routledge.

Cixous, H. and Clément, C. (1986) *The Newly Born Woman*. Minneapolis, MN: University of Minnesota Press.

Clark, A. (1999) *Being There: Putting Brain, Body, and World Together Again*. Cambridge, MA: MIT Press.

Clark, M. (2013) 'HISTGC06: Chinese Film and the Body', MA module descriptor, University College London, www.ucl.ac.uk/chinahealth/teaching/chinese_film_and_the_body (accessed 4 September 2014).

Claxton, G. (2000) 'The Anatomy of Intuition'. In T. Atkinson and G. Claxton (eds), *The Intuitive Practitioner*, 32–52. Buckingham: Open University Press.

Clouser, K.D. (1971) 'Humanities and the Medical School: A Sketched Rationale and Description'. *Medical Education*, 5: 226–31.

Coats, E. (ed.) (2004) *Swallows to Other Continents: Creative Arts and Humanities in Healthcare*. London: Nuffield Trust.

Cohen, S. (2009) 'The Human Whisperer'. *Stanford Alumni*, January/February, https://alumni.stanford.edu/get/page/magazine/article/?article_id=30545 (accessed 18 August 2014).

Coleridge, S.T. (1956) *Biographia Literaria or Biographical Sketches of My Literary Life and Opinions*. London: Everyman's Library.

Colliver, J.A., Conlee, M.J., Verhukst, S.J. and Dorsey, J.K. (2010) 'Reports of the

Decline of Empathy during Medical Education are Greatly Exaggerated: A Re-examination of the Research'. *Academic Medicine*, 85: 588–93.

Connelly, J. (2002) 'In the Absence of Narrative'. In R. Charon and M. Montello (eds), *Stories Matter: The Role of Narrative in Medical Ethics*, 138–40. New York: Routledge.

Cook, H.J. (2010) 'Borderlands: A Historian's Perspective on Medical Humanities in the US and the UK'. *Medical Humanities*, 36: 3–4.

Cooke, M., Irby, D.M. and O'Brien, B.C. (2010) *Educating Physicians: A Call for Reform of Medical School and Residency*. San Francisco, CA: Jossey-Bass.

Coombs, R.H. and Paulson, M.J. (1990) 'Is Premedical Education Dehumanizing? A Literature Review'. *Journal of Medical Humanities*, 11: 13–22.

Cooperrider, D.L. and Whitney, D. (1999) 'Appreciative Inquiry'. In P. Holman and T. Devane (eds), *Collaborating for Change*. San Francisco, CA: Berrett-Koehler.

Corbin, H. (2005) *Time, Desire and Horror: Towards a History of the Senses*. London: Polity Press.

Cork, R. (2012) *The Healing Presence of Art: A History of Western Art in Hospitals*. New Haven, CT: Yale University Press.

Coulter, A. (2002) *The Autonomous Patient: Ending Paternalism in Medical Care*. London: TSO.

Cowan, L. (ed.) (2011) *The Terrain of Comedy*. Dallas, TX: Dallas Institute.

Cowan, B. and Cowan, L. (eds) (2012) *The Prospect of Lyric*. Dallas, TX: Dallas Institute.

Crawford, P., Brown, B., Tischler, V. and Baker, C. (2010) 'Health Humanities: The Future of Medical Humanities?'. *Mental Health Review Journal*, 15: 4–10.

Crawshaw, R. (1975) 'Humanism in Medicine – The Rudimentary Process'. *New England Journal of Medicine*, 293: 1320–22.

Csikszentmihalyi, M. (1999) 'Implications of a Systems Perspective for the Study of Creativity'. In R.J. Sternberg (ed.), *Handbook of Creativity*, 313–36. Cambridge: Cambridge University Press.

Dangerous Minds (undated) '"Illness, Madness and Death": The World of Edvard Munch and "The Scream"'. http://dangerousminds.net/comments/illness_madness_and_death_the_world_of_edvard_munch_and_the_scream (accessed 3 November 2014).

Deleuze, G. (1993) *Essays Critical and Clinical*. London: Verso.

Deleuze, G. and Guattari, F. (2004a) *A Thousand Plateaus*. London: Continuum.

Deleuze, G. and Guattari, F. (2004b) *Anti-Oedipus*. London: Continuum.

Denig, P., Wahlstrom, R., Chaput de Saintonge, M. and Haaijer-Ruskamp, F. (2002) 'The Value of Clinical Judgement Analysis for Improving the Quality of Doctors' Prescribing Decisions'. *Medical Education*, 36: 770–80.

Deranty, J. (ed.) (2010) *Jacques Rancière: Key Concepts*. Durham: Acumen.

Derrida, J. (1968) 'Difference'. http://projectlamar.com/media/Derrida-Difference.pdf (accessed 12 September 2014).

Derrida, J. (1993) 'The Rhetoric of Drugs: An Interview'. *Differences*, 5: 1–25.

Derrida, J. (2000) *Of Hospitality*. Stanford, CA: Stanford University Press.

Derrida, J., Brault, P-A. and Naas, M. (2004) 'The Last of the Rogue States: The "Democracy to Come," Opening in Two Turns'. *South Atlantic Quarterly*, 103: 323–41.

Diamond, D. (2007) *Theatre for Living: The Art and Science of Community-Based Dialogue*. Bloomington, IN: Trafford Publishing.

Dolev, J., Friedlander, L. and Braverman, I. (2001) 'Use of Fine Art to Enhance Visual Diagnostic Skills'. *Journal of the American Medical Association*, 286: 1020–21.

Donoghue, D. (2014) *Metaphor*. Cambridge, MA: Harvard University Press.

Drew, T., Vo, M.L-H. and Wolfe, J.M. (2013) 'The Invisible Gorilla Strikes Again Sustained Inattentional Blindness in Expert Observers'. *Psychological Science*, 24: 1848–53.

Durham University (2009) 'Medical Humanities'. March, www.dur.ac.uk/cmh/medicalhumanities (accessed 24 October 2014).

Durham University (undated) 'Critical Medical Humanities'. www.dur.ac.uk/cmh/themesofenquiry/pecr (accessed 24 October 2014).

Dyrbye, L.N. *et al.* (2008) 'Burnout and Suicidal Ideation among U.S. Medical Students'. *Annals of Internal Medicine*, 149: 334–41.

eä (undated) 'About Us'. www.ea-journal.com/en/about-us/about-ea-journal (accessed 23 October 2014).

Eco, U. (1999) *Serendipities: Language and Lunacy*. London: Phoenix.

Edson, M. (1999) *W;t*. London: Nick Hern Books.

Eggers, D. (2013) *The Circle*, San Francisco, CA: McSweeney's Books.

Eisner, E.W. (1976) 'Educational Connoisseurship and Criticism: Their Form and Functions in Educational Evaluation'. *Journal of Aesthetic Education*, 10: 135–50.

Eisner, E. (1979) *The Educational Imagination*. New York: Macmillan.

Eisner, E. (1998) *The Enlightened Eye*. Upper Saddle River, NJ: Prentice Hall.

Elder, N.C., Tobias, B., Lucero-Criswell, A. and Goldenhar, L. (2006) 'The Art of Observation: Impact of a Family Medicine and Art Museum Partnership on Student Education'. *Family Medicine*, 38: 393–38.

Elias, N. (2000) *The Civilizing Process*. Oxford: Blackwell.

Elkins, J. (1999) *The Domain of Images*. Ithaca, NY: Cornell University Press.

Elkins, J. (2003) *Visual Studies: A Skeptical Introduction*. New York: Routledge.

Elkins, J. (2008) *How to Use Your Eyes*. London: Routledge.

Ellis, B.E. (2005) *Lunar Park*. London: Picador.

Empson, W. (1991) *Seven Types of Ambiguity*. London: The Hogarth Press.

Engel, P.J.H. (2008) 'Tacit Knowledge and Visual Expertise in Medical Diagnostic Reasoning: Implications for Medical Education'. *Medical Teacher*, 30: e184–8.

Engeström, Y. (1987) *Learning by Expanding: An Activity-Theoretical Approach to Developmental Research*. Helsinki: Orienta-Konsultit.

Engeström, Y. (2008) *From Teams to Knots*. Cambridge: Cambridge University Press.

Evans, M. and Finlay, I. (eds) (2001) *Medical Humanities*. London: BMJ Books.

Evans, H.M. and Greaves, D.A. (2001a) 'Medical Humanities at the University of Wales Swansea'. *Medical Humanities*, 27: 51–2.

Evans, H.M. and Greaves, D.A. (2001b) 'Developing the Medical Humanities – Report of a Research Colloquium, and Collected Abstracts of Papers'. *Medical Humanities*, 27: 93–8.

Evans, H.M. and Greaves, D.A. (2002) '"Medical Humanities" – What's In a Name?'. *Medical Humanities*, 28: 1–2.

Ewen, S. (2013) *Global Medical Humanities: Association for Medical Humanities Annual Conference 2013*, 41. Aberdeen: Association for Medical Humanities.

Faulkner, W. (1936) *Absalom, Absalom!* New York: Random House.

Feighny, K.M., Arnold, L., Monaco, M., Munro, S. and Earl, B. (1998) 'In Pursuit of Empathy and its Relation to Physician Communication Skills: Multidimensional Empathy Training For Medical Students'. *Annals of Behavioral Science and Medical Education*, 5: 13–21.

Fennell, E. (1997) 'Categorising Creativity'. *Competence and Assessment*, 23: 7.

Feudtner, C., Christakis, D.A. and Christakis, N.A. (1994) 'Do Clinical Clerks Suffer Ethical Erosion? Students' Perceptions of Their Ethical Environment and Personal Development'. *Academic Medicine*, 69: 670–79.

Fieschi, L., Matarese, M., Vellone, E., Alvaro, R. and De Marinis, M.G. (2013), 'Medical Humanities in Healthcare Education in Italy: A Literature Review'. *Ann Ist Super Sanità*, 49: 56–64.

Fish, D. and Coles, C. (1998) *Developing Professional Judgement in Health Care: Learning Through the Critical Appreciation of Practice*. Oxford: Butterworth Heinemann.

Flexner, A. (1910) *Medical Education in the United States and Canada*. New York: Carnegie Foundation for the Advancement of Teaching.

Fokkelman, J.P. (1987) 'Genesis'. In R. Alter and F. Kermode (eds), *The Literary Guide to the Bible*, 36–55. Cambridge, MA: Harvard University Press.

Fonteyn, M. and Fisher, A. (1995) 'Use of Think Aloud Method to Study Nurses' Reasoning and Decision Making in Clinical Practice Settings'. *Journal of Neuroscience Nursing*, 27: 124–48.

Foucault, M. (1989) *The Birth of the Clinic: An Archaeology of Medical Perception*. London: Routledge.

Foucault, M. (1991) *Discipline and Punish: The Birth of the Prison*. London: Penguin.

Foucault, M. (2002) *Power: The Essential Works of Michel Foucault 1954–1984*, 3rd edn. Harmondsworth: Penguin.

Foucault M. (2005) *The Hermeneutics of the Subject: Lectures at the Collège de France 1981–1982*. New York: Picador.

Foucault, M. (2006) *History of Madness*. London: Routledge.

Fox, E., Arnold, R.M. and Brody, B. (1995) 'Medical Ethics Education: Past Present and Future'. *Academic Medicine*, 70: 761–68.

Frankish, K. (2010) 'Dual-Process and Dual-System Theories of Reasoning'. *Philosophy Compass*, 5: 914–26.

Frank, A.W. (1995) *The Wounded Storyteller: Body, Illness and Ethics*, Chicago, IL: University of Chicago Press.

Franzen J. (2001) *The Corrections*. London: Fourth Estate.

Fredrick, D. (2002) 'Introduction: Invisible Rome'. In D. Fredrick (ed.), *The Roman Gaze: Vision, Power, and the Body*, 1–30. Baltimore, MD: Johns Hopkins University Press.

Freire, P. (1996) *Pedagogy of the Oppressed*. London: Penguin.

Freshwater, D. and Johns, C.J. (eds) (2005) *Transforming Nursing Through Reflective Practice*. Oxford: Blackwell.

Garelick, A.I. (2014) 'Doctors' Health: Stigma and the Professional Discomfort in Seeking Help'. *The Psychiatric Bulletin*, 38: 1.

Gaufberg, E. and Williams, R. (2011) 'Reflection in a Museum Setting: The Personal Responses Tour'. *Journal of Graduate Medical Education*, 3: 546–49.

Gawande, A. (2002) *Complications: A Surgeon's Notes on an Imperfect Science*. London: Profile Books.

Gawande, A. (2008) *Better: A Surgeon's Notes on Performance*. London: Profile Books.

Geertz, C. (1973) *The Interpretations of Cultures*. Boston, MA: Basic Books.

General Medical Council (1993) *Tomorrow's Doctors*. London: General Medical Council.

General Medical Council (2003) *Tomorrow's Doctors: Recommendations on Undergraduate Medical Education*. London: General Medical Council.

General Medical Council (2006) *Good Medical Practice*. London: General Medical Council.

General Medical Council (2007) *The New Doctor*. London: General Medical Council.

General Medical Council (2009) *Good Medical Practice*. London: General Medical Council.

Genn, J.M. (2001) 'Curriculum, Environment, Climate, Quality and Change in Medical Education – A Unifying Perspective'. *Medical Teacher*, 23: 337–44 (part 1), 445–54 (part 2).

Gergen, K.J. (2001) *Social Construction in Context*. London: Sage.

Gibson, J.J. (1979) *The Ecological Approach to Visual Perception*. Boston, MA: Houghton Mifflin.

Ginsburg, S. and Lingard, L. (2006) 'Using Reflection and Rhetoric to Understand Professional Behaviors'. In D.T. Stern (ed.), *Measuring Medical* Professionalism, 195–212. Oxford: Oxford University Press.

Gonzales, L. (2012) *Surviving Survival: The Art and Science of Resilience*. New York: W.W. Norton & Co.

Good, B. (1994) *Medicine, Rationality and Experience: An Anthropological Perspective*. Cambridge: Cambridge University Press.

Good, B.J. (2000) 'Ethnography – in the Subjunctive Mode', paper prepared for Cultural Psychology Meets Anthropology: Papers in Honor of Jerome Bruner, AAA Annual Meetings, San Francisco, CA, 18 November, www.english.ubc.ca/PROJECTS/PAIN/DGOOD.HTM (accessed 4 September 2014).

Goodman, P. (1964) *Compulsory Mis-education*. New York: Horizon Press.

Goodwin, B. (1995) *How the Leopard Changed its Spots*. London: Phoenix.

Gordon, J. (2005) 'Medical Humanities: To Cure Sometimes, to Relieve Often, to Comfort Always'. *Medical Journal of Australia*, 182: 5–8.

Gordon, J.J. and Evans, H.M. (2010) 'Learning Medicine from the Humanities'. In T. Swanwick (ed.), *Understanding Medical Education: Evidence, Theory and Practice*, 2nd edn, 213–26. Oxford: Wiley-Blackwell.

Gorz, A. (2010) *The Immaterial*. London: Seagull.

Grant, K. (2014) 'Dissection Debate: Why are Medical Schools Cutting Back on Cadavers?'. *The Globe and Mail*, 27 Apr, www.theglobeandmail.com/life/health-and-fitness/health/dissection-debate-why-are-medical-schools-cutting-back-on-cadavers/article18296300 (accessed 4 September 2014).

Grant, V.J. (2003) 'Special Theme Brief Article: International – University of Auckland, Faculty of Medical and Health Sciences, Medical Humanities Courses'. *Academic Medicine*, 78: 1072.

Graves, R. (1961) *The White Goddess: A Historical Grammar of Poetic Myth*. London: Faber & Faber.

Greene, G. (1993) *The Ministry of Fear: An Entertainment*. Harmondsworth: Penguin Books.

Greenhalgh, T. and Hurwitz, B. (1999) 'Narrative Based Medicine: Why Study Narrative?'. *British Medical Journal*, 318: 48–50.

Groopman, J. (2007) *How Doctors Think*. Boston, MA: Houghton Mifflin.

Guattari, F. (1995) *Chaosmosis: An Ethico-Aesthetic Paradigm*. Bloomington, IN: Indiana University Press.

Gulbenkian Foundation (1982) *Report on the Arts in Schools: Principles, Practice and Provision*. London: Calouste Gulbenkian Foundation.

Gupta, R., Singh, S. and Kotru, M. (2011) 'Reaching People through Medical Humanities: An Initiative'. *Journal of Educational Evaluation for Health Professions*, 8, www.ncbi.nlm.nih.gov/pmc/articles/PMC3110875 (accessed 23 October 2014).

Haddon, M. (2012) *The Red House*. London: Cape.

Hafferty, F. (2006) 'Measuring Professionalism: A Commentary'. In D.T. Stern (ed.), *Measuring Medical Professionalism*, 281–306. Oxford: Oxford University Press.

Haidet, P. (2007) 'Jazz and the "Art" of Medicine: Improvisation in the Clinical Encounter'. *Annals of Family Medicine*, 5: 164–69.

Hallyn, F. (1993) *The Poetic Structure of the World: Copernicus and Kepler*. New York: Zone Books.

Halpern, J. (2001) *From Detached Concern to Empathy: Humanizing Medical Practice*. Oxford: Oxford University Press.

Hamilton, C., Hinks, S. and Petticrew, M. (2003) 'Arts for Health: Still Searching for the Holy Grail'. *Journal of Epidemiology and Community Health*, 57: 401–2.

Hancock, J., Roberts, M., Monrouxe, L. and Mattick, K. (in press) 'Medical Student and Junior Doctors' Tolerance of Ambiguity: Development of a New Scale'. *Advances in Health Sciences Theory and Practice*, published online ahead of print (PMID: 24841480).

Handfield-Jones, R., Nasmith, L., Steinert, Y. and Lawn, N. (1993) 'Creativity in Medical Education: The Use of Innovative Techniques in Clinical Teaching'. *Medical Teacher*, 15: 3–10.

Hardee, J.T. and Kasper, I.K. (2005) 'From Standardized Patient to Care Actor: Evolution of a Teaching Methodology'. *Permanente Journal*, 9: 79–82.

Harmon, K. (2009) 'Deaths from Avoidable Medical Error More than Double in Past Decade, Investigation Shows'. *Scientific American*, 10 August, www.scientificamerican.com/blog/post/deaths-from-avoidable-medical-error-2009-08-10/?id=deaths-from-avoidable-medical-error-2009-08-10 (accessed 3 November 2014).

Hawhee, D. (2004) *Bodily Arts: Rhetoric and Athletics in Ancient Greece*. Austin, TX; University of Texas Press.

Hawkins, A.H., Ballard, J.O. and Hufford, D.J. (2003) 'Humanities Education at Pennsylvania State University College of Medicine, Hershey, Pennsylvania'. *Academic Medicine*, 78: 1001–5.

Health Development Agency (2000) *Art for Health: A Review of Good Practice in Community-Based Arts Projects and Initiatives which Impact on Health and Wellbeing*. London: Health Development Agency.

Health Service Journal (1999) 'Send in the Clowns'. 22 April, www.hsj.co.uk/news/send-in-the-clowns/29709.article (accessed 5 September 2014).

Heathfield, A. (undated) 'Transfigured Night: A Conversation with Alphonso Lingis'. http://vimeo.com/77410520 (accessed 23 October 2014).

Hennessy, B.A. and Amabile, T.M. (1988) 'The Conditions of Creativity'. In R.J.

Sternberg (ed.), *The Nature of Creativity: Contemporary Psychological Perspectives*, 11–40. Cambridge: Cambridge University Press.

Hill, A. (1945) *Art versus Illness: A Story of Art Therapy*. London: Allen & Unwin.

Hillman, J. (1972a) *The Myth of Analysis: Three Essays in Archetypal Psychology*. New York: Harper & Row.

Hillman, J. (1972b) 'An Essay on Pan'. In W.H. Roscher and J. Hillman, *Pan and the Nightmare: Two Essays*. Dallas, TX: Spring Publications.

Hillman, J. (1992) *Re-visioning Psychology*, 2nd edn. New York: HarperPerennial.

Hillman, J. and Ventura, M. (1993) *We've Had a Hundred Years of Psychotherapy, and the World's Getting Worse*. San Francisco, CA: HarperSanFrancisco.

Hodges, B. (2005) 'The Many and Conflicting Histories of Medical Education in Canada and the USA: An Introduction to the Paradigm Wars'. *Medical Education*, 39: 613–21.

Hodges, B. and Lingard, L. (2012) *The Question of Competence: Reconsidering Medical Education in the Twenty-First Century*. New York: Cornell University Press.

Hogan, H., Healey, F., Neale, G., Thomson, R., Vincent, C. and Black, N. (2012) 'Preventable Deaths Due to Problems in Care in English Acute Hospitals: A Retrospective Case Record Review Study'. *BMJ Quality and Safety*, published online ahead of print http://qualitysafety.bmj.com/content/early/2012/07/06/bmjqs-2012-001159.full.pdf (accessed 3 November 2014).

Hojat, M., Gonnella, J.S., Nasca, T.J., Salvatore, M., Vergare, M. and Magee, M. (2002a) 'Physician Empathy: Definition, Components, Measurement, and Relationship to Gender and Specialty'. *American Journal of Psychiatry*, 159: 1563–9.

Hojat, M., Gonnella, J.S., Nasca, T.J., Salvatore, M., Veloski, J.J. and Magee, M. (2002b) 'The Jefferson Scale of Physician Empathy: Further Psychometric Data and Differences by Gender and Specialty at Item Level'. *Academic Medicine*, 77: S58–60.

Hojat, M., Gonnella, J.S., Mangione, S., Nasca, T.J., Veloski, J.J., Erdmann, J.B., Callahan, C.A. and Magee, M. (2002c) 'Empathy in Medical Students as Related to Academic Performance, Clinical Competence and Gender'. *Medical Education*, 36: 522–7.

Hojat, M., Mangione, S., Nasca, T.J., Vergare, M., Rattner, S., Erdmann, J.B., Gonnella, J.S. and Magee, M. (2004) 'An Empirical Study of Decline in Empathy in Medical School'. *Medical Education*, 38: 934–41.

Hooker, C. (2008) 'The Medical Humanities: A Brief Introduction'. *Australian Family Physician*, 37: 369–70.

Hooker, C. and Noonan, E. (2011) 'Medical Humanities as Expressive of Western Culture'. *Medical Humanities*, 37: 79–84.

Housen, A. (1992) 'Validating a Measure of Aesthetic Development for Museums and Schools'. *ILVS Review: A Journal of Visitor Behavior*, 2: 2–8.

Housen, A. (2002) 'Aesthetic Thought, Critical Thinking and Transfer'. *Arts Learning Journal*, 18: 1–7.

House of Commons Health Committee (2009) *Patient Safety: Sixth Report of Session 2008–2009*. London: The Stationery Office.

Howe, M. (1999) *Genius Explained*. Cambridge: Cambridge University Press.

Hunter, K.M. (1991a) 'Toward the Cultural Interpretation of Medicine'. *Literature and Medicine*, 10: 1–17.

Hunter, K.M. (1991b) *Doctors' Stories: The Narrative Structure of Medical Knowledge*. Princeton, NJ: Princeton University Press.

Huntington, B. and Kuhn, N. (2003) 'Communication Gaffes: A Root Cause of Malpractice Claims'. *Proceedings of the Bayley University Medical Center*, 16: 157–61, www.ncbi.nlm.nih.gov/pmc/articles/PMC1201002 (accessed 4 September 2014).

Hurwitz, B. and Dakin, P. (2009) 'Welcome Developments in UK Medical Humanities'. *Journal of the Royal Society of Medicine*, 102: 84–5.

Illich, I. (1977) *Limits to Medicine: Medical Nemesis and the Expropriation of Health*. Harmondsworth: Penguin Books.

Illich, I. (1985) *H₂O and the Waters of Forgetfulness*. Dallas, TX: Dallas Institute.

Ingrassia, A. (2013) 'Portfolio-Based Learning in Medical Education'. *Advances in Psychiatric Treatment*, 19: 329–36.

Irby, D. (1978) 'Clinical Teacher Effectiveness in Medicine'. *Journal of Medical Education*, 37: 258–61.

Jacques, A., Trinkley, R., Stone, L., Tang, R., Hudson, W.A. and Khandelwal, S. (2012) 'Art of Analysis: A Cooperative Program between a Museum and Medicine'. *Journal for Learning Through the Arts*, 8: 1–9.

Jasani, S. and Sacks, N. (2012) 'Utilizing Visual Art to Enhance the Clinical Observation Skills of Medical Students'. *Medical Teacher*, 35: e1327–31.

Johns, C. (2009) *Becoming a Reflective Practitioner*, 2nd edn. Oxford: Wiley-Blackwell.

Jones, A.H. and Carson, R.A. (2003) 'Medical Humanities at the University of Texas Medical Branch at Galveston'. *Academic Medicine*, 78: 1006–9.

Jones, C. and Galison, P. (eds) (1998) *Picturing Science, Producing Art*. New York: Routledge.

Jones, T., Wear, D. and Friedman, L.D. (eds) (2014) *Health Humanities Reade*. New Brunswick, NJ: Rutgers University Press.

Joyce, J. (1939) *Finnegan's Wake*. London: Faber & Faber.

Kahneman, D., Slovic, P. and Tversky, A. (eds) (1982) *Judgement under Uncertainty: Heuristics and Biases*. Cambridge: Cambridge University Press.

Kaiser, R. (2002) 'Fixing Identity by Denying Uniqueness: An Analysis of Professional Identity in Medicine'. *Journal of Medical Humanities*, 23: 95–105.

Kauffman, S. (1995) *At Home in the Universe: The Search for Laws of Self-Organization and Complexity*. London: Viking.

Kaufman, D.M. and Mann, K.V. (2014) 'Teaching and Learning in Medical Education: How Theory Can Inform Practice'. In T. Swanwick (ed.), *Understanding Medical Education: Evidence, Theory and Practice*, 2nd edn, 7–30. Oxford: Wiley-Blackwell.

Ke, W. (2012) 'Healthcare Reform: Using Medical Humanities as an Alternative Solution'. http://triplehelixblog.com/2012/03/healthcare-reform-using-medical-humanities-as-an-alternative-solution (accessed 8 September 2014).

Kelly, N. (2012) 'What Are You Doing Creatively These Days?'. *Academic Medicine*, 87: 1476.

Kember, D. (2001) *Reflective Teaching and Learning in the Health Professions*. Oxford: Blackwell Science.

Kidd, D.C. and Castano, E. (2013) 'Reading Literary Fiction Improves Theory of Mind'. *Science*, 342: 377–80.

Kidd, M.J. and Connor, J.T. (2008) 'Striving to do Good Things: Teaching

Humanities in Canadian Medical Schools'. *Journal of Medical Humanities*, 29: 45–54.

Kim, M.G. (2004) *Affinity, That Elusive Dream: A Genealogy of the Chemical Revolution*. Cambridge, MA: MIT Press.

Kirklin, D.B. (2002) 'Acquiring Experience in Medical Humanities Teaching: The Chicken and Egg Conundrum'. *Medical Humanities*, 28: 101.

Kirklin, D. (2003) 'The Centre for Medical Humanities, Royal Free and University College Medical School, London, England'. *Academic Medicine*, 78: 1048–53.

Kirklin, D. (2005) 'The Search for Meaning in Modern Medicine'. Doctoral thesis, University College, London, http://eprints.ucl.ac.uk/144687 (accessed 5 September 2014).

Kirklin, D., Duncan, J., McBride, S., Hunt, S. and Griffin, M. (2007) 'A Cluster Design Controlled Trial of Arts-Based Observational Skills Training in Primary Care'. *Medical Education*, 41: 395–401.

Kjær, A.M. (2004) *Governance*. Cambridge: Polity.

Klamen, D. and Williams, R. (2006) 'Using Standardized Clinical Encounters to Assess Physician Communication'. In D.T. Stern (ed.), *Measuring Medical Professionalism*, 53–74. Oxford: Oxford University Press.

Kleinman, A. (1988) *The Illness Narratives: Suffering, Healing and the Human Condition*. New York: Basic Books.

Klugman, C.M., Peel, J. and Beckmann-Mendez, D. (2011) 'Art Rounds: Teaching Interprofessional Students Visual Thinking Strategies at One School'. *Academic Medicine*, 86: 1266–71.

Kneebone, R. (2013a) 'Jazz Musicians Can Teach Surgeons How to Improvise'. 28 May, http://theconversation.com/jazz-musicians-can-teach-surgeons-how-to-improvise-14020 (accessed 25 October 2014).

Kneebone, R. (2013b) 'Looking Deeply: Roger Kneebone at TEDMEDLive Imperial College 2013'. 23 May, www.youtube.com/watch?v=dWtILWOYwpQ (accessed 25 October 2014).

Kneebone, R. and Baillie, S. (2008) 'Contextualized Simulation and Procedural Skills: A View from Medical Education'. *Journal of Veterinary Medical Education*, 35: 595–8.

Kneebone, R., Arora, S., King, D., Bello, F., Sevdalis, N., Kassab, E., Aggarwal, R., Darzi, A. and Nestel, D. (2010) 'Distributed Simulation – Accessible Immersive Training'. *Medical Teacher*, 32: 65–70.

Knight, D. (1992) *Humphry Davy: Science and Power*. Oxford: Blackwell.

Kohn, L.T., Corrigan, J.M. and Donaldson, M.S. (1999) *To Err is Human*. Washington, DC: National Academy Press.

Konrath, S., O'Brien, E. and Hsing, C. (2010) 'Changes in Dispositional Empathy in American College Students over Time: A Meta-Analysis'. *Personality and Social Psychology Review*, 15: 180–98.

Kumagai, A.K. (2008) 'A Conceptual Framework for the Use of Illness Narratives in Medical Education'. *Academic Medicine*, 83: 653–58.

Kumagai, A.K. (2009) 'The Patient's Voice in Medical Education: The Family Centered Experience Program'. *Virtual Mentor*, 11(3): 228–31, http://virtualmentor.ama-assn.org/2009/03/medu1-0903.html (accessed 24 October 2014).

Kumagai, A.K. (2012) 'Acts of Interpretation: A Philosophical Approach to Using Creative Arts in Medical Education, *Academic Medicine*, 87: 1138–44.

Kumagai, A.K. (2013) 'On the Way to Reflection: A Conversation on a Country Path'. *Perspectives in Biology and Medicine*, 56: 362–70.

Kumagai, A.K. and Lypson, M.L. (2009) 'Beyond Cultural Competence: Critical Consciousness, Social Justice, and Multicultural Education'. *Academic Medicine*, 84: 782–87.

Kumagai, A.K. and Wear, D. (2014) '"Making Strange": A Role for the Humanities in Medical Education'. *Academic Medicine*, 89: 973–77.

Kumagai, A., White, C.B., Ross, P.T., Purkiss, J.A., O'Neal, C.M. and Steiger, J.A. (2007) 'Use of Interactive Theater for Faculty Development in Multicultural Medical Education'. *Medical Teacher*, 29: 335–40.

LaCombe, M.A. (1993) 'Letters of Intent'. In H.M. Spiro, M.G. McCrea, E.P. Curnen and D. St James (eds), *Empathy and the Practice of Medicine: Beyond Pills and the Scalpel*, 54–66. New Haven, CT: Yale University Press.

Laerdal Medical (2011) 'Just A Routine Operation'. 6 July, www.youtube.com/watch?v=JzlvgtPIof4 (accessed 25 October 2014).

Lakoff, G. and Johnson, M. (1980) *Metaphors We Live By*, Chicago, IL: University of Chicago Press.

Lakoff, G. and Johnson, M. (1999) *Philosophy in the Flesh: The Embodied Mind and its Challenge to Western Thought*. New York: Basic Books.

Lam, V. (2006) *Bloodletting and Miraculous Cures*. New York: Doubleday.

Lancet (2006) Special Issue on Medicine and Creativity. *The Lancet*, 368: S1–66.

Larkin, P. (2003) 'Annus Mirabilis'. In his *Collected Poems*, 146. London: Faber & Faber.

Lave, J. and Wenger, E. (1991) *Situated Learning: Legitimate Peripheral Participation*. Cambridge: Cambridge University Press.

Law, J. (2006) *Big Pharma: How the World's Biggest Drug Companies Control Illness*. London: Constable.

Leake, C. (1973) 'Humanistic Studies in US Medical Education'. *Journal of Medical Education*, 48: 878–9.

Leigh, A. (1997) 'The Place of Creativity within the Development and Assessment of NVQs and SVQs'. *Competence and Assessment*, 23: 5–6.

Levine, D. and Bleakley, A. (2012) 'Maximising Medicine through Aphorisms'. *Medical Education*, 46: 153–62.

Lippell, S. (2002) 'Creativity and Medical Education'. *Medical Education*, 36: 519–21.

Locke, J. (1975) *An Essay Concerning Human Understanding*, ed. P. Nidditch. Oxford: Clarendon Press.

Lowes, J.L. (1978) *The Road to Xanadu: A Study in the Ways of the Imagination*. London: Pan Books.

Lubart, T.I. (1999) 'Creativity across cultures'. In R.J. Sternberg (ed.), *Handbook of Creativity*, 339–50. Cambridge: Cambridge University Press.

Ludmerer, K.M. (1999) *Time to Heal: American Medical Education from the Turn of the Century to the Era of Managed Care*. Oxford: Oxford University Press.

Luther, V.P. and Crandall, S.J. (2011) 'Ambiguity and Uncertainty: Neglected Elements of Medical Education Curricula?'. *Academic Medicine*, 86: 799–800.

Lyotard, F. (1984) *The Postmodern Condition*. Manchester: University of Manchester Press.

Macleod, C.W. (1985) *Homer: Iliad*. Cambridge: Cambridge University Press.

Macnaughton, J. (2009) 'The Dangerous Practice of Empathy'. *The Lancet*, 373: 1940–41.

Macneill, P.U. (2011) 'The Arts and Medicine: A Challenging Relationship'. *Medical Humanities*, 37: 85–90.

Mamede, S. and Schmidt, H.G. (2004) 'The Structure of Reflective Practice in Medicine'. *Medical Education*, 38: 1302–8.

Mar, R., Tackett, J. and Moore, C. (2010) 'Exposure to Media and Theory-of-Mind Development in Preschoolers'. *Cognitive Development*, 25: 69–78.

Marcum, J.A. (2013) 'The Role of Empathy and Wisdom in Medical Practice and Pedagogy: Confronting the Hidden Curriculum'. *Journal of Biomedical Education*, http://dx.doi.org/10.1155/2013/923810 (accessed 5 September 2014).

Marinetti, F. T. (1909) 'The Futurist Manifesto'. http://vserver1.cscs.lsa.umich.edu/~crshalizi/T4PM/futurist-manifesto.html (accessed 25 October 2014).

Marsh, H. (2014) *Do No Harm: Stories of Life, Death and Brain Surgery*. London: Weidenfeld & Nicolson.

Marshall, R.J. and Bleakley, A. (2008) 'Putting it Bluntly: Communication Skills in the *Iliad*'. *Medical Humanities*, 34: 30–34.

Marshall, R. and Bleakley, A. (2009) 'The Death of Hector: Pity in Homer, Empathy in Medical Education'. *Medical Humanities*, 35: 10–12.

Marshall, R. and Bleakley, A. (2011) 'Sing, Muse: Songs in Homer and in Hospital'. *Medical Humanities*, 37: 27–33.

Marshall, R.J. and Bleakley, A. (2013) 'Lost in Translation: Homer in English; the Patient's Story in Medicine'. *Medical Humanities*, 39: 47–52.

Mattingly, C. and Fleming, M.H. (1994) *Clinical Reasoning: Forms of Inquiry in a Therapeutic Practice*. Philadelphia, PA: F.A. Davis.

Mattingly, C. and Garro, L.C. (eds) (2000) *Narrative and the Cultural Construction of Illness and Healing*. Berkeley, CA: University of California Press.

McDonald, L. (ed.) (2009) *Florence Nightingale: The Nightingale School – Collected Works of Florence Nightingale*. Waterloo, Ontario: Wilfrid Laurier University Press.

McElwee, S. (2013) 'A Rising Empathy Gap Hurts the Poor—But Also the Economy'. 25 October, www.demos.org/blog/10/25/13/rising-empathy-gap-hurts-poor%E2%80%94-also-economy (accessed 23 October 2014).

McGough, J.J., Pataki, C.S. and Suddath, R. (2005) 'Dexmethylphenidate Extended-Release Capsules for Attention Deficit Hyperactivity Disorder'. *Expert Review of Neurotherapeutics*, 9: 437–41.

McKie, R. (2011) 'The Fine Art of Medical Diagnosis'. *The Observer*, 11 September, www.theguardian.com/artanddesign/2011/sep/11/medicine-clues-doctors-art-paintings (accessed 5 September 2014).

McLachlan, J.C. and de Bere, S.R. (2004) 'How We Teach Anatomy Without Cadavers'. *The Clinical Teacher*, 1: 49–52.

McLachlan, J.C., Bligh, J., Bradley, P. and Searle, J. (2004) 'Teaching Anatomy without Cadavers'. *Medical Education*, 38: 418–24.

McManus, I.C. (1995) 'Humanity and the Medical Humanities'. *The Lancet*, 346: 1143–5.

McWilliam, E. (2007) 'Is Creativity Teachable? Conceptualising the Creativity/Pedagogy Relationship in Higher Education'. Paper presented at 30th HERDSA Annual Conference: Enhancing Higher Education, Theory and Scholarship, Adelaide, 8–11 July.

Meza, J.P. and Passerman, D.S. (2011) *Integrating Narrative Medicine and Evidence-Based Medicine*. London: Radcliffe Publishing.

Miller, A. (2013) 'The Art Practicum: Clinical Skills for the Digital Age'. www.medicalfutureslab.org/videos (accessed 5 September 2014).

Mohr, J.C. (2000) 'American Medical Malpractice Litigation in Historical Perspective'. *Journal of the American Medical Association*, 283: 1731–7.

Montgomery, K. (2006) *How Doctors Think: Clinical Judgment and the Practice of Medicine.* Oxford: Oxford University Press.

Moody, R. (2002) *The Black Veil.* London: Faber & Faber.

Moody, N. and Hallam, J. (eds) (1998) *Medical Fictions.* Liverpool: John Moores University.

Moody Medical Library (undated) 'Society for Health and Human Values: Records, (1970–1997)'. www.lib.utexas.edu/taro/utmb/00079/utmb-00079.html (accessed 23 October 2014).

Mooney, R.L. (1963) 'A Conceptual Model for Integrating Four Approaches to the Identification of Creative Talent'. In C.W. Taylor and F. Barron (eds), *Scientific Creativity: Its Recognition and Development*, 331–40. New York: Wiley.

Moore, A.R. (1976) 'Medical Humanities: A New Medical Adventure'. *New England Journal of Medicine*, 295: 1479–80.

Moore, A. (2007) 'Eternal Sunshine'. *The Observer Magazine*, 13 May: 20–29.

Morris, R. (undated) 'Robert Morris'. www.theartstory.org/artist-morris-robert.htm (accessed 25 October 2014).

Muller, D. and Kase, N. (2010) 'Challenging Traditional Premedical Requirements as Predictors of Success in Medical School: The Mount Sinai School of Medicine Humanities and Medicine Program'. *Academic Medicine*, 85: 1378–83.

Murray, J. (2000) *Intensive Care: A Doctor's Journal*, Berkeley, CA: University of California Press.

Murray, J. (2003) 'Development of a Medical Humanities Program at Dalhousie University Faculty of Medicine, Novia Scotia, Canada, 1992–2003'. *Academic Medicine*, 78: 1020–23.

Mylopoulos, M., Lohfeld, L., Norman, G.R., Dhaliwal, G. and Eva, K.W. (2012) 'Renowned Physicians' Perceptions of Expert Diagnostic Practice'. *Academic Medicine*, 87: 1413–17.

Naghshineh, S., Hafler, J.P., Miller, A.R., Blanco, M.A., Lipsitz, S.R., Dubroff, R.P. Khoshbin, S. and Katz, J.T. (2008) 'Formal Art Observation Training Improves Medical Students' Visual Diagnostic Skills'. *Journal of General and Internal Medicine*, 23: 991–7.

Naghshineh, S., Hafler, J.P., Miller, A.R., Blanco, M.A., Lipsitz, S.R., Dubroff, R.P., Khoshbin, S. and Katz, J.T. (2011) 'Commentary: Teaching Creativity and Innovative Thinking in Medicine and the Health Sciences'. *Academic Medicine*, 86: 1201–3.

Nelson, L.H. (ed.) (1997) *Stories and Their Limits: Narrative Approaches to Bioethics.* London: Routledge.

Nendaz, M.R. and Bordage, G. (2002) 'Promoting Diagnostic Problem Representation'. *Medical Education*, 36: 760–66.

Ness, R.B. (2011) 'Commentary: Teaching Creativity and Innovative Thinking in Medicine and the Health Sciences'. *Academic Medicine*, 86: 1201–3.

Neumann, M., Edelhäuser, F., Tauschel, D., Fischer, M., Wirtz, M., Woopen, C., Haramati, A. and Scheffer, C. (2011) 'Empathy Decline and Its Reasons: A Systematic Review of Studies With Medical Students and Residents'. *Academic Medicine*, 86: 996–1009.

Neumann, M., Scheffer, C., Tauschel, D., Lutz, G., Wirtz, M. and Edelhäuser, F. (2012) 'Physician Empathy: Definition, Outcome-Relevance and its Measurement in Patient Care and Medical Education'. *German Journal for Medical Education (MS Z Med Ausbild)*, 29(1): Doc11.

NHS Choices (undated) 'Attention Deficit Hyperactivity Disorder (ADHD)'. www.nhs.uk/conditions/attention-deficit-hyperactivity-disorder/Pages/Introduction.aspx (accessed 27 October 2014).

Nickerson, R.S. (1999) 'Enhancing Creativity'. In R.J. Sternberg (ed.), *Handbook of Creativity*, 392–430. Cambridge: Cambridge University Press.

Nietzsche, F. (1984) *Human, All Too Human*. Lincoln, NE: University of Nebraska Press.

Noel, D. (1986) *Approaching Earth: A Search for the Mythic Significance of the Space Age*. New York: Amity House.

Norman, G.R. and Eva, K.W. (2010) 'Diagnostic Error and Clinical Reasoning'. *Medical Education*, 44: 94–100.

Norman, G.R., Young, M. and Brooks, L. (2007) 'Non-analytic Models of Clinical Reasoning: The Role of Experience'. *Medical Education*, 41: 1140–45.

Nunes, P., Williams, S., Bidyadhar, S. and Stevenson, K. (2011) 'A Study of Empathy Decline in Students from Five Health Disciplines during their First Year of Training'. *International Journal of Medical Education*, 2: 12–17.

Nussbaum, M. (2001) *The Fragility of Goodness: Luck and Ethics in Greek Tragedy and Philosophy*, 2nd edn. Cambridge: Cambridge University Press.

Nussbaum, M. (2010) *Not for Profit: Why Democracy Needs the Humanities*. Princeton, NJ: Princeton University Press.

O'Connell, A. (2011) 'The Times Campaign to Free Ai Weiwei'. *The Times*, 18 May, www.thetimes.co.uk/tto/arts/visualarts/article3022815.ece (accessed 24 October 2014).

Ofri, D. (2013) *What Doctors Feel: How Emotions Affect the Practice of Medicine*. Boston, MA: Beacon Press.

Ofri, D. (undated) 'Creativity in Medicine'. http://danielleofri.com/creativity-in-medicine (accessed 5 September 2014).

Onians, R.B. (1988) *The Origins of European Thought*. Cambridge: Cambridge University Press.

Orr, D. (2000) 'The Counter-culture Fights On'. *The Independent*, 12 May, www.independent.co.uk/voices/commentators/deborah-orr/the-counterculture-fights-on-278197.html (accessed 4 November 2014).

Osler, W. (1932) *Aequanimitas*, 3rd edn. New York: McGraw-Hill.

Ousager, J. and Johannessen, H. (2010) 'Humanities in Undergraduate Medical Education: A Literature Review'. *Academic Medicine*, 85: 988–98.

Owen, W. (1994) *The War Poems of Wilfred Owen*, ed. J. Stallworthy. London: Chatto & Windus.

Padel, R. (1992) *In and Out of the Mind: Greek Images of the Tragic Sel*. Princeton, NJ: Princeton University Press.

Padel, R. (1995) *Whom Gods Destroy: Elements of Greek and Tragic Madness*. Princeton, NJ: Princeton University Press.

Padfield, D. (2003) *Perceptions of Pain*. Stockport: Dewi Lewis.

Page, R. and Thomas, B. (eds) (2011) *New Narratives: Stories and Storytelling in the Digital Age*. Lincoln, NE: University of Nebraska Press.

Palmer, D. (2003) 'Professional Judgement and Clinical Decision-Making'. In D.

Palmer and S. Kaur (eds), *Core Skills for Nurse Practitioners: A Handbook for Nurse Practitioners*, 145–59. London: Whurr Publishers.

Panagia, D. (2010) '"*Partage du Sensible*": The Distribution of the Sensible'. In J.-P. Deranty (ed.), *Jacques Rancière: Key Concepts*, 95–103. Durham: Acumen.

Pauli, H.G., White, K.L. and McWhinney, I.R. (2000) 'Medical Education, Research, and Scientific Thinking in the 21st Century'. *Education for Health*, 13: 15–25 (part 1), 165–72 (part 2), 173–86 (part 3).

Pedersen, R. (2010) 'Empathy development in medical education – A critical review'. *Medical Teacher*, 32: 593–600.

Peirce, C.S. (1931) *Collected Papers, Vol 5*. Cambridge, MA: Harvard University Press.

Pellegrino, E.D. (1972) 'Welcoming Remarks'. In L.L. Hunt (ed.), *Proceedings of the First Session, Institute on Human Values in Medicine*, 3–9. Philadelphia, PA: Society for Health and Human Values.

Pellegrino, E.D. (1974) 'Educating the Humanist Physician: An Ancient Ideal Reconsidered'. *Journal of the American Medical Association*, 227: 1288–94.

Pellegrino, E.D. (1979) *Humanism and the Physician*. Knoxville, TN: University of Tennessee Press.

Pellegrino, E.D. (1984) 'The Humanities in Medical Education: Entering the Post-evangelical Era'. *Theoretical Medicine and Bioethics*, 5: 253–66.

Perry, M., Maffulli, N., Willson, S. and Morrisey, D. (2011) 'The Effectiveness of Arts-Based Interventions in Medical Education: A Literature Review'. *Medical Education* 45: 141–8.

Perse, S.-J. (1961) *On Poetry: Speech of Acceptance Upon the Award of the Nobel Prize for Literature Delivered in Stockholm December 10, 1960*. New York: Bollingen Series.

Peterkin, A. (2012) *Staying Human During Residency Training: How to Survive and Thrive After Medical School*. Toronto: University of Toronto Press.

Peterkin, A. and Brett-Maclean, P. (eds) (forthcoming) *Keeping Reflection Fresh: Top Educators Share Their Innovations in Health Professional Education*. Kent, OH: Kent State University Press.

Peterkin, A. and Risdon, C. (2003) *Caring for Lesbian and Gay People: A Clinical Guide*. Toronto: University of Toronto Press.

Petersen, A., Bleakley, A., Brömer, R. and Marshall, R. (2008) 'The Medical Humanities Today: Humane Health Care or Tool of Governance?'. *Journal of Medical Humanities*, 29: 1–4.

Philipp, R., Baum, M., Mawson, A. and Calman, K. (1999) *Beyond the Millennium: A Summary of the Proceedings of the First Windsor Conference*. London: Nuffield Trust.

Phillip, R., Baum, M., Macnaughton, J. and Calman, K. (2002) *Arts, Health and Well-being*. London: Nuffield Trust.

Phillips, A. and Rakusen, J. (1996) *The New Our Bodies, Ourselves*, UK edn. London: Penguin.

Pilpel, D., Schor, R. and Benbassat, J. (1998) 'Barriers to Acceptance of Medical Error: The Case for a Teaching Programme'. *Medical Education*, 32: 3–7.

Pinar, W. (2012) *What is Curriculum Theory?*, 2nd edn. New York: Routledge.

Pinar, W.F. and Reynolds, W.M. (1992) 'Introduction: Curriculum as Text'. In W.F. Pinar and W.M. Reynolds (eds), *Understanding Curriculum as Phenomenological and Deconstructed Text*, 1–16. New York: Teachers College Press.

Plant, S. (2001) *Writing on Drugs*, 2nd edn. London: Faber & Faber.

Plato (1956) *Meno* trs. W.K.C. Guthrie, in *Protagoras and Meno*. Harmondsworth: Penguin Books.

Platt, F.W. (1979) 'Clinical Hypocompetence: The Interview'. *Annals of Internal Medicine*, 91: 898–902.

Polanyi, M. (1983) *The Tacit Dimension*. Gloucester: Smith.

Polanyi, M. (1998) *Personal Knowledge*. London: Routledge.

Polianski, I.J. and Fangerou, H. (2012) 'Toward "Harder" Medical Humanities: Moving Beyond the "Two Cultures" Dichotomy'. *Academic Medicine*, 87: 121–6.

Polanyi, M. and Prosch, H. (1975) *Meaning*. Chicago, IL: University of Chicago Press.

Popper, K. (2002) *The Open Society and Its Enemies*. London: Routledge.

Potchen, E.J. (2006) 'Measuring Observer Performance in Chest Radiology: Some Experiences'. *Journal of the American College of Radiology*, 3: 423–32.

Pound, P., Britten, N., Morgan, M., Yardley, L. Pope, C., Daker-White, G. and Campbell, R. (2005) 'Resisting Medicines: A Synthesis of Qualitative Studies of Medicine Taking'. *Social Science and Medicine*, 61: 133–55.

Pretorius, R., Lohr, G., McGuigan, D. and Devlin, K. (undated) *Art in Medicine: The Power of Observation*. www.smbs.buffalo.edu/fam-med/files/facDevPpt/011906.pdf (accessed 25 October 2014).

Prideaux, S. (2005) *Edvard Munch: Behind the Scream*. New Haven, CT: Yale University Press.

Quain, R. (1833) *Quain's Dictionary of Medicine*, New York: D. Appleton and Co.

Rakel, D.P., Hoeft, T.J., Barrett, B.P., Chewning, B.A., Craig, B.M. and Niu, M. (2009) 'Practitioner Empathy and the Duration of the Common Cold'. *Family Medicine*, 41: 494–501.

Ramaswamy, R. (2013) 'Theatre of the Oppressed in Medical Humanities'. www.ccdc.in/theatre-oppressed-medical-humanities (accessed 5 September 2014).

Rancière, J. (2006) *The Politics of Aesthetics*. London: Continuum.

Rancière, J. (2010) *Dissensus: On Politics and Aesthetics*. London: Continuum.

Rancière, J. (2013) *Aisthesis: Scenes From the Aesthetic Regime of Art*. London: Verso.

Raphael, L. (2013) 'A Conversation With Linda Raphael'. *Graphic Medicine*, 18 April, www.graphicmedicine.org/a-conversation-with-linda-raphael (accessed 29 October 2014).

Reason, P. (1994) 'Three Approaches to Participative Inquiry'. In N.K. Denzin and Y.S. Lincoln (eds), *Handbook of Qualitative Research*, 324–39. Thousand Oaks, CA: Sage.

Reber, A.S. (1993) *Implicit Learning and Tacit Knowledge: An Essay on the Cognitive Unconscious*. Oxford: Oxford University Press.

Rees, G. (2010) 'The Ethical Imperative of Medical Humanities'. *Journal of Medical Humanities*, 31: 267–77.

Rees-Lee, J. and Kneebone, R. (in press) 'Cutting for a Career: A Discussion of the Domains of Surgical Competence Using Expert Bespoke Tailoring as a Metaphor for Surgical Practice'. *Advances in Health Sciences Education: Theory and Practice*, published online ahead of print.

Reilly, J.M., Ring, J. and Duke, L. (2005) 'Visual Thinking Strategies: A New Role for Art in Medical Education'. www.museum-ed.org/visual-thinking-strategies-a-new-role-for-art-in-medical-education (accessed 5 September 2014).

Reinke, E.E. (2003) 'From the Archives: Liberal Values in Premedical Education'. *Academic Medicine*, 78: 1058 (edited version). Originally published in 1937 in *The Journal of the Association of American Medical Colleges*, 12: 151–6.

Remen, R.N. (2012) 'Well-Being and Idealism'. http://meded.ucsf.edu/wellbeing/well-being-and-idealism (accessed 5 September 2014).

Reynolds, R. and Carson, R. (1976) 'The Place of Humanities in Medical Education'. *Journal of Medical Education*, 51: 142–3.

Rich, B. (2006) 'Breeding Cynicism: The Re-education of Medical Students'. *American Philosophical Association Newsletters*, 6: 24–28.

Ricouer, P. (1990) *Time and Narrative Vol 1*, Chicago, IL: University of Chicago Press.

Riggs, G. (2010) 'Commentary: Are We Ready to Embrace the Rest of the Flexner Report?'. *Academic Medicine*, 85: 1669–71.

Robinson, K. (2006) 'How Schools Kill Creativity'. TED2006 lecture, February, www.ted.com/talks/ken_robinson_says_schools_kill_creativity (accessed 25 October 2014).

Rockhill, G. (2006) 'Jacques Rancière's Politics of Perception'. In J. Rancière, *The Politics of Aesthetics*, 1–6. London: Continuum.

Rodenhauser, P., Strickland, M.A. and Gambala, C.T. (2004) 'Arts-Related Activities across U.S. Medical Schools: A Follow-Up Study'. *Teaching and Learning in Medicine*, 16: 233–9.

Roff, S. and Preece, P. (2004) 'Helping Medical Students to Find Their Moral Compasses: Ethics Teaching for Second and Third Year Undergraduates, *Journal of Medical Ethics*, 30: 487–9.

Rogers, C.R. (2004) *On Becoming a Person*. London: Constable.

Rosenthal, S., Howard, B., Schlussel, Y.R., Herrigel, D., Smolarz, B.G., Gable, B., Vasquez, J., Grigo, H. and Kaufman, M. (2011) 'Humanism at Heart: Preserving Empathy in Third-Year Medical Students'. *Academic Medicine* 86: 350–58.

Roter, D.L. and Hall, J.A. (2006) *Doctors Talking with Patients/Patients Talking with Doctors: Improving Communication in Medical Visits*, 2nd edn. London: Praeger.

Royal College of Physicians and Surgeons of Canada (2013) 'CanMEDS 2015: Stepping Up Emphasis on Leadership Competencies'. *Dialogue* 13(10), October, www.royalcollege.ca/portal/page/portal/rc/resources/publications/dialogue/vol13_10/canmeds2015_leadership (accessed 25 October 2014).

Runco, M. (1996) *The Creativity Research Handbook, Vol. 1*. New York: Hampton Press.

Runco, M. (2006) *The Creativity Research Handbook, Vol. 2*. New York: Hampton Press.

Runco, M. (2011) *The Creativity Research Hanbook, Vol. 3*. New York: Hampton Press.

Sacks, O. (2011) *The Man Who Mistook his Wife for a Hat*. London: Picador.

Salmon, P. and Young, B. (2011) Creativity in Clinical Communication: From Communication Skills to Skilled Communication, *Medical Education*, 45: 217–26.

Sanders, L. (2010) *Diagnosis: Dispatches From the Frontlines of Medical Mysteries*. London: Icon Books.

Sarton, G. and Siegel, F. (1949) 'Seventy-First Critical Bibliography of the History and Philosophy of Science and of the History of Civilization (to October 1947)'. *Isis*, 39: 70–139.

Schaff, P.B., Isken, S. and Tager, R.M. (2011) 'From Contemporary Art to Core Clinical Skills: Observation, Interpretation, and Meaning-Making in a Complex Environment'. *Academic Medicine*, 86: 1272–6.

Schein, S.L. (1984) *The Mortal Hero*. Berkeley, CA: University of California Press.

Schleifer, R. and Vannatta, J.B. (2013) *The Chief Concern of Medicine: The Integration of the Medical Humanities and Narrative Knowledge into Medical Practices*. Ann Arbor, MI: University of Michigan Press.

Schmidt, H.G. and Boshuizen, H.P.A. (1993) 'On Acquiring Expertise in Medicine'. *Educational Psychology Review*, 5: 205–21.

Schön, D.A. (1991) *Educating the Reflective Practitioner: Toward a New Design for Teaching and Learning in the Professions*. San Francisco, CA: Jossey-Bass.

Self, D.J. (1993) 'The Educational Philosophies behind the Medical Humanities Programs in the United States: An Empirical Assessment of Three Different Approaches to Humanistic Medical Education'. *Theoretical Medicine*, 14: 221–9.

Sellers, S. (ed.) (1994) *The Hélène Cixous Reader*. London: Routledge.

Selzer, R. (1996) *Mortal Lessons: Notes on the Art of Surgery*. San Diego, CA: Harcourt.

Selzer, R. (2001) 'Letter from a Young Doctor'. In T.K. Kushner and D.C. Thomasma (eds), *Ward Ethics: Dilemmas for Medical Students and Doctors in Training*, 5–8. New York: Cambridge University Press.

Shankar, P.R. (2008) 'Medical Humanities: Sowing the Seeds in the Himalayan Country of Nepal'. http://medhum.med.nyu.edu/blog/?p=113%22 (accessed 23 October 2014).

Shankar, P.R. (2010) 'Sir Robert Hutchison's Petition and the Medical Humanities'. *International Journal of Medical Education*, 1: 2–4.

Shapiro, J. (2008) 'Walking a Mile in Their Patients' Shoes: Empathy and Othering in Medical Students' Education'. *Philosophy, Ethics, and Humanities in Medicine*, 3: 10.

Shapiro, J. (2011) 'Illness Narratives: Reliability, Authenticity and the Empathic Witness'. *Medical Humanities*, 37: 68–72.

Shapiro, J., Rucker, L. and Beck, J. (2006) 'Training the Clinical Eye and Mind: Using the Arts to Develop Medical Students' Observational and Pattern Recognition Skills'. *Medical Education*, 40: 263–8.

Shapiro, J., Coulehan, J., Wear, D. and Montello, M. (2009) 'Medical Humanities and their Discontents: Definitions, Critiques, and Implications'. *Academic Medicine*, 84: 192–8.

Silverman, M.E., Murray, T.J. and Bryan, C.S. (eds) (2003) *The Quotable Osler*. Philadelphia, PA: American College of Physicians.

Simeon, D. and Abugel, J. (2006) *Feeling Unreal: Depersonalization Disorder and the Loss of the Self*. New York: Oxford University Press.

Skvorecky, J. (1994) *The Bass Saxophone*. New York: Ecco Press.

Slouka, M. (2009) 'Dehumanized: When Math and Science Rule the School'. *Harpers Magazine*, September, http://harpers.org/archive/2009/09/dehumanized (accessed 4 November 2014).

Slouka, M. (2010) *Essays from the Nick of Time: Reflections and Refutations*. Minneapolis, MN: Graywolf Press.

Smajdor, A., Stöckl, A. and Salter, C. (2011) 'The Limits of Empathy: Problems in Medical Education and Practice'. *Journal of Medical Ethics*, 37: 380–83.

Smith, D.W. (2005) 'Critical, Clinical'. In C.J. Stivale (ed.), *Gilles Deleuze: Key Concepts*, 182–93. Stocksfield: Acumen.

Snow, C.P. (1959) 'The Rede Lecture 1959'. http://s-f-walker.org.uk/pubsebooks/2cultures/Rede-lecture-2-cultures.pdf (accessed 30 October 2014).

Snow, C.P. (1963) *The Two Cultures: and A Second Look*. Cambridge: Cambridge University Press.

Spence, D. (1987) *The Freudian Metaphor*. New York: W.W. Norton.

Spiro, H.M., McCrea, M.G., Curnen, E.P., Peschel, E. and St James, D. (eds) (1993) *Empathy and the Practice of Medicine: Beyond Pills and the Scalpel*. New Haven, CT: Yale University Press.

Stafford, B.M. (1993) *Body Criticism: Imaging the Unseen in Enlightenment Art and Medicine*. Cambridge, MA: MIT Press.

Starfield, B. (2000) 'Is US Health Really the Best in the World?'. *Journal of the American Medical Association*, 284: 483–5.

Staricoff, R.L. (2004) *Arts in Health: A Review of the Medical Literature*. London: Arts Council England.

Staricoff, R.L. (2006) 'Arts in Health: The Value of Evaluation'. *Perspectives in Public Health*, 126: 116–20.

Stern, D.T. (ed.) (2006) *Measuring Medical Professionalism*. Oxford: Oxford University Press.

Sternberg, R.J. (ed.) (1988) *The Nature of Creativity: Contemporary Psychological Perspectives*. Cambridge: Cambridge University Press.

Sternberg, R.J. (ed.) (1999) *Handbook of Creativity*. Cambridge: Cambridge University Press.

Sternberg, R.J. and Lubart, T.I. (1999) 'The Concept of Creativity: Prospects and Paradigms'. In R.J. Sternberg (ed.), *Handbook of Creativity*, 3–15. Cambridge: Cambridge University Press.

Strawson, G. (2004) 'Against Narrativity'. *Ratio*, XVII: 428–52.

Stuckey, H.L. and Nobel, J. (2010) 'The Connection Between Art, Healing, and Public Health: A Review of Current Literature'. *American Journal of Public Health*, 100: 254–63.

Tatum, J. (2004) *The Mourner's Song: War and Remembrance from the Iliad to Vietnam*. Chicago, IL: University of Chicago Press.

Taylor, C.W. (1988) 'Various Approaches to and Definitions of Creativity'. In R.J. Sternberg (ed.), *The Nature of Creativity: Contemporary Psychological Perspectives*, 99–124. Cambridge: Cambridge University Press.

Thomas, C. (2005) 'Ellis Writes Himself into Suburbs'. *San Francisco Chronicle*, 14 August, www.sfgate.com/default/article/Ellis-writes-himself-into-suburbs-2647761.php (accessed 4 November 2014).

Thompson, C. and Dowding, D. (2002) *Clinical Decision Making and Judgement in Nursing*. Edinburgh: Churchill Livingstone.

Torrance, E.P. (1988) 'The Nature of Creativity as Manifest in its Testing'. In R.J. Sternberg (ed.), *The Nature of Creativity: Contemporary Psychological Perspectives*, 43–75. Cambridge: Cambridge University Press.

Truog, R.D., Browning, D.M., Johnson, J.A. and Gallagher, T.H. (2011) *Talking with Patients and Families about Medical Error*. Baltimore, MD: Johns Hopkins University Press.

Twenge, J.M. and Campbell, W.K. (2009) *The Narcissism Epidemic: Living in the Age of Entitlement*. New York: Free Press.

Uglow, J. (2002) *The Lunar Men: The Friends Who Made the Future 1730–1810*. London: Faber & Faber.

Ulrich, R., Zimring, C., Quan, X., Joseph, A. and Choudhary, R. (2004) 'The Role of the Physical Environment in the Hospital of the 21st Century'. www.healthdesign.org/chd/research/role-physical-environment-hospital-21st-century (accessed 6 September 2014).

UMKC (undated) 'The Sirridge Office of Medical Humanities and Bioethics'. http://med.umkc.edu/docs/alumni/MEDICAL-HUMANITIES-PROGRAM-EXPANSION-final-3-6-13.pdf (accessed 23 October 2014).

Ursitti, C. (2008) 'The Phenomenology of Olfactory Perception: An interview with Cara Ursitti'. *Art and Research*, 2 (Summer), www.artandresearch.org.uk/v2n1/ursitti.html (accessed 5 September 2014).

Van Wyck, H.B. (1951) 'Humanities in Medical Education'. *Canadian Medical Association Journal*, 64: 254–60.

Veloski, J. and Hojat, M. (2006) 'Measuring Specific Elements of Professionalism: Empathy, Teamwork, and Lifelong Learning'. In D.T. Stern (ed.), *Measuring Medical Professionalism*, 117–46. Oxford: Oxford University Press.

Verghese, A. (1992) 'Soundings'. *Granta*, 39: 81–90.

Verghese, A. (1994) *My Own Country: A Doctor's Story of a Town and its People in the Age of AIDS*. New York: Simon & Schuster.

Verghese, A. (1999) *The Tennis Partner*. London: Vintage.

Verghese, A. (2007) 'Bedside Manners'. *Texas Monthly*, February, www.texasmonthly.com/content/bedside-manners (accessed 4 November 2014).

Verghese, A. (2009) *Cutting for Stone. London:* Chatto & Windus.

Verghese, A. (2011) 'A Doctor's Touch'. www.ted.com/talks/abraham_verghese_a_doctor_s_touch (accessed 18 August 2014).

Verghese, A. (undated) 'Stanford Initiative in Bedside Medicine'. http://medicine.stanford.edu/education/stanford_25.html (accessed 6 September 2014).

Vollmann, W.T. (2007) *Poor People*, 3rd edn, New York: Ecco Press.

Wallace, D.F. (1996) *Infinite Jest*. London: Abacus.

Wallace, D.F. (2001) *Brief Interviews with Hideous Men*. London: Abacus.

Ward, S. (1999) 'Send in the Clowns'. *Health Service Journal*, 109: 11–12.

Warner, J.H. (2011) 'The Humanising Power of Medical History: Responses to Biomedicine in the 20th Century United States'. *Medical Humanities*, 37: 91–6.

Wassersug, J.D. (1987) 'Teach Humanities to Doctors? Says Who?'. *Postgraduate Medicine*, 82: 317–18.

Way, E.C. (1994) *Knowledge Representation and Metaphor*. Oxford: Intellect.

Wayne, S., Dellmore, D., Sena, L., Jerabek, R., Timm, C. and Kalishman, S. (2011) 'The Association between Tolerance of Ambiguity and Decline in Medical Students' Attitudes towards the Underdeserved'. *Academic Medicine*, 86: 877–82.

Wear, D. (2009) 'The Medical Humanities: Toward a Renewed Praxis'. *Journal of Medical Humanities*, 30: 209–20.

Wear, D. and Aultman, J.M. (2005) 'The Limits of Narrative: Medical Student Resistance to Confronting Inequality and Oppression in Literature and Beyond'. *Medical Education*, 39: 1056–65.

Wear, D., Kumagai, A., Varley, J. and Zarconi, J. (2012) 'Cultural Competency 2.0: Exploring the Concept of "Difference" in Engagement With the Other'. *Academic Medicine*, 87: 752–8.

Weatherall, D.J. (1994) 'The Inhumanity of Medicine'. *British Medical Journal*, 309: 1671–2.

Weill Cornell Medical College (undated) 'Guidelines for Case Presentations'. http://weill.cornell.edu/education/curriculum/third/med_gui_cas.html (accessed 27 October 2014).

Weiss, P. (2005) *The Aesthetics of Resistance*. Durham, NC: Duke University Press.

Welch, G., Schwartz, L.M. and Woloshin, S. (2011) *Over-Diagnosed: Making People Sick in the Pursuit of Health*. Boston, MA: Beacon Press.

Wellberry, C. and McAteer, R.A. (forthcoming) 'The Art of Observation: A Pedagogical Framework'. *Academic Medicine*.

Wershof Schwartz, A., Abramson, J.S., Wojnowich, I., Accordino, R., Ronan, E.J. and Rifkin, M.R. (2009) 'Evaluating the Impact of the Humanities in Medical Education'. *Mount Sinai Journal of Medicine*, 76: 372–80.

Weston, G. (2009) *Direct Red: A Surgeon's Story*. London: Jonathan Cape.

Weston, G. (2013) *Dirty Work*. London: Vintage Books.

White, C., Kumagai, A., Ross, P.T. and Fantone, J. (2009) 'A Qualitative Exploration of How the Conflict Between the Formal and Informal Curriculum Influences Student Values and Behaviors'. *Academic Medicine*, 84: 597: 603.

Wible P. (2014) 'How to Get Naked with Your Doctor: Dr Pamela Wible at TEDxSalem'. www.youtube.com/watch?v=5cvHgGM-cRI (accessed 6 September 2014).

Williams, I. (2014) *The Bad Doctor: The Troubled Life and Times of Dr Iwan James*. Brighton: Myriad Editions.

Wilmer, H.A. (1968) 'The Doctor–Patient Relationship and Issues of Pity, Sympathy and Empathy'. *British Journal of Medical Psychology*, 41: 243–8.

Winnicott, D.W. (1971) *Playing and Reality*. Harmondsworth: Penguin.

Wispé, L. (1991) *The Psychology of Sympathy*. Dordrecht: Kluwer.

Woods, A. (2011) 'The Limits of Narrative: Provocations for the Medical Humanities'. *Medical Humanities*, 37: 73–8.

Woods, A. and Whitehead, A. (eds) (forthcoming) *Edinburgh Companion to the Medical Humanities*. Edinburgh: University of Edinburgh Press.

Xyrichis, A. and Ream, E. (2008) 'Teamwork: A Concept Analysis'. *Journal of Advanced Nursing*, 61: 232–41.

Yenawine, P. (1997) 'Thoughts on Visual Literacy'. In J. Flood, S.B. Heath and D. Lapp (eds), *Handbook of Research on Teaching Literacy through the Communicative Visual Arts*, Basingstoke: Macmillan Library Reference, 845–60. Reprint available at http://vtshome.org/system/resources/0000/0005/Thoughts_Visual_Literacy.pdf (accessed 4 September 2014).

YoungMinds (2013) 'Mental Health Statistics'. www.youngminds.org.uk/training_services/policy/mental_health_statistics (accessed 27 October 2014).

Index